# PRIMARY LOW VISION CARE

**Rodney W. Nowakowski, OD, PhD**

Professor
School of Optometry/The Medical Center
University of Alabama at Birmingham
Birmingham, Alabama

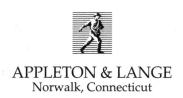

APPLETON & LANGE
Norwalk, Connecticut

Copyright © 1994 by Appleton & Lange
Paramount Publishing Business and Professional Group

94 95 96 97 98 / 10 9 8 7 6 5 4 3 2 1

Prentice Hall International (UK) Limited, *London*
Prentice Hall of Australia Pty. Limited, *Sydney*
Prentice Hall Canada, Inc., *Toronto*
Prentice Hall Hispanoamericana, S.A., *Mexico*
Prentice Hall of India Private Limited, *New Delhi*
Prentice Hall of Japan, Inc., *Tokyo*
Simon & Schuster Asia Pte. Ltd., *Singapore*
Editora Prentice Hall do Brasil Ltda., *Rio de Janeiro*
Prentice Hall, *Englewood Cliffs, New Jersey*

Library of Congress Cataloging-in-Publication Data

Nowakowski, Rodney W.
    Primary low vision care / Rodney W. Nowakowski.
        p.      cm.
    Includes bibliographical references.
    ISBN 0-8385-7980-9
    1. Low vision—Treatment.    I. Title.
    [DNLM: 1. Vision, Subnormal—rehabilitation. WW 140 N946p 1994]
    RE91.N69    1994
    617.7′12—dc20
DNLM/DLC
for Library of Congress                                        94-8438

Acquisitions Editor: Cheryl L. Mehalik
Designer: Penny Kindzierski
Art and photography: Rodney W. Nowakowski

PRINTED IN THE UNITED STATES OF AMERICA

ISBN 0-8385-7980-9

90000

9 780838 579800

To my parents,
Hazel Conlon Nowakowski and Rodney Edward Nowakowski,
for all those things that give special meaning to the word *family,*
and to my wife Deborrah,
who has given me love and support
beyond all reasonable expectations.

# CONTENTS

# Contents In Detail

# PREFACE

This text is intended for primary vision care practitioners, students, and residents who are seeking an introduction to low vision rehabilitation. It is my goal that those who would like to provide some degree of rehabilitative care, but are not doing so presently, will feel comfortable including at least some aspects of this specialty care in their practices after reading the text.

The overall organization of the text is meant to have a logical flow similar to the actual sequence of clinical evaluation and management: introduction → case history → examination → diagnostic trial of devices → prescription of devices → other management options → case examples, and finally, some personal experiences to reflect on some of the lessons learned. This sequence should assist the reader in developing a structured approach to the fundamentals of providing low vision care as well as an organized perspective of vision impairment, its potential effect on an individual's life, and what management options exist.

Management, to a large extent, involves prescribing optical assistive devices. I know, from long experience, that some students and practitioners are reluctant to learn more about low vision care because of the perception that it requires a detailed understanding of complex optics. Although some knowledge of optical principles is necessary, the principles are not as complex as many believe. For those who are interested, I have tried to develop them in a simple and straightforward manner with many detailed and clinically applicable examples. It is often the derivation of formulas that appears relatively intimidating, rather than their clinical applications. Therefore, the chapters devoted to optical theory and prescribing optical devices (Chapters 10 to 15) are organized so that a reader may skip the detailed information concerning the derivations and simply see how they are applied clinically by reading the examples and chapter summaries. (There, I said it—but it wasn't easy!) For similar reasons, I have tried to limit the references to those that are most germane yet give sufficient additional reading suggestions to anyone who seeks more information.

I have assumed that most readers will be either an optometrist or ophthalmologist, or one in training, and will be familiar with the related basic theories of clinical optics, vision, and clinical procedures. For that reason, there is no discussion about how to perform traditional clinical tests; instead, the text focuses on how to make adaptations that may be helpful if the person being examined is visually impaired. I have also assumed that the reader is knowledgeable about management of the disease causing the vision impairment. Topics in this regard are not included because they are not part of the intended scope of the book. This text is not about ocular disease per se but rather about rehabilitation of the resultant visual loss.

For the most part, I have purposely avoided a discussion of the specific parameters of optical devices that are currently available. The reason is simple—design, availability, and price change frequently, as do manufacturers. The occasional mention or illustration of a specific product or manufacturer has been made to emphasize a specific point and should not be construed as an endorsement, nor should the exclusion of others be considered the opposite. Chapter 31 includes a sufficient number of resources to allow the reader to order catalogues and learn what specific products are generally available.

Vision rehabilitation is a unique and rewarding form of clinical care. It offers an opportunity to make a significant difference in the lives of those in need. I hope the knowledge gained from this text will allow you to share in this wonderful experience.

During the past 19 years it has been my good fortune to work closely with many people who contributed generously to my knowledge in clinical care and vision rehabilitation, and/or to the development of the Low Vision Clinics at the UAB School of Optometry in The Medical Center of the University of Alabama at Birmingham, and at the Alabama Institute for Deaf and Blind in Talladega, Alabama. I would particularly like to acknowledge the special contributions of Henry B. Peters, Randy Jose, Vasha and Bill Rosenblum, Jerry Thompson, Larry Alexander, G. Gayle Stephens, Tom Raasch, Robert Kleinstein, Brad Wild, Adam Gordon, Jimmy Bartlett, Jennie Phillips, Lynn Hazard, Pat Kilgore, Brenda Watkins, Mary Jean Sanspree, Pam and Terry Graham, Janice and Jack Hawkins, Charles Johnson, Bob McBride, and George McFaden. Thank you.

*Rod Nowakowski*

# CHAPTER I

# VISION IMPAIRMENT AND ITS REHABILITATION

*People with impaired vision display a highly variable degree of function that is not predictable from standard clinical measures such as visual acuity or visual field. Because of this fact, attempts to define levels or categories of visual impairment (such as "low vision," "legal blindness," and "moderately" or "severely" impaired vision) based on clinical measures have proven unsatisfactory. Unfortunately, since there is no accepted battery of functional tests to determine functional impairment, visual acuity and visual field continue to be the most often used tests for establishing the level of impairment. Visual acuity is invariably the measure used in studies to determine the prevalence and incidence of vision impairment and/or legal blindness. Little information is available concerning the number of people who have a visual field restriction. The goal of vision rehabilitation is to allow a person to use his or her remaining vision in the most effective manner and to adapt to the loss of vision in order to live as normal a lifestyle as possible.*

## LOW VISION

The term *low vision* implies some reduction in visual acuity and/or visual field. Because there is no national definition of low vision or vision impairment other than legal blindness, studies to determine the prevalence and incidence of vision impairment have used a variety of acuity levels as the point at which one

might be classified as having low vision. Performance is a more realistic criterion for determining a disability level. Therefore, it is better to avoid specifying
any particular visual acuity or visual field size and to use a functional definition
instead; for example, a fighter pilot with a visual acuity of 20/70 might be functionally impaired, whereas a waiter might perform very well with that same
level of vision. Thus, low vision can be defined as vision that is not adequate for
the person's needs. In this regard a cardiac surgeon might be considered visually impaired, under certain circumstances, since the suturing of small coronary
vessels requires the use of a magnifying device. By the same token, everyone is
visually impaired for some tasks. Consequently, it is possible to think of visual
impairment as a continuum with no discrete cutoff points.

A significant restriction in visual field, regardless of visual acuity, should
also qualify a person as having low vision, but, as will be seen in the studies
summarized later, visual fields have not typically been measured in epidemio-
logical studies to determine the prevalence of vision impairment.

## LEGAL BLINDNESS

Legal blindness is one subcategory of vision impairment. Federal and state aid
to the blind was instituted in the United States in the 1930s, and this necessitated the development of a standard definition for blindness. The American
Medical Association presented a definition for *economic blindness* that was
modified and adopted as the definition for legal blindness with the passage of
the Social Security Act in 1935.[1] The general definition of legal blindness used
in the United States is that the best corrected visual acuity in the better eye is
less than or equal to 20/200 or, if the visual acuity in that eye is better than
20/200, that the visual field is less than or equal to 20 degrees in the widest diameter.[1, 2] A person can therefore be legally blind based on either reduced acuity or reduced visual field. There are two key points in this definition. First, the
acuity must be the best corrected acuity of the better eye. Often one hears
someone say, *"I am legally blind without my glasses."* This is a nonsensical
statement. There is no definition of legal blindness without best correction.
Second, since the better eye is considered the determining factor, it doesn't
matter what the acuity of the other eye is. In other words, both eyes must meet
the field or acuity criterion in order for a person to be declared legally blind; for
example, a person with best corrected visual acuities of 20/4000 right eye and
20/190 left eye is not legally blind because the better eye is better than 20/200.

This example introduces another interesting point and occasional
dilemma. The usual Snellen charts have a rather large gap between some letter
sizes; for example, between 20/100 and 20/200. Anyone whose visual acuity
falls between these two values can only read the 200-foot letters on the chart
and is automatically classified as legally blind. Under such circumstances, many

people now classified as legally blind really are not, according to a strict inter-pretation of the definition; however, since it is standard and accepted clinical practice to use such charts, these persons do meet the definition in terms of how the test is, and has been, typically given. Perhaps a more realistic definition based on the traditional method of determining visual acuity would have been "best corrected acuity less than 20/100." In any case, the clinician should be aware that a stringent measurement of visual acuity may unclassify a patient as legally blind, eliminate some available benefits, and cause considerable change in a lifestyle to which that person may have become accustomed over many years. It is also worth noting that the definition, as usually stated, does not spec-ify the conditions for testing. Visual acuity is variable and is affected by many factors, such as ambient room illumination, delayed adaptation to changes in il-lumination, motivation, target contrast, and time given to respond. Visual field measurements are similarly affected by target size, speed of presentation for ki-netic testing, and background or ambient illumination. This creates some po-tential for latitude that is consistent with the fact that some states allow the practitioner to make a judgment based on the overall effect of the vision impair-ment regardless of the visual acuity or visual field. This permits an individual to be declared legally blind who, for example, has multiple visual deficits, the cu-mulative effect of which reduces his or her functional ability to a level consis-tent with legal blindness in the examiner's professional opinion, even though the exact definition might not be met in terms of visual acuity or visual field.

Approximately 25% of those who are legally blind, and only about 17% of the newly blind,[2] are estimated to have no useful vision. It is therefore not ap-propriate to think of those who are legally blind as being truly blind. The lead-ing cause of new blindness is probably age-related retinal degeneration, with diabetic retinopathy being a close second and perhaps first for some specific age groups. Hereditary conditions are responsible for almost 15% of legal blind-ness according to the National Society for the Prevention of Blindness. The most frequent hereditary cause is the group of disorders known as retinitis pig-mentosa, which accounts for 5% of the prevalence and 3% of the incidence of legal blindness.[2]

## EPIDEMIOLOGY OF BLINDNESS AND VISUAL IMPAIRMENT

Accurate data on the epidemiology of blindness and visual impairment for the United States do not exist since there is no national program requiring registra-tion of those with blindness and visual impairments and there have been rela-tively few well-designed population-based studies. For many years the best available data came from the Model Reporting Area, which is still often quoted. The Model Reporting Area (MRA) was established in 1962 by the National Insti-tute of Neurological Diseases and Blindness and was discontinued in 1971. The

MRA was composed of states that maintained a registry for the blind. At the onset there were nine such states; when the MRA was discontinued in 1971 by the National Eye Institute, which had become its sponsor, there were 16 member states. This continues to be the largest segment of the U.S. population for which such statistics have been gathered, but the data are now quite dated and extrapolation to the United States at large is difficult. One problem with extrapolation is that there is no certainty with respect to the completeness of the registers for parameters such as age, race, and diagnostic categories. The data have been summarized in detail in a monograph from the National Society to Prevent Blindness (NSPB).[2] The total number of individuals in the United States who were legally blind was estimated to be approximately one-half million (498,000), with an annual incidence of 46,600. The NSPB also estimated the total number of visually impaired individuals, based on the Health Interview Survey (HIS) conducted by the National Center for Health Statistics in 1977, as 11.4 million. This figure included the legally blind. The number of severely visually impaired persons was estimated at approximately 1.4 million. The definition of *visually impaired* was "some difficulty seeing with one or both eyes even when wearing glasses," and the definition of *severely visually impaired* was "unable to read newspaper print even with glasses."

The HIS had a number of faults of its own. It was a survey; therefore, the figures were based on personal interviews, not examinations, and individuals were allowed to report on other household members. The results consequently represent *perceived* visual problems from the interviewee's point of view. All persons included were noninstitutionalized, which meant that nursing home residents (who, along with other institutionalized populations, have high rates of visual impairment) were excluded. The definitions of visual impairment were arbitrary, and there was no way to exclude those who might function normally with new glasses or simple optical aids.

The data from the 1977 HIS and the 1984 Supplement on Aging (SOA), which corrected some of the problems with the HIS, were reassessed in 1993 by Nelson and Dimitrova.[3] They applied the age-specific rates from these two studies to the 1990 decennial census using the 1977 HIS for persons under age 45 and the 1984 SOA for people aged 45 and older. They estimated the total number of persons with (perceived) severe visual impairment to be 4,293,360, with an average rate of 17.3 per 1,000. Those who reported being "blind in both eyes" represented 12% of the total, or 515,000. The rate for younger people, aged 17 and under, was estimated to be 1.5 per 1,000 compared to 210.6 per 1,000 for those 85 and over.

A supplemental questionnaire was included in the 1988 National Health Interview Survey[4] that addressed child health problems. The vision conditions asked about were blindness in one eye, blindness in both eyes, crossed eyes, and any other trouble seeing. Again, the information gathered was based on an interview concerning perceived health problems. An adult was asked to respond for one child, selected at random, in the household. The final sample included 17,110 children under the age of 18. The prevalence of blindness and vision impairment was 12.7 cases per 1,000. This higher rate, compared to the figure given above, reflects the fact that the former survey addressed "severe vision impairment" and the latter included "blindness with vision impairment" (any trouble seeing). The rates by age, weighted to reflect the 1988 population, were 10.3 per 1,000 under age 10 and 16 per 1,000 for those 10 to 17 years of age.[5]

A population-based study[6] for legal blindness among 10-year-old children, conducted in Atlanta, Georgia, found a prevalence of 6.8 per 10,000. Legal blindness was determined by a review of records at schools, service agencies, and hospitals. Rates were based on an estimated population of 89,534 10-year-old children in the metropolitan Atlanta area during the years 1985 to 1987. Most of the conditions causing legal blindness in this population were congenital, yet the diagnosis of severe vision loss was not usually documented until after the age of four years.

## The Framingham Eye Study

The Framingham Eye Study[7] was a population-based study begun in 1973 to determine the epidemiology of ocular pathology in local residents of Framingham, Massachusetts. The study population consisted of a subset of those survivors who had participated in the Framingham Heart Study.[8] Best corrected visual acuities were measured on 2,477 individuals among a study population of 2,940 aged 52 to 85 years. The rate of legal blindness, as defined in the United States, was 8.9 (0.89%) per 1,000 persons. The authors did not define visual impairment, but the percentage of people with a best corrected acuity worse than 20/40 in the better eye was 3.3%. The percentage of individuals with some degree of visual impairment increased with age, and the rates for legal blindness and visual impairment were higher in women than men. Unfortunately, the Framingham Eye Study lacked data on race-specific rates and on individuals older than 85 years of age.

It is also important to know that examiners are not necessarily accurate in assessing visual acuities levels for those who are visually impaired, especially if they are not experienced in working with this population. Gresset et al.[9] found considerable disparity in the classification of visual impairment between general practitioners and low vision specialists when both examined the same population of elderly subjects. They attributed the discrepancy, at least in part, to the lack of standardized methods for assessing visual acuity in those who are visually impaired.

Several recent population-based studies with well-designed protocols are summarized in the text following. The determination of visual impairment and legal blindness in these studies was based on visual acuities only and not visual fields and was determined for adults only, the youngest included age being 40.

## The Beaver Dam Eye Study

Beaver Dam, Wisconsin, was chosen for this study[10] because it had a large, stable, geographically defined population that had participated actively in a previous study of diabetic retinopathy. Best corrected visual acuities were obtained for 4,926 individuals 43 to 86 years of age. A standardized refraction and corrected acuities were obtained with a Humphrey 530 refractor. The refractive finding was placed in a trial frame, and acuities were reassessed following the protocol used in the Early Treatment Diabetic Retinopathy Study[11] with logMAR acuity charts (see Chapter 4). If the acuity was 20/40 or worse, another refraction was performed and the acuity reassessed. Visual impairment was defined as "none" (better than 20/40), "mild" (20/40 to 20/63), "moderate" (20/80 to 20/160), or "severe" (20/200 or worse).

The percentage of legally blind subjects among the entire study group was 0.5%, while 4.7% were visually impaired but not legally blind, and 5.2% had some degree of visual impairment including legal blindness. Best corrected visual acuity declined with increasing age. Visual impairment, including legal blindness, increased from 0.8% among those aged 43 to 54 to 21.1% of those 75 years of age or older. Legal blindness increased from 0.1% of those aged 43 to 54 to 2.0% of those who were 75 years of age or older. Visual impairment and legal blindness rates for those aged 75 and older were higher for those who resided in nursing homes than for those who did not and were higher for women than for men.

## The Baltimore Eye Survey

The Baltimore Eye Survey[12] (BES) was the first study to determine blindness and visual impairment rates among an urban, multiracial population in the United States. Eligible subjects were nontransient residents 40 years of age or older and were examined during the period from January 1985 through November 1988. Those who completed an initial enrollment interview received a vision screening that included an automated refraction or, when this was not possible, a retinoscopic and/or manual refraction. Data were collected on 5,300 people with approximately equal numbers of blacks and whites. Two definitions for both visual impairment and blindness were reported. Visual impairment was defined as either visual acuity less than 20/60 in accordance with the World Health Organization (WHO) or less than 20/40, which is a typical requirement for driving in the United States. Legal blindness was defined as either worse than 20/400 in accordance with the WHO or 20/200 or worse as defined in the United States. The authors analyzed data for the presenting acuity as well as for the best corrected acuity. The analyses reviewed here refer to the data corresponding to the better eye with best correction. Visual impairment and blindness, regardless of the definition used, increased with age in both groups. The overall age-adjusted rates were approximately twice as high for blacks compared to whites. Unlike the Beaver Dam Study, there was no difference in the prevalence of either blindness or visual impairment with respect to sex. The authors projected their data to the estimated 1985 population and estimated that more than 3 million persons were visually impaired, 890,000 of whom would be legally blind according to the definition used in the United States.

## The Mud Creek Valley Study

The Mud Creek Valley Study[13] (MCVS), in contradistinction to the BES, was conducted in a rural valley in the Appalachian hills of southeastern Kentucky. This was a population-based study of 1,136 subjects 40 years of age or older. All of the subjects were white. There were 527 men and 609 women. Subjects were initially screened for visual acuity with current correction. Those with an acuity worse than 20/60 in either eye underwent a complete examination, including refraction. Again, the WHO and U.S. definitions for legal blindness were used in the data analysis. Low vision was defined as a best corrected acuity worse than 20/60 in the better eye, but not legally blind. Monocular visual impairments were determined but are not summarized here. The prevalence of legal blindness by the U.S definition was 1.1%, and the prevalence of low vision, but not legally blind, was 2.2%. These percentages were based on the estimated U.S. population in 1985. Both legal blindness and low vision were associated with age, but there was no statistically significant difference associated with gender.

## Summary of Population-Based Studies for Adults

The four studies summarized above give a basis for estimating a range of persons, aged 40 and up, with visual impairment in the United States, but such estimates must still be viewed with some caution because these studies were not consistent with respect to the age ranges studied, the racial composition, or the socio-economic status of the subjects. Unfortunately, there are no equivalent recent studies for younger age groups.

Virtually all of the estimates given for prevalence and incidence of vision impairment, in these and other studies, are based on measures of visual acuity and not visual field. A significant visual field loss is also debilitating and may be remediated to some extent by techniques referred to as "visual field enhancement." Visual field enhancement is the subject of Chapter 18.

All studies agree that rates of visual impairment and blindness increase significantly with age. For example, the NSPB figures reported that more than 50% of both the visually impaired and the legally blind were persons aged 65 and over. The aging population is increasing both in numbers and as a percentage of the total population. Within its own ranks, the aging population is growing older, that is, the percentages of the oldest age groups are increasing.[14] There were 30,984,000 people aged 65 or older in 1989,[15] and this represented 12.45% of the total population of 248,762,000. It is estimated[14] that until 2010 the population aged 65 and older will increase 1.2% per year, and by 2030 this age group will total 65.6 million, which will then represent 21.8% of the population. The overall ratio of elderly females to elderly males is 3:2. The ratio increases within the older age groups. In brief, there is a clear trend toward increasing numbers of older persons in the United States, primarily women, who are blind and/or visually impaired. This problem of vision impairment among those who are older is exacerbated by the fact that other health problems are also more common with age. This makes vision rehabilitation both more complex and more difficult. An additional barrier to providing effective rehabilitation to the elderly is the fact that a significant number of them are impoverished. In 1987, 12.2% of the elderly were below the poverty level.[14]

The age-based entitlement programs such as Medicare and Social Security, established when life expectancy was less than 60 years (it is now greater than 65), will be unable to support the increasing numbers of elderly recipients much beyond the year 2020 unless there is significant change in their funding base.[16] Future health care funding and specialization training for health care providers must reflect these trends in order to provide for this growing population of people with very special needs.

In spite of the aging trend for the prevalence and incidence of visual impairment and blindness, approximately 97% of the annual federal costs of blindness (approximately $4 billion in 1990) is accounted for by expenditure on working-aged adults.[17] The federal expenditure for a working-aged American has been estimated at $11,896 per person-year including income assistance programs, health insurance programs such as Medicare and Medicaid, and tax losses from lowered potential earnings.[17]

## VISION REHABILITATION

When good functional vision can be restored (for example, through cataract extraction), that is the goal and the process ends. The people who require low vision rehabilitation, however, are those for whom there is currently no restorative process. The goal for these individuals is to help them to use their remaining vision in the most advantageous manner to achieve as independent a lifestyle as possible. It is important that this be communicated carefully in order to avoid the disappointment of false expectations. A frank approach is appropriate in which the person is told, *"I cannot give you back the vision that you have lost. What I will try to do is to help you to use your remaining vision more effectively."* This is consistent with the characteristics others have used to describe the rehabilitation process as shown in the following two quotes: "The hallmark of Rehabilitation Medicine practice, therefore, is its functional approach, which seeks to redress or substitute for disability and minimize handicap,"[18] and ". . . rehabilitation is predicated on a set of factors—adaptation, coping, and adjustment—rather than cure."[19]

There are different settings in which the rehabilitative process might take place. One such setting is a large clinic that offers the expertise of a multidisciplinary staff. The staff might include social workers, orientation and mobility instructors, psychologists, and others in addition to vision specialists. This is the right setting for some patients but probably not for most. The majority of routine vision care is provided in the private practice setting, and it is reasonable to assume that the majority of low vision rehabilitation could take place there also.

When the vision loss is severe and/or the needs of the individual are such that the multidisciplinary setting is appropriate, the private practitioner may still serve as the primary entry point to the system and a key participant in the process. If there are adequate separate resources available locally to which the patient can be referred, then the private practitioner might remain the case coordinator and facilitate the overall process by being aware of, and taking advantage of, these resources. Opportunities exist for private practitioners to engage in low vision care at a variety of levels, within the framework of their own degree of expertise and confidence.

The rehabilitative process is the subject of the chapters that follow. As a brief introduction, however, rehabilitation starts by discovering the problems faced by the patient as a result of the loss of vision and then proceeds to find the means to ameliorate them. One treatment option is to prescribe optical devices that provide magnification. Some examples are hand-held magnifiers, high power bifocal adds, and miniature telescopes mounted in spectacles. The prescription of optical devices, however, is only one aspect of the rehabilitative process. Other therapeutic considerations include the prescription of nonoptical aids such as illumination systems, counseling, lessons in independent travel, and training in the activities of daily living; for example, people with difficulty moving about the environment will benefit from training by an orientation and mobility specialist who can provide lessons in safe travel for persons with all degrees of vision loss including total blindness. A rehabilitation teacher can come into the home and provide training in how to cook safely and how to organize possessions in order to make activities of daily living, such as eating, dressing, and grooming, easier to accomplish. Other professionals who might be involved in the rehabilitative process include occupational therapists, social workers, teachers, child life specialists, vocational rehabilitation counselors, and psychologists.

## SUMMARY

From the statistics given in the preceding sections, it is clear that there are many people who are visually impaired, with useful residual vision, needing more than routine vision care. It is this population (and specifically, those for whom there is no restorative procedure) that will be addressed in this text.

These individuals, regardless of their exact visual level, will be considered to be visually impaired or to have *low vision*. The specialized area of vision care for this population is known as *low vision rehabilitation*. The rehabilitation process may involve many other professional specialties.

## REFERENCES

1. Goldstein H: *The Demography of Blindness Throughout the World.* New York, American Foundation for the Blind, 1980, pp 4-5.
2. Operations Research Department. *Vision Problems in the United States.* New York, National Society to Prevent Blindness, 1980.
3. Nelson KA, Dimitrova E: Severe visual impairment in the United States and in each state, 1990. *J Vis Impair Blind* 87(3):80-85, 1993.
4. Adams PW, Halfon N, Budetti PP: Current Estimates from the National Health Interview Survey: United States, 1988. *Vital and Health Statistics.* Series 10, No.173. Hyattsville, MD, National Center for Health Statistics, 1990.
5. Newacheck PW, Taylor WR: Childhood chronic illness: Prevalence, severity and impact. *Am J Pub Health* 82:364-371, 1992.
6. Drews CD, Yeargin-Allsopp M, Murphy CC, Decoufle P: Legal blindness among 10-year-old children in metropolitan Atlanta. Prevalence, 1985-1987. *Am J Pub Health* 82:1377, 1992.
7. Kahn HA, Leibowitz HM, Ganley JP, Kini MM, Colton T, Nickerson RS, Dawber TR: The Framingham eye study: I. Outline and major prevalence findings. *Am J Epidem* 106(1):17-32, 1977.
8. Gordon T, Kannel WB: The Framingham, Massachusetts, Study, twenty years later, in II Kessler, Levin ML (eds): *The Community as an Epidemiologic Laboratory. A Casebook of Community Studies. II.* Baltimore, Johns Hopkins Press, 1970, pp 123-144.
9. Gresset J, Vachon N, Simonet P, Bolduc M: Discrepancy in the evaluation of visual impairment of elderly low-vision patients by general eye care practitioners and by low-vision practitioners. *Optom Vis Sci* 70:39-44, 1993.
10. Klein R, Klein BEK, Linton KLP, De Mets DL: The Beaver Dam eye study: Visual acuity. *Ophthalmol* 98(8):1310-1315, 1991.
11. *Early Treatment Diabetic Retinopathy Study (ETDRS). Manual of Operations.* Baltimore, EDTRS Coordinating Center, University of Maryland, Department of Epidemiology and Preventive Medicine, 1980.
12. Tielsch JM, Sommer A, Witt K, Katz J, Royall RM: Blindness and visual impairment in an American urban population: The Baltimore eye survey. *Arch Ophthalmol* 108:286-290, 1990.
13. Dana MR, Tielsch JM, Enger C, Joyce E, Santoli JM, Taylor HR: Visual impairment in a rural Appalachian community. *JAMA* 264(18):2400-2405, 1990.
14. U.S. Bureau of the Census, Current Population Reports, Series P-23 No. 159, *Population Profile of the United States: 1989.* Washington, D.C., U.S. Government Printing Office, 1989.

15. U.S. Bureau of the Census, *Statistical Abstract of the United States: 1991* (111th edition). Washington, D.C., 1991.
16. Olshansky SJ, Carnes BA, Cassel CK: The aging of the human species. *Sci Amer* 268(4):46–52, 1993.
17. Chiang YP, Bassi LJ, Javitt JC: *Milbank Q* 70:319, 1992.
18. Mayer NH: Evaluation, in Kaplan PE, Materson RS (eds): *The Practice of Rehabilitation Medicine.* Springfield, IL, Charles C. Thomas, 1982, p 3.
19. Russell MV: Clinical social work, in Goodgold J (ed): *Rehabilitation Medicine.* St. Louis, C.V. Mosby Company, 1988, p 944.

## ADDITIONAL READING

Kirchner C: *Data on Blindness and Visual Impairment in the U.S.,* 2 ed. New York, American Foundation for the Blind, 1988.
The visual system, in *Guides to the Evaluation of Permanent Impairment,* 3 ed (Revised). Chicago, American Medical Association, 1990, pp 162–171.

# CHAPTER II

# PSYCHOSOCIAL ASPECTS OF VISION IMPAIRMENT

*There are many myths and misunderstandings about vision impairment and, especially, blindness. These contribute to the difficulties faced by anyone with impaired vision who is trying to adapt psychologically to the vision loss or trying to function normally in a sighted world. Clinicians will be able to relate more humanely to persons who are visually impaired if they have some degree of understanding of how vision impairment affects individuals beyond the measured loss of visual acuity or visual field.*

## THE LOSS OF VISION

Vision impairment can be congenital or adventitious, the latter meaning acquired. The adjustment to blindness in a sighted world is different in each case. The adjustment to any loss of sight depends on many factors, such as etiology, rate of progression, stability, and extent of the loss. Very different psychological effects must result between a loss caused by an unfortunate accident versus one caused by an intentional assault or between a loss from congenital syphilis versus congenital toxoplasmosis. The loss of vision can be rapid, as in trauma, or slowly progressive, as in the loss of sight from retinitis pigmentosa. In the former case, the loss is an immediate fact; in the latter, it can be a dreaded eventuality, monitored with daily reminders, such as the onset of nightblindness with every setting sun. Each patient responds in unique ways based on his or her personality and the parameters of the vision loss.

Common stages of reaction to any adventitious and significant loss may be:

- Shock . . . . . . . . . . . . . . . . *Oh my God!*
- Denial . . . . . . . . . . . . . . . . *This can't be happening to me.*
- Anxiety . . . . . . . . . . . . . . . *Now what will I do?*
- Anger . . . . . . . . . . . . . . . . *I don't deserve this.*
- Depression . . . . . . . . . . . *I'll never again be a worthwhile person.*
- Acceptance . . . . . . . . . . . *I guess I might as well get used to it.*
- Adjustment . . . . . . . . . . . *I'm going to make the most of it.*

An individual may not progress through all of these stages, particularly those of acceptance and adjustment. Some examples of indicators of poor adjustment are continual unwarranted hope for recovery, unnecessary or exaggerated displays of dependence, personal devaluation, social reclusion, lack of motivation, prolonged depression, continued denial, and exaggerated blind behaviorisms.

The consequences of lost vision may explain some of the reactions to it. There is, for example, a loss of confidence in one's remaining senses without the ability to verify a message visually. *"Is the sound of cloth rustling just the curtains moving in the breeze or a mouse running across the floor?" "Is that odor of smoke coming from my neighbor's outdoor grill, or is my apartment on fire?"* Vision contributes to communication by allowing us to interpret facial expressions, gestures, body language, and lip movements. None of these is available to the severely visually impaired. Our sense of independence depends on the ability to drive, which is lost or curtailed with a loss of vision. The ability to continue in a chosen occupation may vanish along with financial security, the sense of a meaningful role in society, and the ability to provide for the retirement years. All of these losses, and others, may diminish one's self-concept, and that can become the greatest loss of all. The provider of low vision care will encounter patients with many types of vision loss and all degrees of reaction to that loss. Referral to others who can help the patient deal with the loss of vision should always be a consideration but should never be an assumed necessity.

## THE FEAR OF BLINDNESS

A fear of blindness is shared by most of us, second only to cancer and perhaps recently to AIDS. It is not difficult to imagine how a fear of blindness might have originated with the first humans on earth. Because defense against natural enemies depended on the ability to see, early humans were most vulnerable in the absence of light. The inability of humans to see well in the dark made them easy prey for large carnivores with keen night vision. In mythological tales, blindness was often interpreted as a sign of divine disfavor. The ancient Greeks believed that blindness was caused by gods against mortals who displeased them. The idea that light is good and darkness is not is reinforced by Biblical references such as Genesis 1:4, *"And God saw the light, that it was good: and God divided the light from the darkness."* Wasn't the dark also good? The implication is that it was not. Lucifer, "son of the morning," was transformed to the angel of darkness when he fell from heaven (Isaiah 14:12) to become the embodiment of evil. The notion of darkness has been equated with death in recurring Biblical references such as Job 10:21, *"The land of darkness and the shadow of death";* Psalms 107:10, *"Such as sit in darkness and in the shadow of death";* and Luke 1:79, *"To give light to them that sit in darkness and in the shadow of death."*

## BLINDNESS VIEWED AS A CURSE OR AS PUNISHMENT

In order to explain the unexplainable, mythologies often interpreted blindness as a sign of divine disfavor. Zeus allegedly punished Phineus because he was cruel to his sons or, for inappropriate use of his gift of prophecy, by blinding him and sending the Harpies to pollute his food.[1] Tiresias was blinded in one account by Athena because he had seen her nude while bathing and in another, by Hera, for judging against her in a dispute with Zeus.[2] Zeus, in turn, gave him the gift of prophecy, a skill often associated with blindness in myths.

Blindness has also been associated with guilt. Oedipus, in overwhelming guilt for committing patricide and incest, tore out his own eyes. Autoenucleation continues to this day. In a review of the medical literature Krauss et al.[3] found 19 cases of bilateral self-enucleation and 31 cases of unilateral self-enucleation. The acts had been performed with fingers, scissors, and even a meat hook. As the stimulus, some patients cited guilt over a misdeed and referenced the Biblical passage Matthew 5:29, *"... if thy right eye offends thee, pluck it out...."* The authors presented a contemporary case report of a 29-year-old woman who, feeling guilty over an extramarital affair, walked onto the beach, removed her right eye with her fingers, and walked to a nearby house where help was called.

## BLINDNESS ASSOCIATED WITH SUPERHUMAN POWERS

In direct contrast to the view of blindness as a curse or punishment is the notion that those who are blind are endowed with special sensory gifts. This idea is surely a result of the fact that historically some individuals who were blind survived and succeeded against overwhelming odds. From this arose the belief that they were endowed with a superhuman command of the nonvisual senses or that nature compensated for their loss of sight by endowing them with extra talents such as an exceptional memory, superkeen senses of touch, hearing, and smell, and even the gift of prophecy. To this day popular belief holds that the blind have superhuman powers such as a sixth sense, facial vision, and exceptionally acute senses. One can see a contemporary example of how these ideas are perpetuated in the television series Kung Fu, first popular in the 1970s and recently revitalized. Master Ho, a blind master of the Kung Fu martial art, could hear a grasshopper walking at his feet and could defend against the strike of an enemy by seeming to sense the position of the antagonist and his weapon. Unfortunately, losing one's sight is not compensated for by the development of any special senses. Helen Keller sought to dispel the myth that persons who are visually impaired are somehow different from others beyond the mere loss of sight as evidenced in an eloquent statement made in 1904, *"A blind man can do nothing less and nothing more than what a person with five senses can do, minus what can be done only with the eye."*[4]

## STEREOTYPIC VIEWS: THE MUSICIAN AND THE HELPLESS BEGGAR

Most people have had little sustained contact with individuals who are blind or severely visually impaired. The ones they are most familiar with are those seen on television—usually talented musicians such as Ray Charles, Stevie Wonder, and Ronnie Milsap. It is no wonder that there exists a popular notion that all or most blind people are musically talented. They are not. The other exposure to blindness that most people are likely to have and remember is seeing the street-corner beggar with dark glasses, holding out a cup for donations. The author once asked a class of 18 graduate students studying rehabilitation counseling to draw a picture of a blind man as an introductory exercise to learning about stereotypes. The result was 16 figures with a cane and/or dark glasses and two with a guide dog. No one drew a picture of a person with no stigmatizing characteristics.

Some totally self-sufficient blind persons even report having had gifts of money stuffed in their hands or pockets when using public transportation. Such stereotypic views of helplessness were, and are, enhanced by the lack of resources for education and rehabilitation that would allow those who are visually impaired to learn to live independently. The first true schools for those who were blind did not come into existence until the late 18th century in Europe and early 19th century in the United States. Even at that, the U.S. school was called the New England *Asylum* for the Blind.

Helen Keller was a strong advocate for public assistance in helping those who are visually impaired to become independent. When she addressed the First Annual Meeting of the Massachusetts Association for Promoting the Interests of the Adult Blind, she stated, *"Remember too, that when a man loses his sight he does not know himself what he can do. He needs someone of experience to advise him."*[4]

## THE SOCIAL STIGMATA OF BLINDNESS

One disability is often unjustly associated with others. Such associations may begin inadvertently or be taken out of context, but with the reinforcement of repetition, these associations may become accepted as true. Such is the case with blindness and ignorance or blindness and helplessness as the following literary quotations bear witness. These quotations demonstrate that misconceptions can be held literally over centuries; that is precisely how they become ingrained in our society.

### Blindness and Ignorance

I know my soul hath power to know all things
Yet she is blind and ignorant in all:
    Sir John Davies, Nosce Teipsum (1599), *st.* 44

Blind and naked ignorance
Delivers brawling judgements, unashamed . . .
    Alfred, Lord Tennyson, Idylls of the King (1859–1885), Merlin and
    Vivien, *l.* 662

Now you know—that's the happy existence you wanted to go back to. Ignorance and blindness.
    Thornton N. Wilder, Our Town (1938)

### Blindness and Helplessness

They be blind leaders of the blind. And if the blind lead the blind, both shall fall into the ditch.
    The Holy Bible, Matthew 15:14

An unstable pilot steers a leaking ship, and the blind is leading the blind straight to the pit.
    St. Jerome (c. A.D. 4th century), Letter 7

A fairer lady there never was seen
Than the blind beggar's daughter of Bethnal Green.
    Anonymous, The Beggar's Daughter of Bethnal Green, *st.* 33

## Social Reinforcement of Blind Stigmata

It has been proposed that those who are blind are forced into a stereotypic role by the same processes of socialization that have formed us all and that blindness is therefore a learned social role.[5] There is nothing inherent in the condition of blindness that requires a person to be dependent or helpless, nor is there anything about it that would lead one to become assertive and independent. If significant people in a blind person's life reinforce the idea of helplessness by doing everything for them, then helplessness will be a self-fulfilling prophecy. Agencies, while trying to help, can actually reinforce this socialization process by lumping together people who are blind, directing them into stereotypic occupations such as piano tuning or broom winding, and limiting their social interaction with the sighted world.

It is regrettable that people with disabilities are also frequently stigmatized or dehumanized by the use of inappropriate descriptive terminology. It is common to see references to "the blind" or "the visually impaired." This feature, or their disease, becomes their most prominent identifying factor rather than the fact that they are people who happen to have an impairment or disability. One term used in the past for what we now refer to as *low vision* was "subnormal vision." This is clearly not an appropriate term. No one wishes to be considered subnormal in any respect, nor is it proper to suggest that they might be just because they are visually impaired.

Just as blindness is a stigma, the disease, more than any other personal trait, may identify the individual in medical settings. Unfortunately, disease identifiers often become a part of some clinicians' vocabulary. This practice must be eliminated. There are no "myopes," "aphakes," or "albinos"—just *people* who have myopia, aphakia, or albinism.

## SUMMARY

Those who are blind have been viewed as blessed with superhuman gifts or punished, by self or others, for misdeeds. Such beliefs have laid the groundwork for both the fear of blindness that most share and the stereotypic views of blindness or of people who are blind that, again, probably most people share. It has been suggested that the leading cause of "blindness" is the definition.[6] Therefore, the definition itself, when attached to an individual, may become a social liability because of the misperceptions and insensitivities of those who are not visually impaired.

The medical setting should be a safe haven from the stigmata of blindness. It is incumbent on clinicians to make sure that this is the case by accepting those who are visually impaired as what they are—people—by using appropriate terminology and by understanding some of the psychosocial aspects of vision impairment.

# REFERENCES

1. Oswalt SG: *Concise Encyclopedia of Greek and Roman Mythology.* Chicago, Follet, 1969, p 238.
2. Van Aken ARA: *The Encyclopedia of Classical Mythology.* Englewood Cliffs, NJ, Prentice-Hall, Inc., 1965, p 143.
3. Krauss HR, Yee RD, Foos RY: Autoenucleation. *Surv Ophthalmol,* 29(3):179–187, 1984.
4. Keller H: *Our Duties to the Blind: A Paper.* Boston, Thomas Todd, 1904.
5. Scott RA: *The Making of Blind Men: A Study of Adult Socialization.* New York, Russell Sage Foundation, 1969.
6. Goldstein H: *The Demography of Blindness Throughout the World.* New York, American Foundation for the Blind, 1980, p 4.

# ADDITIONAL READING

Hollins M: *Understanding Blindness.* Hillsdale, NJ, Lawrence Erlbaum Associates, 1989.
Koestler FA: *The Unseen Minority: A Social History of Blindness in the United States.* New York, David McKay Co., 1976.
Schulz PJ: *How Does it Feel to be Blind? The Psychodynamics of Visual Impairment.* Los Angeles, Muse-Ed Company, 1980.
Trevor-Roper PD: *The World Through Blunted Sight: An Inquiry Into the Influence of Defective Vision on Art and Character.* New York, Bobbs-Merrill, 1970.

# CHAPTER III

# THE PATIENT INTERVIEW

*There is no getting around it—sooner or later, and usually it is sooner, the clinician has to talk with the patient. Prior to that first exchange, all things are possible. What is possible afterwards depends on the effectiveness of the communication that takes place. Effective communication is central to the rehabilitation process and will be emphasized throughout this text. Direct patient-doctor communication begins with the interview, although impressions are being formed prior to that based on indirect communication; such as the patient's perception of the physical surroundings, the courtesy of the office staff, and how long he or she had to wait.*

## THE CASE HISTORY

What is traditionally called the "case history" is really only one component of the patient interview. The interview has been divided into a three-function approach by Cohen-Cole: gathering data to learn about the patient's problem in order to understand it, developing rapport and responding to the patient's emotions, and educating patients about their problems and motivating them to adhere to the prescribed treatment.[1] It is the first of these that is customarily referred to as the case history.

The traditional categories of a medical case history that are familiar to the clinician as well as the advanced student include the chief complaint, the history of the present illness, the current health status, past medical history, the family medical history, the social/personal history, and the review of systems. The general medical case history format is appropriate for the initial interview of a person with impaired vision when supplemented by questions related to the vision impairment. This general medical format is reviewed briefly below. Areas of emphasis unique to persons who are visually impaired are presented in more detail.

## The General Medical Format for the Case History

The *source(s) of the history* should be recorded and may include the patient, friends, relatives, or other care givers. Who contributes to the case history may reveal insight into the patient's degree of independence and ability to interact with others.

The *chief complaint* (CC) is a statement in the patient's own words concerning the purpose for the visit. It is typically concise; for example, *"My vision is so bad that I can't read the newspaper."*

The *history of the present illness* (HPI) is a narrative paragraph in which the details and chronology of the chief complaint are described. This portion of the history is recorded in the interviewer's words and is not a direct quote of the patient. It may include previous diagnoses, duration, stability, severity, and previous treatment including prior experience with low vision rehabilitation. The emphasis is on the chronology.

The *past medical history* (PMH) refers to significant medical problems in the remote past and need not cover details elicited in the history of the present illness or current health status. Included here are hospitalizations, immunizations, significant injuries and illnesses, and surgeries. The *past ocular history* is part of the past medical history and is logically included here, although some practitioners may prefer a separate indicator such as POH.

The *general health* or *current health status* (GH) covers present medical conditions not covered by the chief complaint or past medical history. Current medications, both prescribed and self-selected, are included here and may have a separate indicator such as MEDS.

The *family medical history* (FMH) is concerned with the immediate family and may be best accomplished by drawing a pedigree to elicit familial and genetic problems. A three-generation pedigree including the parents, the patient, and his or her offspring is typically sufficient unless a strong hereditary history is uncovered. Significant medical conditions, age, and cause of death are indicated directly on the drawing. Pedigree construction is covered in Chapter 25. Some clinicians prefer a separate category for *family ocular history,* but it is part of the family medical history and should be included here even if it has a separate indicator such as FOH.

The *social and personal history* emphasizes occupation, hobbies, living status, education, risk factors such as habits, and functional aspects of daily living activities. The aspects of visual function are described in greater detail below.

The *review of systems* (ROS) is meant to be a means of picking up pertinent health information that was omitted, on purpose or by oversight, in the preceding portions of the interview. It is a systematic review that should not take long to complete if the rest of the history was appropriately productive. It is possible to use a form that lists the various systems as a reminder of what to ask about, but another means of recalling the systems is simply to view the patient and think of the various systems, from head to toe, that are right there in front of you. The ROS is also directed by the examiner's understanding of the pathophysiology of disease processes so that appropriate systems are asked about relative to the patient's current and past medical problems. For example, a history of long-standing insulin-dependent diabetes suggests the possibility of peripheral neuropathy, nephropathy, or skin lesions that are recalcitrant to healing, and it would therefore be logical to inquire about the associated systems.

## Special Considerations for Persons with Impaired Vision

*The Chief Complaint Versus the Main Goal.* A comprehensive low vision evaluation may take several visits. In order to keep patients motivated, it is important to address their main goal, at least superficially, during the first visit. The main goal should be elicited specifically by asking, *"If you could choose one area in which you could be helped visually, what would it be?"* The response should be distinguished from the chief complaint. The statement *"I want to read"* is not a chief complaint but rather a goal. Identify and separate the chief complaint and the main goal. Clinicians should be prepared for the two common responses: *"I want to read"* and *"I want to drive."* These are activities everyone wants to perform because of their importance to daily activities. Some people will state that they want to read merely because they associate that activity with good vision. Further questioning might reveal that they never read books or newspapers and don't plan to now. There are other important reading tasks though, such as reading price tags, bills, and letters. When these activities are elicited as specific goals, it is possible to use appropriate examples during the diagnostic evaluation of optical devices. Therefore, samples of these items should be available in the examination room.

*The Social and Personal History.* Social and personal information plays an important role in the management of the patient. It may reveal the need for care from additional professionals or that he or she is still adapting to the vision loss and is not yet ready to try prosthetic devices. This portion of the patient interview is devoted to understanding the patient as a person and how the vision impairment affects his or her life. Typical components include place of birth, schooling, people with whom they live, past and current occupations, leisure activities, where they live currently, interaction with family members, and typical daily activities. A broad opening question is *"Tell me some things about yourself.*" More specific questions might be: *"How has this eye problem affected your home life?" "Who can you turn to for help?" "Who lives in your house?" "What are you like as a person?" "How would your friends describe you as a person?"*

The social history is one of the more neglected components of the patient interview. It is probably true that some clinicians actively avoid this area because they feel uncomfortable dealing with highly charged emotional issues that may be revealed. When the clinician makes an effort to understand the patient as an individual, it sets the tone for a better relationship. Such an expression of interest may make the person more responsive to testing and more compliant with recommended treatment. An in-depth understanding of all the individual's problems allows a more humane approach to medical care, and this ultimately results in the provision of better care.

*Visual Function.* The goal in this aspect of the interview is to relate the illness to functional aspects of the person's life. This portion of the interview may be covered in the social and personal history or as a separate category. The physical evaluation, which follows the case history, involves the precise measurement of many visual abilities such as visual acuity and the extent of the visual field. The determining factor for the person's ultimate rehabilitation, however, is the visual function regardless of measured levels of visual acuity and/or visual field. Not all people with the same visual acuity demonstrate the same level of visual function, nor should they be expected to. A person with 20/200 acuity from a cataract has a much different visual sense than someone who is also 20/200, but from age-related maculopathy. Their visual abilities may appear the same quantitatively but can be very different qualitatively. Other factors that may affect visual function include diminished color perception, reduced contrast sensitivity, glare, and visual field restrictions.

The clinician can obtain a sense of someone's functional ability by asking certain specific questions. Good examples are questions about activities of normal daily function and the current life situation. The home setting may have important implications concerning functional ability and potential problems. One might inquire whether or not the home has stairs, what the lighting is like, and whether or not the person lives alone. Activities within the home that might be problematic include cooking, cleaning, grooming, care for dependents, use of the telephone (dialing and directory listings), and the ability to identify medications. Activities of daily living outside the home to be addressed include driving, mobility, grocery shopping, banking, the ability to identify friends' faces, the ability to see in differing levels of illumination, problems with glare, photophobia, and the ability to identify denominations of paper money. Broad questions are *"What activities are you no longer able to perform?"* and, on a more positive note, *"What activities do you enjoy (that can still be performed)?"* A description of daily activities within the home or on the job may reveal areas where vision enhancement can improve function even though they were not mentioned as specific goals.

Some examples of useful questions both general and specific are:

- *How do you spend your day?* or *Describe a typical day in your life.*
- *What was your day like yesterday?*
- *What would it have been like if you could see better?*
- *Are you able to cook for yourself?*
- *Are you able to go grocery shopping?*
- *Can you read your personal mail or bills?*
- *What size print are you able to read (headlines, price tags, large print books)?*
- *Do you see better in bright or dim illumination?*
- *Can you recognize your friends' faces?*
- *Are you able to shave, apply makeup, clean fingernails, and so forth?*
- *Can you use the public transportation system?*
- *Can you identify the denominations of paper money?*

**The Prognosis for Successful Rehabilitation.** Other questions that help to establish the prognosis for successful rehabilitation relate to the extent, duration, and stability of the vision loss. A recent loss implies that the person may not have adjusted to the fact of the loss and is still interested only in a total restoration to normal visual function. He or she may still seek some experimental surgery or other treatment, no matter how bizarre, and cling to the hope of an eventual cure. This is normal behavior for a period of time. Until an individual accepts that the vision loss is permanent, he or she is less likely to employ assistive devices such as those offered by the low vision specialist.

A severe loss of vision implies a poorer prognosis for rehabilitation, as does a condition that is not stable. Both are more difficult to adapt to, and a variable condition also makes the prescription of assistive devices somewhat more difficult because the devices must be adaptable to varying visual levels. As a general rule, the best prognosis is associated with a long-standing, stable, moderate loss of vision. Careful questioning during the case history should give the examiner some feel for the prognosis for success and hence the approach to take in the examination; for example, those with a poorer prognosis might benefit from a slower process and more counseling with respect to the condition and the available treatment options.

**Previous Exposure to Low Vision Rehabilitation.** It is important to ask about experiences with prior low vision examinations. If there were none, now is a good time to explain how this examination is going to be different from previous eye examinations. This creates an opportunity to begin motivating the patient. The examiner may explain that additional tests will be performed and special devices demonstrated that may help the patient to use his or her remaining vision more effectively. Many people with a visual impairment have had multiple examinations for their vision loss, all of which were very much the same, and, at the conclusion of each, they were told that nothing else could be done for them. This forms a negative mind-set that is difficult to overcome.

If patients are familiar with the concepts of low vision, vision rehabilitation, and low vision examinations, the clinician should next ask about the experiences they have had; for example, what therapy was prescribed, what devices they have tried, how those devices did or did not help them, whether the devices were professionally prescribed or self-prescribed, and what type(s) of training they received. This can save time by directing the examination in appropriate directions and can avoid the embarrassment of prescribing the same magnifier they have at home but forgot to mention.

## MENTAL STATUS ASSESSMENT

Since many visually impaired people are older and some have age-related neurological disorders that affect vision, the assessment of mental status becomes an important aspect of the evaluation. While assessment of mental status is often considered part of the neurologic evaluation, it may be accomplished, at least in part, during the interview, particularly with respect to the patient's ability to recall recent and past events. Inability to recall information directs the examiner to perform a careful assessment of mental status during the physical examination. Deficiencies discovered in the mental status will certainly affect the rehabilitative effort and direction. The minimal aspects are an assessment of the individual's orientation with respect to time, place, and person. There are several excellent texts covering mental status assessment.[1-3]

A brief outline of the assessment of mental function may be remembered with the help of the acronym FROMAJE (function, reasoning, orientation, memory, arithmetic, judgment, and emotion). Questions posed to the patient should not require a simple "yes" or "no" answer. Function may be elicited with the broad question *"Tell me something about your daily activities."* Specific questions may be *"When do you get up and go to bed? Do you get dressed, fix your own meals, keep your own checkbook, pay your bills, shop, use the phone directory, and so forth? How is your disposition (mood)?"* This latter question opens the door for investigation of anger, worry, and such things as intrusive uncontrollable thoughts. Reasoning refers to the ability to interpret some degree of abstraction such as proverbs or similarities and differences. *"What is meant by a stitch in time saves nine? How are an apple and an orange similar?"* Orientation should be ascertained for time, place, and person, the order in which loss of orientation typically occurs. Ask questions such as *"What day (month, year) is it? Do you ever get turned around, mixed up, lost? Do you ever forget people's names?"* Memory should be tested for recent and past events as well as new memory. *"What did you eat today? How did you get to the clinic? Who is our president? Name the past three presidents."* (It is wise to ask questions to which the clinician knows the answer!) New memory refers to immediate recall. *"Repeat these three digits back to me. Remember these three (unrelated) things. I'll ask you about them later (5 minutes) in the exam—dog, car, umbrella."* Arithmetic ability is tested by asking the patient to "make change" in a hypothetical example or to count backwards by nines or sevens, starting at 100. Judgment is assessed by posing hypothetical situations such as *"What would you do if . . . you saw a fire in the wastebasket, found an addressed letter on the sidewalk, found someone breaking into your home?"* Proverbs with a moral element may also be used. *"What is meant by the saying, do unto others as you would have others do unto you?"* Emotion is assessed primarily by observation of the patient. Does he or she seem irritable, depressed, sad, inappropriately cheerful, fearful, paranoid, or apathetic?

A brief mental status test that can be scored is the Mini-Mental State Examination (MMSE).[4, 5] The capacity of the MMSE to distinguish patients with clinically diagnosed dementia or delirium from those without when the score is 23 or less (of 30 possible) has a sensitivity of 87%, a specificity of 82%, a 39.4% false positive ratio, and a 4.7% false negative ratio.[4]

## INTERVIEW TECHNIQUES

### Circumstances of the Interview

The interview sets the stage for the doctor-patient relationship and influences the prognosis for a successful outcome. The circumstances of the interview can be controlled to ensure a good initial impression. The manner in which the provider introduces him- or herself to the patient should reflect a degree of concern and respect. The use of a patient's first name should be granted by the patient and not assumed by the examiner. Both parties should be seated in a manner that ensures mutual respect. Chairs should be at eye-to-eye height so the doctor does not appear to be domineering or superior. Seating should be as comfortable as possible for the initial interview to allow the patient to relax and concentrate on the recall of important details. Lighting should be neither dim nor bright, and seating should be arranged so that light from windows does not obscure the person's view of the doctor's face. Note taking, while necessary, should not be obtrusive. Main points should be recorded as necessary, and the remainder filled in later when the history is recorded in the record. The interviewer should be alert to inconsistencies in the patient's responses such as a statement of well-being by a patient whose clothes are disheveled or who smells of urine. Sufficient time should be taken to ensure that the patient does not feel rushed and is therefore less likely to omit important details.

The case history is traditionally the first part of the examination, and it is here that the clinician can assure a success-oriented examination by establishing a positive attitude for the process. Case histories often dwell, partially by necessity, on the problems the person is experiencing. This emphasis can be averted to some extent by eliciting some of the things that he or she is able to do in spite of the loss of vision and by using positive words or phrases such as *"Tell me how well you can see,"* as opposed to *"Tell me how poor your vision is."*

## How to Phrase Interview Questions

Although open-ended questions such as *"How do you spend your day?"* are usually preferred, the clinician should ask detailed questions if the patient's responses are vague or general. Homebound patients might respond that they spend the day at home and have no functional difficulty. If they engage in hobbies, watch television, clean the house, and perform other typical activities, they could have a nice lifestyle. By asking specifically what they do, however, the clinician might learn that the day is spent sitting in a chair staring out the window or staring at a television that they can't really see. They may say they are able to prepare their own meals but in reality have tuna fish three times a day because these cans are easy to distinguish at the supermarket. They may have a "surprise" soup each evening because all soup cans look the same even though the contents are different. A specific question such as *"Tell me what you had for breakfast this morning"* may elicit a more informative response. They may express no difficulty with mobility because everyone can move about familiar surroundings. The clinician can propose a hypothetical situation: If the patient were dropped off downtown, would he or she be able to find the way around an unfamiliar store or get home using the public transportation system? Specific questioning, as in the previous examples, should provide a good profile of the person's functional abilities and perhaps even the motivation to deal with the vision loss. This knowledge gives direction to the examination and to the consideration of various treatment options.

There are certain techniques of facilitation that assist in maintaining the flow of the interview. *Reflection* is used when the patient pauses and the interviewer does not wish to inject a thought or opinion but wants to encourage the person to continue. Reflection is aptly named in that the interviewer reflects back the last thought or concern; for example, *"It felt like the worst pain you had ever had . . . ,"* and pauses until the description resumes. No one really ever understands precisely how someone else feels, and it is therefore not appropriate to say so; however, *empathy* should be expressed to let the patient know the interviewer has some regard for the depth of his or her expression of emotion or emotional experiences. One might express empathy by saying *"That must have been a difficult time for you"* or *"I can see how that might have upset you."*

At the conclusion of the case history it is important to allow the patient to add something that may have been omitted or forgotten when the appropriate area was covered earlier. *"Is there anything else you would like to tell me?"*

## EMOTIONALLY CHARGED INTERVIEWS

The interview may be an emotionally charged encounter in which questions about the vision loss and how it has affected the person's lifestyle, career, family, hopes, and aspirations may lead to tears. If this occurs, it is not appropriate to abandon the patient. Emotional support may be offered in the form of handing the patient a tissue and remaining in the room until his or her composure is regained.

Patients may also harbor strong feelings of anger, sadness, or frustration. These feelings may be directed against medical providers, family members, or others. The clinician must be prepared to listen attentively and offer appropriate support and, if indicated, referral for counseling or other therapy.

It is often informative to ask what the person thinks has caused his or her vision loss. People may have incorrect ideas that have caused them unnecessary concern over many years. Other family members or health providers may be blamed for conditions that they couldn't possibly have caused, yet the patient believes otherwise. If it is possible to uncover hidden bitterness or misconceptions, it may contribute to an improved patient attitude and a better prognosis for success if patients are given a factual understanding of the true etiology of their vision loss. Everyone has the right to be fully informed about his or her health and medical care, and it is the responsibility of health care providers to be sure that patients have all the appropriate factual information to allow them to understand their condition and make informed decisions about how they will deal with it.

## EXAMPLE CASE HISTORIES

The following case histories are given as examples from an initial visit. The histories are from actual patients, but the identifying information is fictitious. As the case histories are read, some thought should be given to what additional information should be solicited and how the information given would direct the physical examination; specifically, what the main problems are, what the patient's goal is, and how these aspects would be addressed as well as, hopefully, remediated. Management aspects related to ocular disease are omitted from the discussion since they are not within the scope of this text.

The first example is a rather typical case history in terms of the details. It represents an older woman who is visually impaired and who has been told there is nothing more that can be done for her. Her prognosis, however, appears to be good based on her functional abilities. The second example is more complex. That patient has a severe vision problem and has been examined previously at a low vision clinic but was unable to use the devices that were prescribed for him.

## CASE HISTORY EXAMPLE NO. 1

*Patient:* Ms. Christine Grant, DOB: February 4, 1910

*Source of History:* Patient and female companion

*CC:* "Can't really see anything."

*HPI:* Her left eye has been "weak" as long as she can remember, and her vision with the right eye began to deteriorate about one year ago. She saw a retinal specialist last July or August; he said she had "hardening of the arteries" and there was no treatment. She received a recall card recently but did not return to the clinic since she had been told that there was nothing to be done. She is uncertain if her left eye was poor as a child. She does not know her actual diagnosis for either eye but knows she has cataracts that were described as mild and removal was not recommended. A friend suggested that she come to this clinic for another opinion.

*GH:* Fine, except for arthritis, for which she occasionally takes Bufferin. She takes no other medications and says that medicines tend to make her sick. Her only known allergy to medication is to sulfa drugs. She denies diabetes and hypertension. She has never smoked and occasionally has a glass of wine before going to bed.

*PMH:* She had an appendectomy in 1945 and denies other hospitalizations or serious illnesses. She has never had an eye disease or eye injury and has worn bifocals for many years.

*FMH:* Both her parents died in their 60s from "natural causes." She has six siblings who are all living and in good health with the exception of one brother who has adult onset diabetes. She is the only one with any eye problem. She has only two children, both of whom are married and live out of state. Her son has adult onset diabetes, and her daughter has no known medical problems.

*SOCIAL/FUNCTIONAL:* Her husband was killed in WWII, and she never remarried. She lives alone and says she has no difficulty with daily activities, yet she is unable to grocery shop without assistance and spends her day listening to the TV. She is able to cook and knows when food is getting overcooked by the smell. She occasionally plays cards with her four sisters and two brothers. She can almost see large print cards but needs help. She is unable to read any of the newspaper except for the headlines. Her financial affairs are taken care of by her daughter, although she maintains control over the account. She is unable to read her bank statement or see her checks. She likes to knit but is generally unable to do so unless there is bright outdoor light. Her light bulbs at home are 100-watt. Her main GOAL is to be able to see better in order to read recipes and attend to her personal affairs. She has not tried magnifiers and has never been to a low vision clinic.

*ROS:* She denies problems with ears, heart and blood vessels, GI, thyroid, lungs, and skin. She has been told that she has "mild osteoporosis." She generally feels energetic but limited by her vision. She has taken a mild tranquilizer in the past for "nerves" but does not do so presently. She appears alert, and her affect appears normal.

## DISCUSSION

This woman appears to have a good prognosis for being helped. She has useful residual vision as indicated by her ability to read headlines and knit if there is bright enough light. She has maintained some independence in her lifestyle and has family support and interaction. She may be helped by cataract extraction if her lenses are more opacified than suggested in the history. She reported that brighter illumination is helpful, yet she only has 100-watt bulbs in her lamps at home. She has areas of difficulty that were discovered by specific questioning; for example, she reported no problems with daily activities, yet it was revealed that she was unable to grocery shop and only knew when her food was done by detecting a scorched odor. This demonstrates the value of asking specific questions when answers to broad or open-ended questions do not provide adequate detail.

# CASE HISTORY EXAMPLE NO. 2

*Patient:* William Nixon, DOB: December 8, 1915

*Source of History:* Patient and daughter

*CC:* "Poor vision in each eye."

*HPI:* He has a history of macular degeneration for seven years, but his vision has worsened significantly in the past 12 months. In general, he experiences fluctuations in his vision. It dims and then returns over a period of days. When this first occurred last year, he was examined by a retinal specialist, who had seen him previously, and he ordered an MRI and thought it revealed a mass on the lateral rectus muscle of the right eye. He referred Mr. Nixon to a neurologist for consultation, who reviewed the MRI and a CT scan with "several" radiologists; they decided that the MRI did NOT show a mass and the CT scan was normal. A SED rate at that time was described as normal, but the value is not remembered. There was apparently some mention that the MRI was not well done, which contributed to the erroneous suggestion of a retrobulbar lesion. There was no diagnosis, and no treatment was recommended. His vision has now decreased to the point that it interferes with virtually everything he wants to be able to do.

*PMH:* Hospitalized in May of 1990 for "kidney failure." He believes it began as a urinary tract infection. Prior to that he had "felt bad," and an internist prescribed two types of antibiotics (unknown). He had a sonogram (type unknown) and was hospitalized for 5 days approximately 2 weeks after the symptoms began. He responded to IV antibiotics and was released. During that stay he reports having "elevated liver enzymes, normal blood pressure, and increased blood gases." He also reported markedly decreased vision. An eye specialist examined him in June and found that his vision was decreased from prior examinations, the right more than the left, but no active pathology was found and no treatment was recommended. He had successful cataract surgery with IOL implantation O.D. in 1986 and O.S. in 1987. There have been no other surgeries. He has never broken a bone and has no history of head trauma or other serious illnesses.

*FMH:* His father died of a "heart attack" at age 65 and his mother died following a "stroke" at age 78. He has a brother with macular degeneration;

there are no other siblings. He has two children, a daughter who is 59 years old and a son who is 60. Both are in good health.

*GH:* He describes his current health as good. He takes Carafate every 2 days for indigestion and Peri-Colace "rarely" for constipation; he has been told to take one baby aspirin every other day but doesn't do it. He has been told that he has "liver stones." He has an appointment to see his internist next month for routine follow-up.

*SOCIAL/PERSONAL:* He is retired and lives alone in a retirement home. His wife died seven years ago. He has a son and daughter who live in town. He volunteers one day a week at a hospital where he takes phone messages. He rarely drinks and has never smoked. He takes no nonprescription drugs.

*VISION FUNCTION:* He is unable to read any size print. He has been to a low vision clinic and received training in eccentric viewing but says it was not particularly helpful. He has a closed-circuit television but is unable to use it successfully. He has tried various magnifiers, but they do not help him. He has bifocals that he wears consistently, although they make little difference in his vision. He is able to play bridge with large print cards and with some assistance from a sighted partner. He does not cook for himself since all meals are provided at the retirement home. He can recognize some faces if they are 10 to 15 feet away. He takes daily walks, but in the past year they have shortened in distance and he feels less secure when he is by himself. His main GOAL is to be able to see better for playing bridge and reading the newspaper.

*ROS:* General constitution is described as deteriorated compared to one year ago. GI system is positive for constipation and hiatal hernia. He denies problems with his thyroid, heart, ears, or vascular system. Mental: His daughter states that he was disoriented last week. She visited him on Sunday, and he did not know what day it was. She attributes this to the fact that there are no activities at the home on Sunday and this gives him no frame of reference. She recalls having called him earlier to remind him that there was only a noon meal to be served there and to be sure to remember to eat, but he forgot. She also reports that he plays bridge very well; although he can't see the cards in the "boot," he can recall them easily after being told what they are. He denies difficulty with recalling names of familiar people. He describes one episode last winter of falling out of bed at night and finding that he had apparently been in his bed backwards. He admits to being embarrassed about this incident and can't imagine how he got reversed.

## DISCUSSION

This case history raises a number of points for consideration regarding the anticipated course of vision rehabilitation. These will become clearer as the reader progresses through the text, but some are worth enumerating briefly at this point. Mr. Nixon has a relatively long-standing condition but appears to have had difficulty adapting to it since he has had a number of assistive devices prescribed for him, none of which are being used. This may reflect the fact that his vision is not stable or that his vision loss is particularly severe and he has not adjusted to it. It is also possible that inappropriate devices were prescribed and/or he was not taught how to use them effectively. The onset of his macular degeneration corresponds to the loss of his wife, and he may continue to grieve both. There is also some question raised by his daughter about his mental status. It is possible that this will interfere with successful use of assistive devices. He has a clear goal, which is helpful in giving direction to the evaluation of optical devices. If it turns out that he really is unable to use optical devices successfully for reading, he might enjoy recorded books or the Radio Reading Service available through the Public Broadcasting Service.

Other aspects of rehabilitation that should be considered for him would be training by an orientation and mobility instructor to improve his travel skills. This would allow him to continue to enjoy walking, which would assist him in maintaining his physical condition. Even though meals are provided for him, he might enjoy being able to fix snacks or occasional meals for himself. These skills could be taught by a rehabilitation teacher and an occupational therapist. They could also address other aspects of daily activities that are not revealed in the case history such as attending to personal hygiene and organizing and caring for his personal belongings.

## SUMMARY

The patient interview may be the single most important component of the doctor-patient encounter. It initiates the personal relationship and establishes the tone of future interaction. The information elicited gives direction to the physical examination and helps the clinician decide about the course of therapy and how to lessen the impact of the disease on the individual's life. The manner in which the information is elicited forms the basis of the patient's initial impression of the clinician. A poor impression at this point is not easily reversed.

## REFERENCES

1. Cohen-Cole SA: *The Medical Interview: The Three Function Approach.* St. Louis, Mosby Year Book, 1991.
2. Bates B: *A Guide to Physical Examination and History Taking,* 5 ed. Philadelphia, J. B. Lippincott Company, 1991.
3. Morgan L Jr., Engel GL: *The Clinical Approach to the Patient.* Philadelphia, W. B. Saunders Company, 1969.
4. Anthony JC, LeResche L, Niaz U, et al.: Limits of "Mini-Mental State" as a screening test for dementia and delirium among hospital patients. *Psych Med* 12:397–408, 1982.
5. Folstein MF, Folstein S, McHugh PR: Mini-Mental State: A practical method for grading the cognitive state of patients for the clinician. *J Psych Res* 12:189–198, 1975.

## ADDITIONAL READING

DeGowin RL: *DeGowin & DeGowin's Bedside Diagnostic Examination,* 5 ed. New York, Macmillan Publishing Company, 1987.

Folstein MF, Anthony JC, et al.: Meaning of cognitive impairment in the elderly. *J Am Geriatr Soc* 33(4):228–235, 1985.

Sapira JD: *Bedside Diagnosis.* Baltimore, Urban & Schwazenberg, 1990.

Spenser MP, Folstein MF: The Mini-Mental State Examination, in Keller PA, Ritt LG: *Innovations in Clinical Practice: A Source Book* 4:305–310, 1985.

# CHAPTER IV

# ASSESSMENT OF VISUAL ACUITY

*A success-oriented examination begins with establishing good rapport during the initial patient interview and is continued by ensuring that the patient can succeed in reading the first several letters or lines of letters presented in the visual acuity measurement. The case history should have revealed to the examiner some idea of the patient's visual ability; it is therefore easy to select letters of the appropriate size for the first attempt at an acuity measurement. If in doubt, start with the largest letters held near the person. This technique might give an individual with small central fields some difficulty, but, again, a good case history should have raised this suspicion and testing could begin at a greater distance.*

*Not every patient is able to read an acuity chart. Other tests should be available for examining infants, those who are cognitively impaired, and those who for any reason cannot be tested in the traditional manner.*

*It is important to obtain an accurate acuity whenever possible for several reasons: it establishes a baseline from which to monitor the ocular pathology; it is used to predict the strength of optical devices that will be required to achieve the person's goals; and it is often requested by other agencies to establish legal blindness, driving privileges, job eligibility, and school program placement. In spite of all these good reasons for measuring a person's visual acuity, the result is of little or no value in determining how a person functions visually in real life settings, which is the ultimate measure of how the vision problem affects his or her lifestyle. Two patients, each with 20/100 acuity, one from cellophane maculopathy and one from nuclear sclerosis, have the same quantitative acuity but may have different qualitative acuities and, therefore, very different functional abilities. Functional differences may be due to differences in contrast sensitivity, glare sensitivity, motivation, and numerous other factors not specifically tested for when visual acuity is measured in the standard manner, although these same factors may affect the measurement of visual acuity in the clinical setting. Visual acuity is a dynamic function and varies with such factors as the test*

> *setting, illumination, attention, doctor-patient rapport, and target contrast. Finally, visual acuity is a clinical measurement of the person's ability to read letters or numbers under artificially controlled conditions of contrast and lighting. This task has no real parallel in most daily activities.*

## DISTANCE VISUAL ACUITY

The clinician should make every effort to allow the patient to read something on the chart. The patient might be very encouraged by any degree of success in reading even a few letters, and it may be the first time this has happened since the vision impairment began. To accomplish this, the examiner must have a portable chart with large optotypes of many sizes. The typical Snellen chart is flawed in this regard in that there are large gaps for which there are no appropriately sized letters; for example, there are seldom letters between the 100- and 200-foot sizes and between the 200- and 400-foot sizes. Because of this, a patient whose visual acuity is 20/120 is automatically recorded as achieving only 20/200, which is the next largest size. This presents a potentially serious situation in which the acuity could decrease from 20/120 to 20/200, yet the examiner measures 20/200 in both cases and misses an important clue to active pathology.

As evidenced by the large variety of available charts, there are diverse opinions about what optotypes, spacing, and size progression make the most appropriate test of visual acuity. A good chart should have optotypes of equal legibility, have tasks of equivalent difficulty on each line (that is, the same number of letters with the same relative spacing), and have a consistent relative change in optotype size between all lines. Such a chart was devised by Bailey and Lovie[1] using a geometric progression of 0.1 log unit between lines. It is available in both distance and near forms. Because the progression of letter sizes and spacing is based on the logarithm of the minimum angle of resolution, the chart is referred as a logMAR chart (Figure 4–1). One "chart" that should not be used is the examiner's hand. "Counts fingers" is never an acceptable measure of visual acuity. Counting fingers is not quantifiable and is not a consistent measure from one examination to the next. Fingers come in different sizes, colors, and spacing. If the patient can count fingers, some letters on the chart can also be read, and he or she should be allowed to succeed at this task.

When the patient is truly unable to read any size letter at any distance, there are some other notations that are used as an indication of visual ability. These are "form perception," "motion perception," "light perception only" (LPO), and "light perception with projection" (LPP). LPP implies that the patient can both detect a light source and indicate its location, whereas LPO indicates the ability to detect only that light is present or absent. None of these

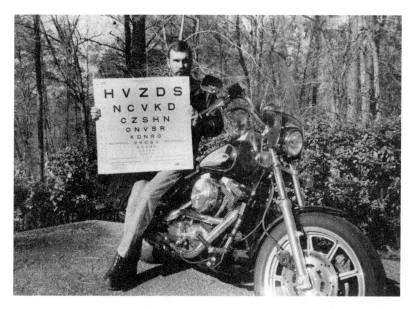

**Figure 4–1.** A distance visual acuity card based on the logMAR principle in which there is a logarithmic relationship between letter sizes, letter spacing, and line separation from one row of letters to the next. Also shown are the author and friend.

descriptors is quantifiable in the usual sense, but at least they give some indication of the patient's level of visual function. It is helpful to know that a person can detect and localize light, for example, since this can be a useful skill for mobility. Anyone who is unable to detect even a bright light source is said to have "no light perception" (NLP).

Distance acuities are often reported in metric notation with 6 meters as the test distance equivalent to 20 feet. These two distances are close but are not precisely the same. Six meters is equivalent to 19.685 feet. This creates a small discrepancy in the sizes of "equivalent" metric letters versus foot letters as shown on Example 4–1. It is important to know the size that a given acuity symbol should be in order to verify that an acuity card is printed accurately.

■ *Example 4.1.* Compare the sizes of a 20-foot letter and a 6-meter letter.

By definition, a 20-foot letter subtends $5'$ arc at a distance of 20 feet. The size can be determined trigonometrically as follows, where the opposite side is the letter height and the adjacent side is the test distance:

$$\text{Tangent } 5' = \text{Opposite side/Adjacent side}$$
$$\text{Tangent } 5' = x/20 \text{ feet}$$
$$0.00145 = x/20 \text{ feet}$$
$$(0.00145)(20) = x$$
$$0.029 \text{ feet} = x$$

The same calculation for metric units is as follows:

$$\text{Tangent } 5' = \text{Opposite side/Adjacent side}$$
$$\text{Tangent } 5' = x/6 \text{ meters}$$
$$0.00145 = x/6 \text{ meters}$$
$$(0.00145)(6) = x$$
$$0.0087 \text{ meters} = x$$

There are 2.54 centimeters per inch; therefore, 0.029 feet is equivalent to 8.84 mm (0.029 ft $\times$ 12 in/ft $\times$ 2.54 cm/in $\times$ 10 mm/cm = 8.8392 mm). There are 1,000 mm per meter; therefore, 0.0087 meters is equivalent to 8.7 mm (0.0087 m $\times$ 1,000 mm/m = 8.7 mm). These two letter sizes differ by only 0.14 mm, and, for a compromise, the average of the two is approximately 8.75 mm.

If a clinician has an acuity chart and wonders if it was calibrated for a certain test distance such as 10 feet versus 20 feet, he or she need only measure the height of the indicated equivalent 20-foot letter. If the card was calibrated for a test distance of 20 feet, the letter should be 8.75 mm tall. If the card had been calibrated for use at 10 feet, the "20-foot" equivalent letter size would be 4.4 mm tall (8.75 mm/2 = 4.375 mm).

Since 6 meters is essentially the same as 20 feet, acuities can be expressed in an equivalent manner by comparing the quotient of the test distance and the letter size; for example, 20/20 = 1= 6/6, or 20/200 = 0.1 = 6/60. The reciprocal of the quotient is considered to be approximately the smallest angular subtense that can be resolved, also referred to as the minimum angle of resolution (MAR). The quotient of 20/20 is 1, and its reciprocal (1/1) is also 1, indicating a resolution ability of 1'of arc. The quotient of 20/200 is 0.1, and its reciprocal (1/0.1) is 10, indicating a resolving capacity of only 10'of arc. Table 4–1 shows the equivalent metric and English notations for a variety of acuity levels.

## NEAR VISUAL ACUITY

Just as there are many charts for assessing distance acuity, there are also many different charts for near, some of which have significant faults. The clinician should avoid near test cards that have letter sizes indicated in Jaeger or point notation. Neither system has internal consistency in that they are not linear, and neither has external consistency in that letters of the same indicated size may actually be of different sizes on different cards.[2] While the near Snellen system is linear and has consistent size, it has its own problem, which stems from user error. Near acuities are often recorded as "20/100 at 10 inches." This statement is hard to interpret; for example, it is possible that the examiner had a card that was calibrated for some specific distance, such as 16 inches, but held it at 10 inches. If that is true, it becomes a challenge to determine what the acuity really was. It is also possible that the examiner really had a card calibrated for 10

**TABLE 4–1. A comparison of English and metric letter sizes representing the same minimum angle of resolution (MAR).**

| | MAR and Letter Size Designation | | | | | | | | | | | | |
|---|---|---|---|---|---|---|---|---|---|---|---|---|---|
| English | 20 | 40 | 50 | 60 | 80 | 100 | 120 | 140 | 160 | 200 | 250 | 300 | 400 |
| Metric | 6 | 12 | 15 | 18 | 24 | 30 | 36 | 42 | 48 | 60 | 75 | 90 | 120 |
| MAR | 1 | 2 | 2.5 | 3 | 4 | 5 | 6 | 7 | 8 | 10 | 12.5 | 15 | 20 |

Example: 20/60 is equivalent to 6/18 and represents a MAR of 3′ of arc.

inches and the patient read the reduced Snellen near equivalent of the 100-foot letter. Unless the examiner has recorded the distance for which the card was calibrated, it is not possible to determine the true acuity.

One near system that is very appealing and avoids the problems mentioned above is the metric, or M, system. The standard is the 1M letter, which by definition subtends an angle of 5′of arc when located 1 meter (1,000 mm) from the eye. The tangent of 5′arc (0.00145) is equal to the opposite side ($x$) divided by the adjacent side (1,000 mm), and therefore a 1M letter is calculated to be 1.45 mm tall as follows:

$$\text{Tan } 5' = x/1{,}000 \text{ mm}$$
$$0.00145 = x/1{,}000 \text{ mm}$$
$$(0.00145)(1{,}000 \text{ mm}) = x$$
$$1.45 \text{ mm} = x$$

The M system is linear, so a 2M letter is exactly twice as large as a 1M letter. The patient is tested at any preferred or desired distance, and the acuity is recorded as a fraction with the test distance in meters as the numerator and the smallest letter size read as the denominator. If the patient reads the 6M letters at 40 cm, the acuity is recorded as 0.4/6M. If the patient reads the 12M letters at 5 cm, the acuity is recorded as 0.05/12M. This notation is entirely unambiguous in that the test distances and letter sizes are exact. Because the charts are constructed of specific letter sizes and are not calibrated for a certain distance, a 6M letter, or any given letter, is the same size on every chart if it was printed accurately (not all charts are; see below). An additional advantage of using metric notation for near is that it allows for easy transition in the calculation of adds since they are expressed in diopters with metric focal lengths. Any near chart that the examiner finds useful, such as a logMAR chart or a chart with continuous text, can be labeled in metric notation if it does not come that way from the manufacturer. One simply measures the letter sizes carefully with a contact lens comparator or similar device and records the M size on the card. It is not necessary to consider any distance conversion since this is not an equivalent letter system, such as the reduced near Snellen equivalent, but rather an absolute measurement of letter size. The M size is determined by dividing the size of the letter, measured in millimeters, by 1.45, the size of a 1M letter in millimeters (Table 4-2).

It is occasionally stated in the literature that a 1M letter is approximately equal in size to the reduced Snellen equivalent of 20/50. This type of statement simply compounds the confusion of reduced Snellen equivalents and serves as a good example of why this concept is best avoided. If such a comparison must be made, then the distance at which this is true must be specified, since any size letter will subtend a different visual angle at different distances. One useful comparison is that a 1M letter is approximately the size of lower-case newspaper print; because of this, a reasonable initial clinical goal is to enable the patient to read 1M print at any distance. However, the eventual goal is to enable the patient to read precisely what he or she wants to read, keeping in mind that acuity cards are quite different from real world examples of print that people must use on a daily basis. Some of the differences are in contrast, font, and texture. Near visual acuities are typically measured with cards that have several letters on a line and fairly widely spaced lines, which presents an easier task than reading continuous text in a book or newspaper in which the letters are closer together, lines are spaced closer to one another, and the print and paper quality are not designed to give maximum contrast. It is therefore common for a person to read smaller letters on an acuity chart than can be read on a page with continuous text from a book or newspaper. This point will be emphasized again later in the text when considering the diagnostic trial and prescription of optical devices for near.

**TABLE 4-2. A conversion table for determining M size based on letter height measured in millimeters.**

| M Size | Height (mm) | M Size | Height (mm) |
|--------|-------------|--------|-------------|
| 0.5 | 0.73 | 8.0 | 11.60 |
| 0.8 | 1.16 | 9.0 | 13.05 |
| 1.0 | 1.45 | 10.0 | 14.50 |
| 1.5 | 2.18 | 11.0 | 15.95 |
| 2.0 | 2.90 | 12.0 | 17.40 |
| 2.5 | 3.63 | 13.0 | 18.85 |
| 3.0 | 4.35 | 14.0 | 20.30 |
| 3.5 | 5.08 | 15.0 | 21.75 |
| 4.0 | 5.80 | 16.0 | 23.20 |
| 4.5 | 6.53 | 17.0 | 24.65 |
| 5.0 | 7.25 | 18.0 | 26.10 |
| 5.5 | 7.98 | 19.0 | 27.55 |
| 6.0 | 8.70 | 20.0 | 29.00 |
| 6.5 | 9.43 | 21.0 | 30.45 |
| 7.0 | 10.15 | 22.0 | 31.90 |

Example: A 6.0 M letter is 8.7 mm tall.

It is not always safe to assume that acuity cards were printed accurately. Romano[3] found that the popular "Rosenbaum Pocket Vision Screener" had optotypes that were, on the average, 50% bigger than they should have been for the indicated size. It is easy to assure that any card is labeled accurately by measuring the letter sizes carefully and recording the M size on the card. Distance charts should be verified in a similar manner.

## ALTERNATIVE TECHNIQUES FOR THE ASSESSMENT OF VISUAL ACUITY

It is not always possible to measure visual acuity in the traditional manner in which the patient verbally signifies recognition of a symbol. This may be true for infants, children, those who are cognitively impaired, and others. Children who are capable of communicating but who have not learned numbers or the alphabet can be tested with cards that have alternative symbols such as pictures of common objects. There are many such cards available.

If the patient is simply hearing impaired, he or she can sign the response. It is an easy matter for the clinician to learn enough signs to assess the responses. A certified interpreter, preferably one who has experience in the medical setting, should be present for total communication, but it promotes a better patient-doctor relationship if the clinician shows some ability to communicate with signs.

If the patient can recognize symbols but has difficulty communicating the response either verbally or with signs, it may be possible to match symbols as an indicator of recognition. The patient has a set of symbols in his or her lap or nearby and matches the test symbol by pointing to the correct match. If near acuity is being assessed with single cards, the patient may use an enlarged set for matching and place the test symbol over the appropriate match. When children are to be examined, it helps if they have had an opportunity to practice at home or in school before the actual examination.

The technique of assessing visual acuity from preferential looking (PL) with commercially available hand-held cards is very useful for infants[4] as well as preverbal children who are visually impaired. The cards are rectangular and have a target, such as vertical stripes, on one side and no target in the corresponding area on the opposite side. The examiner presents the card by holding it in front of his or her face and peering through a small hole in the center to see which side the patient attends to. The peephole is used to ensure that the examiner's face is covered, which prevents it from becoming the primary object of the patient's attention. Multiple cards are used, each with stripes of a different angular subtense. The test is performed at a relatively near distance such as 50 cm, and the result is correlated to an equivalent visual acuity. Because the test distance is short, even a small variation in where the card is held is relatively large; therefore, considerable care must be used to maintain the correct viewing distance or the visual acuity may be significantly over- or underestimated. The main advantage of this test is that the patient is observed for visual attention and need not respond in any other manner. It has been shown that operant conditioning may be used to increase the number of children who may be assessed with this technique. One study, in which the subjects were children with severe and multiple impairments, used encouragement to look at the largest target and then reinforced a correct response with a reward such as music, food, or a toy.[5]

A visual evoked response (VER), also referred to as a visual evoked potential (VEP) or visual evoked cortical potential (VECP), may be measured as an objective assessment of visual acuity but requires expensive equipment and an experienced operator. A number of studies have shown good correlation between the VER and other tests of visual acuity,[6] but some caution must be observed in assuming that a given response correlates to a specific acuity. The VER measures the electrical response from the surface of the visual cortex (area 17). While a normal response is suggestive of vision, it does not verify that vision is actually taking place; for example, there is at least one case of a young male having a normal VER who was totally blind.[7] Computerized tomography demonstrated that he had suffered virtually complete destruction of areas 18 and 19 of the occipital cortex with the exception of the primary visual projection area (area 17). Occipital evoked potentials of normal amplitude were generated by diffuse light flashes, alternating checkerboard patterns, and sinusoidal grating patterns of low spatial frequency.

The test parameters for the VER may have to be altered for children with certain visual impairments; for example, Bane and Birch[8] found that the use of a horizontal bar VEP stimulus was more successful for children with nystagmus than the typical checkerboard pattern. In spite of the limitations mentioned above, the VER has a definite role in the assessment of visual acuities for patients who cannot be tested in other ways.

## SUMMARY

The precise determination of a patient's visual acuity is necessary for monitoring the ocular pathology and, as will be shown in later sections, for determining the magnification of the optical devices to be demonstrated to the patient. On the other hand, visual acuity is not always correlated with visual function, and there can be a large difference between the objective measurement and the subjective impression based on the functional abilities of the patient. The diagnostic trial and prescription of optical devices is guided by, and based on, visual acuity but is directed towards improving visual function.

# REFERENCES

1.  Bailey IL, Lovie JE: New design principles for visual acuity letter charts. *Amer J Optom Physiol Opt* 53(11):740–745, 1976.
2.  Jose RT, Atcherson RM: Type size variability for near point acuity tests. *Amer J Optom Physiol Opt* 54:634–638, 1977.
3.  Romano PE: Optotype distortion on the "Rosenbaum Pocket Vision Screener." *Annal Ophthalmol* 21:362–363, 1989.
4.  Teller DY: The forced choice preferential looking procedure: A psychophysical technique for use with human infants. *Infant Behavior Development* 2:135–153, 1979.
5.  Gerushat DR: Using the acuity card procedure to assess visual acuity in children with severe and multiple impairments. *J Vis Impair Blind* 86(1):25–27, 1992.
6.  Gotlob I, Fendick MG, Guo S, Zubkov AA, Odom JV, Reinecke RD: Visual acuity measurements by swept spatial frequency visual evoked cortical potentials (VCEPS): Clinical applications in children with various visual disorders. *J Ped Ophthalmol Strab* 27:40–47, 1990.
7.  Bodis-Wollner I, Atkin A, Raab E, Wolkstein M: Visual association cortex and vision in man: Pattern-evoked occipital potentials in a blind boy. *Sci* 198(4317):629–631, 1977.
8.  Bane MC, Birch EE: Forced-choice preferential looking and visual evoked potential acuities of visually impaired children. *J Vis Impair Blind* 86(1):21–24, 1992.

# ADDITIONAL READING

Colenbrander A, Fletcher DC: Visual acuity measurements in low vision patients. *J Vis Rehab* 4(1):1–9, 1990.

Ferris FL, Kassoff A, Bresnick GH, Bailey IL: New visual acuity charts for clinical research. *Am J Ophthalmol* 94:91–96, 1982.

Sloan L, Brown DJ: Reading cards for selection of optical aids for the partially sighted. *Am J Ophthalmol* 55(6):1187–1199, 1963.

# REFRACTION

Each patient should be examined carefully to determine the best correction of any refractive error. This is fundamental to the diagnostic trial and prescription of optical devices and must be performed first. The theory of refraction remains the same for a person who is visually impaired as for one who is normally sighted, but the techniques used are often modified, of necessity, to assist the patient in providing subjective responses. It should not be assumed that someone who has had a recent eye examination had his or her refractive error corrected accurately, nor should it be assumed that the glasses he or she is wearing are the best correction. People with extremely high refractive errors are often undercorrected by complacent or unskillful refractionists, and this should be anticipated when a new patient is encountered. It is also not unusual that patients present to the clinic wearing someone else's glasses, which they have found to be preferable to their own, at least under some circumstances.

It is assumed that the reader is already familiar with the fundamentals of refraction. Therefore, this chapter is devoted simply to techniques that may assist in the testing of those who are visually impaired.

## REFRACTION TECHNIQUES

### The Target

A projected chart usually lacks sufficient contrast to be seen by many visually impaired patients and limits the target distance to 20 feet since most examination rooms are arranged for patients with normal or near normal visual acuity. If the patient has a moderate impairment, this arrangement might work satisfactorily. If not, then a portable target that can be located at any desired distance is required. The target can be hung from a simple stand or even propped against the wall, with a table or stool used to provide sufficient height. Several relatively inexpensive portable acuity charts are available. A music stand makes an inexpensive and adjustable support for these charts, and an adjustable lamp can be used to provide the appropriate illumination.

## The Trial Frame Refraction

The phoropter is convenient to use but has two drawbacks for some who are visually impaired: it is hard to align properly for those who view eccentrically, and it is not possible to make larger lens power changes smoothly when the patient has difficulty discriminating the difference between ±0.25 diopter. The demonstration of a 1.00 D change creates the following sequence, *"Which is better, one, or* [click-click-click-click] *two?"* Meanwhile, four lenses flash by; if the choice is repeated, the total is eight, twelve, and so on. A ±1.00 D lens can be held in front of the phoropter, but if that is necessary, the phoropter has lost its advantage. The trial frame avoids both of these problems to some extent since it moves with the patient if the head is turned slightly for eccentric viewing and the examiner can select any power lenses for refining the prescription dependent upon the patient's ability to discriminate power changes. The trial frame also more closely simulates the final form in which ophthalmic lenses are prescribed and is therefore a more realistic situation for testing. It may be cumbersome at first, but with practice a trial frame refraction can be performed smoothly and rapidly.

The trial frame should be carefully adjusted on the patient's face prior to starting the refraction. It should be inspected from the side to adjust the pantoscopic tilt, from the front to ensure that it is level and centered before the eyes, and from the top, by tilting the patient's chin down, to make sure that the vertex distance is equal on each side.

Trial lenses are customarily marked with their back vertex power but have an effective power that changes relative to their distance from the eye. As a general rule, trial lenses used for the spherical component of the refractive correction should be placed in the back cell of the trial frame and the cylinders in the front. If high power lenses are placed in the forward cells, the distance of these cells from the back cell is great enough to induce a significant effective power difference if the vertex distance of the glasses is different. The final prescription from a trial frame refraction should be determined by placing the trial frame in a lensometer to measure the back vertex power of the combined lenses. Whenever possible, if two or more spherical lenses are in the cells of the trial frame, they should be replaced with a single lens of the resultant power in the back cell, again to minimize problems induced by effective power. There is, however, one exception to this rule. The lens aperture is smaller for higher power lenses, usually +6 or more, and it might occasionally be helpful to combine two lower power lenses in order to have a larger aperture. This is especially true for those who view eccentrically.

The trial frame should be supported with one hand while lenses are inserted or removed with the other. This stabilizes the trial frame and is more comfortable for the patient. A hand-held cross-cylinder may be used to determine the cylindrical correction, and the axis can be refined and/or verified by allowing the patient to turn the knob that rotates the cylinder. Once the refraction is completed, the vertex distance should be recorded. A careful measurement of the resultant lens power should be determined by placing the trial frame in a lensometer rather than calculating the sum of the powers of the individual lenses. This is particularly true if there are several lenses in the cells and if the final power is high. A significant error may be induced by adding the individual lenses and not compensating for the effective power difference due to their location in the various cells of the trial frame. This is avoided by using the lensometer since it measures the resultant back vertex power in the spectacle plane and that is what is prescribed for the patient.

■ **Example 5.1.** A tired clinician corrects a patient's refractive error with a +12.50 DS in the front cell of a trial frame and prescribes that as the patient's best correction. Assume that the front cell is 8 mm from the back cell and the back cell corresponds to a vertex distance of 7 mm, which is where the corrective lens will be when the glasses are dispensed. What lens located 7 mm from the eye would have the same effective power as the +12.50 lens at 15 mm from the eye?

Figure 5–1 shows that both lenses must focus parallel light in the same plane, which in this case is at the far point of the eye; therefore, the lens closer to the eye ($F_2$) must have a shorter focal length ($f_2$), and it must be equal to $f_1 - d$, where d is the difference in vertex distances (15 mm $-$ 7 mm). By substitution and a little algebraic manipulation (line 3), the following result is obtained:

$$F_2 = 1/f_2$$
$$F_2 = 1/(f_1 - d)$$
$$F_2 = F_1/F_1[1/(f_1 - d)]$$
$$F_2 = F_1/(1 - dF_1)$$

This should look familiar as one of the formulas used to determine lens effectivity.[1-3] For this example, $F_1$ is + 12.50, and $F_2$ is determined from the formula above:

$$F_2 = F_1/(1 - dF_1)$$
$$F_2 = +12.50/(1 - 0.008(+12.50))$$
$$F_2 = +12.50/(0.9)$$
$$F_2 = +13.89$$

A +12.50 lens that corrected the eye in the front cell would have to be replaced by a +13.89 D lens placed in the back cell; otherwise, there will be an

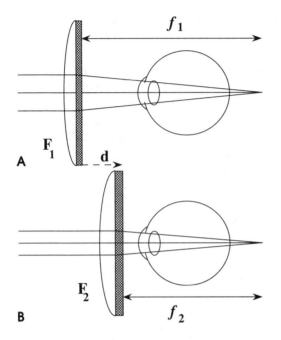

**Figure 5–1.** Any lens has an effective power that varies depending on its position relative to the eye; for example, both F$_1$ and F$_2$ correct the ametropia by bringing light to focus at the far point of the eye but must have different powers in order to do so because of their different relative positions. A convex lens, as in this example (**A**), must be replaced by one of higher power (shorter focal length) when positioned closer to the eye (**B**).

error greater than 1.25 D. Errors induced in this manner are reduced by placing the spherical component in the back cell and, when there is more than one lens in the trial frame, by reading the resultant power in a lensometer.

## Refracting Over Spectacles

For patients who have a high refractive error, it is preferable to have a "refracting set" of spectacles in high powers to serve as diagnostic lenses and to perform an over refraction rather than using a trial frame and trial lenses.[4] If the patient already has glasses, these may serve as the diagnostic lenses. Refracting sets were used frequently before the advent of the intraocular lens implant when patients were rendered aphakic by cataract extraction and required high plus spectacle prescriptions. The purpose of a refracting set is to allow the clinician to choose a frame and lenses that are as close as possible in all dimensions, including lens style and power, to that which the patient will wear for his or her own prescription. This allows the diagnostic frame to be adjusted precisely to the patient's face, with the same pantoscopic tilt and vertex distance as will be in the final prescription. The ideal lenses to have in the frame would be as close as possible to those that correct the patient's refractive error, and they would have a lens separation that corresponded to the patient's interpupillary distance. Since it is not possible to have an unlimited number of diagnostic spectacles, the clinician must purchase a limited set designed for aphakia or design one that seems appropriate based on his or her experience. Clip-on lens holders such as the Halberg or Janelli clips are used to hold the auxiliary lenses during the over refraction. A hand-held cross-cylinder is used to determine the cylindrical correction. Once the refraction is completed, the result should be determined by placing the spectacles, with the auxiliary lens holders, in a lensometer and reading the resultant power. Just as described above for the trial frame, a significant error can be induced if one simply adds the powers of the individual lenses without compensating for the effective power difference caused by placing a trial lens in the lens holder as opposed to having it in the spectacle plane (see Example 5-1).

A refracting set used for patients who have high myopia or hyperopia should be composed of several frames that are similar or identical to that which will be prescribed for the patient, with lenses of approximately $\pm 12.00$ sphere O.U. Each spectacle should have a different lens separation so one can be chosen that is close to the patient's interpupillary distance. The value of a refracting set diminishes the more one allows the prescribed lens and frame format to differ from that of the diagnostic set.

## Ancillary Refraction Techniques

When the refraction is difficult, the examiner can rely on several ancillary techniques to confirm or direct the process. Retinoscopy is of value if the media is clear but can also assist when the media is less clear if it is performed at a closer distance than customary (so-called "radical retinoscopy"). This gives a brighter reflex, and the examiner need only compensate optically for the closer testing distance. Retinoscopy bars are useful for a quick determination of the approximate best spherical correction if retinoscopy itself cannot be performed, since a large number of lenses, over a broad range of powers, can be shown to the patient without the necessity of selecting them sequentially from the trial lens set.

There are a number of visually impaired patients who are that way because they have extremely high refractive errors that are either uncorrected or undercorrected. When retinoscopy is not possible and patients are not responsive to lens choices, there is always the possibility that they are so far out of focus that the lenses shown make no appreciable difference. When this is suspected, large lenses, both plus and minus, can be tried to avoid missing an extremely large refractive error. A plus or minus lens on the order of 20 diopters should make things look worse for virtually all patients except that rare person with 20 diopters of uncorrected refractive error who seemed equivocal over $\pm 0.50$ diopter for the obvious reason. The examiner can work toward plano in five diopter steps to cover a broad range of powers quickly.

Keratometry can be used to determine high astigmatism, at least at the corneal level, and can give a starting point for determining the astigmatic correction with respect to both amount and orientation. The stenopaic slit is also useful when there is high astigmatism. It is a relatively simple device to use for obtaining a starting point about which to refine the correction. A pinhole might detect uncorrected refractive error, but the decreased illumination through it can have a neutralizing effect on its usefulness with some visually impaired patients.

Some clinicians advocate a telescopic refraction in which the patient is refracted while viewing through a telescope. The theory is that a more accurate result comes from the patient's ability to distinguish greater detail. The same result is achieved more easily by using a larger target or a shorter viewing distance and compensating for any induced accommodation. A good reason not to do a telescopic refraction to determine a patient's spectacle correction is the potential for error introduced by the vergence amplification of the telescope. Conversely, if a patient uses a fixed focus telescope at a near distance, it may be necessary to perform a telescopic refraction, specifically to determine if a lens is required to compensate for the vergence amplification. Vergence amplification is discussed in the section devoted to telemicroscopes in Chapter 10.

The patient's current glasses typically are used as a starting point for the refraction, and it is reasonable to do so; however, when faced with a vision loss that is uncorrectable, patients often try other people's glasses and may bring these to the exam. The patient may have old glasses, not brought to the examination, that were prescribed before the media became opacified. These can certainly provide a reasonable estimate if there is no reason to suspect a large change in refractive error based on the etiology of the vision loss.

If an automated refraction can be performed, it may serve as a confirmation of a difficult retinoscopy or refraction, or as an alternative to the traditional refraction when the latter cannot be accomplished.

Two observations during the health assessment can also occasionally assist in determining the refractive error. The lens setting on the direct ophthalmoscope when viewing the patient's fundus gives a clue about the refractive error if the examiner is aware of his or her customary setting for emmetropic patients. Distorted anatomy, noted ophthalmoscopically, can signal significant astigmatism.

Observation of the patient with respect to habitual reading distance and use of current spectacles can provide several clues about uncorrected refractive error; for example, a near reading distance may indicate uncorrected myopia, and repositioning or tilting of spectacles may indicate an attempt to adjust the effective power of the correction or to alter cylindrical power.

## Correlation of Best Corrected Visual Acuities

The best corrected distance and near visual acuities should be approximately equivalent. When they are not, the examiner must attempt to ascertain the reason. Substantially better acuity at near than at distance might be indicative of uncorrected myopia, just as much poorer acuity at near can indicate uncorrected hyperopia. There are also physiologic reasons, such as pupillary constriction and light intensity, that may account for acuities being better or worse than expected. The predicted performance with optical devices, as will be seen in later chapters, is based on the patient's best corrected reference acuity, and their actual performance should always be compared to the predicted level. When performance is not close to that which was predicted, one possible explanation is an uncorrected or miscorrected refractive error.

## The Ocular Condition and Refractive Expectations

Certain refractive errors are characteristic for some ocular conditions. Hyperopia with significant astigmatism is common with oculocutaneous albinism, just as astigmatism is expected with keratoconus and hyperopia with aphakia. A patient with Marfan syndrome or homocystinuria might have a dual refractive error secondary to a subluxated lens. The Marfan syndrome is also associated with myopia presumably secondary to elongation of the globe caused by this disorder of connective tissue.

## SUMMARY

Any improvement in visual acuity is worth pursuing, and it begins with correction of the refractive error. Many people who present with impaired vision will have an improvement with just a careful refraction. The refraction may be time consuming, and it may be difficult to determine an endpoint since reading is slower and discrimination between lens choices is more difficult with impaired vision.

The systematic approach to demonstrating and prescribing optical devices that will be presented in later chapters is dependent on predicting what power will accomplish the patient's stated goals, but performance cannot be accurately predicted if the patient's refractive error has not been completely corrected. It's worth repeating—optical enhancement of visual function begins with a careful refraction.

## REFERENCES

1. Ogle KN: *Optics,* 2 ed. Springfield, IL, Charles C. Thomas, 1968, pp 113–114.
2. Keating MP: *Geometric, Physical, and Visual Optics.* Boston, Butterworths, 1988, p 88.
3. Jalie M: *The Principles of Ophthalmic Lenses,* 2 ed. London, C. F. Hodgson & Son Limited, 1972, p 296.
4. Benton CD Jr, Welsh RC: *Spectacles for Aphakia.* Springfield, IL, Charles C. Thomas, 1966.

## ADDITIONAL READING

Freed B: Refracting the low vision patient. *J Vis Rehab* 1(4):57–61, 1987.

# CHAPTER VI

# ASSESSMENT OF VISUAL FIELDS

A careful measurement of visual fields is important and necessary for all visually impaired patients for accurate diagnosis, for functional assessment, for classifying someone as legally blind based on a field restriction, for determining legal driving status, and as a baseline for monitoring future change. The extent and type of visual field loss is also important in the selection of which types of optical aids are considered and, of course, to determine if field enhancement is a form of therapy that may be beneficial for the patient (Chapter 18). Even if the field cannot be assessed with the customary threshold stimulus or illumination level, it should still be measured by any means that works (Examples 6–1 and 6–2). The result, although not comparable to other methods, serves as a baseline standard for that patient in order to monitor future change.

As with refraction, it is assumed that the reader is already familiar with the fundamentals of visual field assessment. Therefore, this section is devoted to techniques that may assist in the testing of those who are visually impaired.

## FIELD ASSESSMENT TECHNIQUES

Some automated perimeters have special strategies for those with vision impairments, and when automated fields can be performed, that is emerging as the preferred method. If reduced acuity or poor fixation precludes the use of an automated perimeter, then fields may still be assessed with the Goldmann style perimeter, the tangent screen, the Amsler grid, and/or by confrontation. The principles of field assessment are the same as for persons with normal visual acuity, but it may be necessary to use different illumination levels, target sizes, and/or special techniques for maintaining fixation for those with central scotomas. The latter is discussed in the section that follows.

Whenever the visual field test parameters are different from those normally used, they should be carefully recorded in order to establish a baseline from which future deviation can be measured. An inexpensive light meter may be used to measure the approximate illumination level used on a tangent screen or other test apparatus that does not have a built-in, quantifiable illumination control.

Children and infants may be difficult to test with any sense of accuracy, but even gross results can be informative. Two people may be required in order to test a child's visual field, one behind with a stimulus and one in front to maintain fixation by attracting the child's attention. The objects used by each person may be lights of different colors, toys, finger puppets, or anything that works. If lights are used, the examiner should be careful to note whether the child actually sees the light source or the light shining on an object elsewhere in his or her field of view. If the child cannot respond verbally, careful observation will indicate when his or her attention is attracted to the peripheral target. It may be necessary to repeat the test many times until the examiner feels confident with the result. Observation, in addition to or in place of a formal test, may give information about a child's apparent useful field. Behaviors such as head turns, posture, ambulation around objects, and attention drawn to moving objects all suggest the extent of the visual field.

## Techniques for Maintaining Central Fixation

Patients with central scotomas have difficulty maintaining fixation since they must localize the central fixation point within the scotoma. If they are told to look at the fixation point, the unobservant clinician may find that they have an enlarged blind spot instead of a central scotoma. This is because the patient did as instructed and viewed eccentrically in order to see the fixation point. Correct fixation may be helped by placing a large "X" across the fixation point with white tape (Figure 6–1A). The patient is instructed, *"Look as if the center of your missing area is right where the two parts of the 'X' would cross."* The tape used by hairdressers works well since it pulls off of the tangent screen easily without damaging it. Alternatively, the patient may be instructed, *"Look as if you still had your central vision and direct that spot toward the point where the bars of the 'X' would cross."*

Another approach to maintaining central fixation with the tangent screen is to mark the physiological blind spot with a light-colored target (Figure 6–1B) and instruct the patient to keep that target hidden within the blind spot. This helps maintain central fixation without the need for the patient to imagine the intersection of a cross over the central fixation point. Any time the patient de-

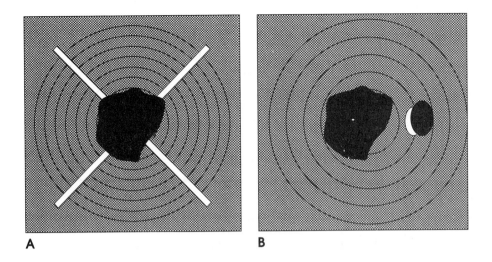

**A**                                    **B**

**Figure 6–1.** (**A**) White tape can be used on the tangent screen to form a fixation target for someone with a central scotoma. The person is instructed to look "as if" he were looking precisely where the two lines would intersect. (**B**) An alternative technique, the blind spot method, uses a lightly colored marker placed over the location of the blind spot. The person is instructed to look straight ahead and maintain a point of fixation that keeps the colored marker hidden from view.

tects the colored spot, it is apparent that fixation has shifted, and with practice one can learn to maintain central fixation in spite of a central scotoma. Variations on this "blind spot technique" have been described by Harrington,[1] Heijl and Krakau,[2] and Ehrnst.[3]

The Amsler grid is typically used to detect metamorphopsia, but it, or any similar chart, may also be used to assess the extent of a significantly limited visual field or a central scotoma. Some patients may find it easier to respond to the Amsler grid than to the tangent screen or an automated perimeter. The "blind spot technique" described above has also been used for maintaining central fixation with a grid similar to the Amsler grid.[4] Even if the patient's acuity is not sufficient to detect the grid, he may still be able to respond to a stimulus that is moved into view across the page. It is only necessary to know the distance at which the test is performed in order to calculate the extent of the visual field in degrees. Examples 6–1 and 6–2 show how the calculation is made.

■ **Example 6–1.** A clinician uses a black piece of cardboard as the background for a field test and a white hat pin for the stimulus. The patient maintains steady fixation at a marked spot and has a field that measures 4 cm to the right of fixation in the horizontal meridian. If the test was performed at a distance of 22 cm from the eye, what is the extent of this visual field in degrees for that portion of the horizontal meridian?

Solution: The extent of the field in degrees is found by using the tangent function just as it is used with the "tangent" screen to determine where to place the circles that represent 5°, 10°, and so on. The angle formed at the eye by imaginary lines from the point of fixation and the edge of the visual field can be considered part of a right triangle. The adjacent side is 22 cm and the opposite side is 4 cm; therefore:

$$\text{Tan } x° = \text{Opposite side/Adjacent side}$$
$$\text{Tan } x° = 4/22$$
$$\text{Tan } x° = 0.18182$$

and:

$$\text{Arctan } (0.18182) = 10°19' \text{ or approximately } 10°$$

■ **Example 6–2.** A clinician who is to serve as an expert witness in a lawsuit would like to know if a child's visual field is restricted to the extent that he could be declared legally blind with reasonable certainty. The only way the child is responsive is with two brightly colored finger puppets as targets. He fixates one at 2 feet, and the other is moved in from each side until it is 4″ from the first, at which point the child suddenly attends to the second target. If the linear extent of the field is therefore presumed to be 8″, what is the angular extent of the visual field in this meridian?

Solution:

$$\text{Tan } x° = \text{Opposite side/Adjacent side}$$
$$\text{Tan } x° = 4″/24″$$
$$\text{Tan } x° = 0.1666666 \ldots$$

and:

$$\text{Arctan } (0.1667) = 9°29'$$
$$9°29' \times 2 = 18°58'$$

These two examples may seem somewhat contrived, but they serve to show that a field assessment could be made, and quantified, under special circumstances if necessary. To avoid the calculations used in Example 6-1, it is necessary to use a grid that has been calibrated for a specific test distance, such as the Amsler grid, and hold it at that distance when testing.

## Training Prior to Field Assessment

When patients have difficulty responding appropriately for an accurate assessment of the visual field, it may be possible to obtain a measurement at another time after several practice sessions in between. This approach is helpful with children who may do much better after practice sessions with larger, easier targets and repeated explanations of the procedure. If the clinician simply abandons the test when the child cannot respond appropriately, it may never be possible to obtain a reasonable field assessment at future visits.

## SUMMARY

Visual field assessment is an indispensable part of the initial evaluation. The extent of the remaining field is used to monitor active pathology, determine legal blindness, recommend orientation and mobility training, select specific optical devices, and determine if field enhancement is to be pursued. A patient with severely impaired visual fields may have considerable difficulty responding appropriately to the test; for some, it may not be possible to obtain anything but a gross estimate of the visual field. It is acceptable to try and fail, but it is not acceptable to omit this important part of the evaluation.

## REFERENCES

1. Harrington DO, Drake MV: *The Visual Fields,* 6 ed. St. Louis, The C. V. Mosby Company, 1990, pp 48–50.
2. Heijl A, Krakau CET: An automated static perimeter, design and pilot study. *Acta Ophthal* 53:293–310, 1975.
3. Ehrnst SF: The blind spot method: A technique for maintaining fixation of age-related maculopathy patients during visual field examination. *J Vis Rehab* 1(2):41–45, 1987.
4. Potter JW, Wild BW: A new self-assessment test for age-related macular degeneration patients. *So J Optom* 4(2):15–17, 1986.

# SPECIAL TESTING

The value of special tests such as electrodiagnosis or tests for color discrimination is well established for the diagnosis and monitoring of ocular conditions but is less clear for vision rehabilitation. Similarly, tests for contrast sensitivity have an emerging role in ocular diagnosis and may play an important role in vision rehabilitation that has not yet been firmly established. This is primarily due to the fact that little can be done to correct or enhance deficits in contrast sensitivity, color perception, or visual functions other than visual acuity and visual field. There are circumstances, however, in which these and other special tests may be helpful to the design and implementation of the vision rehabilitation plan.

## ASSESSMENT OF COLOR VISION

Although there is no means of restoring color perception, it is important to know how a person's color vision is affected in order to provide appropriate counseling concerning daily activities. This is perhaps most evident for school-aged children who may have many educational activities that require color discrimination. It is important that each teacher be informed of a child's color discrimination problem in addition to any reduction in his or her visual acuity and/or visual field. Color perception is important in career selection and function for adolescents and adults. While it is not expected that the vision rehabilitation specialist will serve as the primary career counselor, he or she will certainly attend to this aspect of the patient's life to some extent and will communicate with those who do have primary responsibility in this area.

Ophthalmic filters may affect one's color discrimination (see Chapter 19). How these might affect a patient's visual performance must be considered when filters are prescribed. Tests of color perception performed while the patient wears the filter can serve to document the clinical effect and can serve as a useful demonstration to the patient that color perception is affected by the filter even though the results may be difficult to relate to daily activities.

When a color deficiency is found, suggestions can be made to assist in areas where color discrimination is helpful; for example, strongly contrasting colors might be used to enhance the visibility of table settings, throw rugs, or even food on a plate because of the difference in contrast as opposed to hue. Additional suggestions are given in Chapter 24.

## Tests for Color Perception

Standard tests for color perception may not be suitable for people who have impaired visual acuity and/or severely limited visual fields. Miyakawa et al.[1] showed that performance on standard test plates, by normal subjects whose vision was blurred with lenses, required a visual acuity of 0.3 to 0.1, or 20/67 (6/20) to 20/200 (6/60). Arrangement tests required minimum acuity of 0.20 to 0.05, or 20/100 (6/30) to 20/400 (6/120). Those with actual ocular disease might be expected to do even worse since the disease process could affect color discrimination and also might make a given acuity functionally worse than that created by simple lens blur. A logical alternative might be to use tests that are enlarged, and this has been tried; for example, enlarged versions of the D-15 have been used by some investigators.[2] Such alternatives might give clinically useful information, but they have not been adequately standardized. As mentioned above, it has not yet been established how to relate diminished color discrimination on any particular test to visual function and specific rehabilitative therapy.

## CONTRAST SENSITIVITY

Reduced contrast sensitivity can add significantly to the visual disability, but patients may not complain of this specifically since it is not a commonly understood visual function as is acuity or color perception. However, their complaint may be suggestive if it includes decreased ability to read materials that are known to have poor contrast, such as the newspaper compared to textbooks, or if they complain of "dim" vision. Contrast sensitivity can be measured clinically with several relatively inexpensive charts, and the result is a simplified contrast sensitivity curve. While this is not as accurate as a curve derived from testing with computer-generated patterns displayed on a cathode ray tube, the result still has clinical utility when it can be performed. Some persons with significantly impaired vision may not be able to discern any of the patterns, and this limits the usefulness of the available charts. The test may be performed monocularly and binocularly.

Reduced contrast sensitivity is more easily measured than treated. With few exceptions there is little that can be done to enhance contrast. The one device that allows contrast to be modified effectively is the closed circuit television. This device should be considered, regardless of acuity, when decreased contrast sensitivity is a major feature of the patient's visual limitation. Yellow filters have been used for many years in an attempt to improve contrast. Some patients respond very favorably, but there is presently no body of research that allows the clinician to prescribe filters in a rational manner based on clinical measurements of the patient's visual system. Reduced contrast sensitivity may also be ameliorated to some extent by modifying lighting. The measured contrast of reading materials may serve to indicate which tasks a person can or cannot accomplish based on his or her contrast sensitivity function and visual acuity. One study of the contrast for common reading materials reported newspapers to have approximately 60 to 70% contrast, several popular magazines ranged from 70.7 to 79.3%, whereas acuity cards and laser print were 92.2% and 94% respectively.[3]

A significantly better contrast sensitivity function measured under binocular conditions may indicate that binocular optical devices should be given greater emphasis; this is discussed further in the section devoted to binocularity with microscopes in Chapter 13. Even when little can be done to modify the effect of reduced contrast sensitivity, it serves as a clinical measure of the patient's disability, and in this regard it serves as baseline information to monitor changes that may not manifest in other clinical tests. It may also be used to counsel patients concerning their particular visual disability and how it affects their visual function.

## ELECTRODIAGNOSTIC TESTS

The electroretinogram (ERG), electrooculogram (EOG), and the visual evoked potential (VEP) have an established role in the diagnosis and monitoring of ocular disease. They can also be useful in making estimates about visual potential for patients who cannot be tested in other ways. The VER can be used to estimate visual acuity or to reassure parents or care givers that a child or infant seems to have visual potential. This latter aspect might not seem an important application, but it is. Much of what is accomplished in vision rehabilitation depends on the attitude of the patient and significant others in his or her life. When parents of a severely visually impaired child or infant can be told that a child appears to have visual potential by showing that there is a recordable response at the level of the superficial visual cortex, this can encourage them to pursue vision stimulation and visually related activities more actively.

A recordable response from the ocular structures associated with the electroretinogram and electrooculogram may serve a similar purpose in those who have opacified media or are otherwise difficult to test, but it is more tenuous to make a connection with vision since these two tests are indicative of function within the eye and not the brain. A recent study by Berson et al.,[4] however, found that ERG amplitudes correlated significantly with whether or not a person with retinitis pigmentosa drove during the day or night, walked unaided at night, or was currently employed. These activities were significantly related statistically to the 30-Hz cone ERG amplitude. This study result raises the possibility of using some electrodiagnostic tests as predictors of functional ability.

Even if no immediate value is apparent from the results of electrodiagnostic tests, it may be possible to encourage the patient or others that functioning ocular structures may one day be useful if new treatments are discovered. However, when discussing the results of electrodiagnostic tests, the clinician should temper his or her remarks carefully to avoid giving false hopes yet should strive to be as positive as possible since hope can influence attitude, which, in turn, makes a large difference in how the individual and his or her significant others adjust and adapt to a visual impairment. There is nothing wrong with hoping for future developments that will cure disease unless that hope pervades the patient's or family's life to the point that they do not actively pursue normalizing their present lifestyle to the maximum extent possible.

## GLARE TESTING

Glare may be only an annoyance or may actually be disabling. Questions about glare and the degree to which it affects the patient should be included in the case history, usually in the section related to vision performance. There are several devices available for testing glare disability in the office such as the Brightness Acuity Tester available from Mentor. The basic principle is to expose the patient to a source of glare and measure any reduction in visual acuity caused by that exposure. This necessitates that the patient's acuity be adequate to read some of the the letters provided, which is not always possible for those with significantly reduced acuity.

Glare testing may preclude other testing for a period of time if the patient is temporarily disabled from the test, and that should be considered when determining where in the examination sequence glare tests are performed.

Glare may be modified, if not controlled, by adjusting the light source producing the glare and/or by prescribing ophthalmic filters or other light-restricting devices such as pinhole glasses, visors, hats with wide brims, and typoscopes. Unfortunately, the prescription of individual devices is based more on trial and error than on any scientific rationale related to the results of the actual glare tests.

## OCULAR HEALTH EVALUATION

The ocular health evaluation is not a "special test," and a detailed discussion is not within the scope of this work. However, some considerations about when it is performed relative to the overall evaluation are worth considering at this point.

It is important to address the patient's main goal as soon as possible in order to maximize his or her interest in the examination process. However, if an exact diagnosis of the patient's condition has never been made or confirmed, or if the ocular health has not been assessed within a reasonable time, or if the chief complaint suggests active pathology, this clearly becomes the priority at that visit. Dilation of the pupils, as well as the high levels of illumination associated with fundus examination and biomicroscopy, may render the patient unable to function visually at his or her maximum level for hours or days. This precludes the demonstration of optical devices at the same visit. If the initial visit does not involve the demonstration of assistive devices, it is helpful if the patient has a clear understanding, as early in the encounter as possible, that a reappointment will be necessary for this part of the evaluation. This will avoid disappointment if certain aspects of the main goal are not addressed at that visit.

The practitioner must not let the appearance of the patient's pathology influence his or her judgment about the prognosis for the successful use of residual vision. The appearance of the eye often does not correlate with visual function, and the practitioner must always seek the maximum visual performance without being influenced by the apparent severity of the ocular condition evident on clinical examination.

To some extent, the person's diagnosis, apart from the acuity level or extent of the visual field, directs the examiner in deciding what types of assistive devices should be considered; for example, a variable or progressive condition such as insulin-dependent diabetes may suggest that devices with variable magnification should be the first consideration.

## SUMMARY

The special tests described in this chapter have a useful role in defining the limitations imposed by the visual impairment from a clinical perspective, but, with the exception of glare control, there are limited possibilities for using the results to modify the rehabilitation therapy. This will change as research contributes new means of assessing visual function and determining how it is affected by specific disorders, as well as how it may be remediated by specific forms of therapy.

## REFERENCES

1. Miyakawa N, Ichikawa K, Ichikawa H: Studies of methods of testing acquired color vision defects: 1. The effects of visual acuity. *Folia Ophthalmologica Japonica* 35:1597–1603, 1984.
2. Sloane M, Kuyk T, Owsley C, Ernst S, Nowakowski R: The effect of relative size magnification of Farnsworth D15 color chips on color assessment in low vision patients. Noninvasive Assessment of the Visual System. Technical Digest Volume Series 7. Washington, D.C., Optical Society of America, 1989, pp 140–143.
3. Cohen JM: Contrast of common near point reading materials. *J Vis Rehab* 7:2–4, 1993.
4. Berson EL, Rosner B, Sandberg MA, Hayes KC, Nicholson BW, Weigel-DiFranco C, Willett W: A randomized trial of vitamin A and vitamin E supplementation for retinitis pigmentosa. *Arch Ophthalmol* 111:761–772, 1993.

## ADDITIONAL READING

Knoblauch K, Fischer M: Low vision issues in color vision, in Rosenthal BP, Cole RG (eds): A structured approach to low vision care. *Problems in Optometry* 3(3): 449–461, 1991.
Waiss B, Cohen JM: Glare and contrast sensitivity for low vision practitioners, in Rosenthal BP, Cole RG (eds): A structured approach to low vision care. *Problems in Optometry* 3(3):443–448, 1991.

# COMMUNICATION

*Effective communication is the cornerstone of a successful doctor-patient relationship and must be continuous throughout the encounter. However, there are several points in the examination process at which communication plays a particularly pivotal role: the interview, the point at which initial testing has been completed and before assistive devices are demonstrated, and the point at which the final therapeutic plan is presented.*

*Several benefits derived from effective communication skills[1] include:*

*1. The ability to gather a good case history*
*2. The establishment of a therapeutic foundation*
*3. A lowered risk for litigation[1, 2, 3]*

## COMMUNICATING CONFIDENCE

One obstacle to effective communication in the area of vision rehabilitation may be the practitioner's lack of confidence in his or her own skills. If he or she is ill at ease with his or her abilities in this area, it will soon be apparent to the patient. This erodes the potential for therapeutic intervention. Anyone can communicate confidence if he or she *is* confident. It is easy to gain confidence by increasing one's scope of practice slowly and sequentially; for example, one can start to become involved in vision rehabilitation by first prescribing high adds such as bifocals and microscopes and referring the patient elsewhere for more complex services until additional skills are developed.

## COMMUNICATING FINDINGS AND THE TREATMENT PLAN

After the initial testing of acuity, refraction, and special tests, the clinician has assembled the data that will direct the next phase of the examination—the demonstration and prescription of assistive devices. Before doing that, the clinician can make the patient a partner in the process by conveying his or her impressions based on the initial data gathered and by providing an overview of what happens next. The patient's response at this point gives an indication of his or her willingness to proceed in the recommended direction.

If the visit included an assessment of any aspect of ocular health or if there are questions about it, the findings or impressions must be clearly conveyed to the patient at that point. Each of us has the right to know as much as possible about our health status, and it is incumbent upon the practitioner to provide the patient with a clear explanation of the diagnosis and the prognosis. Many patients are satisfied with nothing more than understanding their condition. Some also seek periodic information on advances in research that may be applicable to them. The practitioner should be prepared to give an overview of recent research developments that is positive yet does not raise false hopes.

Patients who understand their ocular condition typically have a better prognosis for successful rehabilitation. Patients who do not understand that their condition is permanent may still seek a miracle cure or believe their condition will improve in the near future. They are not yet prepared to utilize their remaining vision or prosthetic devices successfully.

At first, some, or maybe even all, patients are overwhelmed with the amount of information they receive concerning the diagnosis, management, and prognosis for their ocular condition, the various options available for vision rehabilitation, instructions about using optical and nonoptical appliances, instructions about environmental adaptations to employ at home and in the work place, the long-term prognosis, and the recommended follow-up schedule. Printed materials are very useful for conveying general information about selected eye diseases and can serve as a source of review for patients and their families at home. An excellent source of information for the patient to review as often as desired is a tape recorded interview. This has been tried with cancer patients,[4] and it was found that audio recordings were well accepted and that the taped interviews were frequently reviewed, usually with family and friends. The investigators found that although patients believed they understood the diagnosis and treatment plan, most felt that they obtained additional information and a clearer understanding about their care by listening to the recordings at home with family and/or friends.

Patient characteristics and communicative styles definitely influence the amount of information given in a medical consultation. An analysis of audiovisual recordings of 41 physician-patient consultations in a family practice clinic revealed that information regarding diagnosis and health matters was primarily related to the patient's anxiety, education, and question-asking, while information regarding treatment was primarily related to the patient's question-asking and expression of concerns.[5]

The need for better communication, such as written instructions or recorded consultations, can be seen in the area of patient compliance with a therapeutic regimen. Patient perceptions of treatment goals were studied by surveying 54 individuals with type II NIDDM and obesity.[6] Their physicians were also surveyed to determine the degree of congruence between patient and health care provider. The investigators found a 53% discrepancy rate in the area of overall treatment goals. A 57% and 43% rate of discrepancy was found for the specific goals of weight loss and blood glucose levels, respectively.

Patient satisfaction with the care provided depends in part on being able to ask questions. Patients who are encouraged to write down their questions in advance of the visit or who feel that they are openly encouraged by the clinician to ask questions during the visit are more likely to be satisfied.[7] It is easy to suggest to patients that they write down their questions for a future visit or even for the first visit if an information sheet is mailed to them prior to the first appointment.

Question-asking is related to the length of the interaction and the perceived time available with the clinician.[8] A clinician who can successfully give the impression of being unhurried and totally involved with that individual will have a more successful interaction.

An investigation of 115 pediatric consultations[9] revealed two interesting findings. First, parents who were less satisfied received more directives and proportionally fewer patient-centered utterances from the care giver than did those parents who were more satisfied. Second, the clinicians' use of statements that were patient-centered was predictive of parents' perceptions of the clinicians' interpersonal sensitivity and partnership building, yet the amount of information physicians provided was unrelated to judgments of their informativeness. In other words, it was not how much was said but how it was said.

## DISCUSSING THE FUTURE

At some point, most patients or their family members ask about research that might lead to a cure or other restorative process. It is important to be familiar with current research and to be able to present an optimistic overview without giving false expectations and without allowing the patient to reject the rehabilitative process while hoping for an imminent breakthrough. Some of the most exciting current research centers around genetic disorders and includes detecting gene loci, sequencing genes, and gene therapy. There have been recent advances in a number of genetic disorders that affect vision. Retinitis pigmentosa

(RP) is a good example. When a person with RP asks about genetic research, the author presents an overview similar to the following:

There are many active researchers in this area, and there is a strong financial basis to support their activities thanks to the Retinitis Pigmentosa Foundation and other groups and individuals who are very active in soliciting funds to support research. Some exciting recent developments include the identification of specific gene mutations that are associated with retinitis pigmentosa in some families. The discovery of a specific gene mutation is very important because that is the first step in understanding what actually goes wrong to cause the disease. The next step is to learn what that gene is supposed to do normally and how the mutation affects that process. Once that is known, it is possible to investigate treatment. For example, if the gene controls the manufacture of a specific compound, such as an enzyme, it may be possible to make that enzyme artificially and replace it in the body. One day it might even be possible to repair the gene or introduce a substitute gene into the cells of the eye that will act in the normal manner. A few years ago this may have sounded like science fiction, but, in fact, similar accomplishments have been made for other diseases in animals and in some cases for humans. Another exciting area of research is in retinal cell transplantation. In animal studies, cells have been transplanted, and they not only lived but appeared to function in a natural manner. Of course, for this to lead to vision, it would be necessary for these cells to make the correct connections with the brain. It is not yet clear how this might be accomplished. We do know, though, that the body did it once when the eye was first being formed, and it may be possible to find a way that allows it to do so again.

I maintain a computerized listing of patients so they can be contacted if a new development is announced that might be beneficial to them. I invite you to call me whenever you have any questions concerning something you have heard about or read about. Because of these recent research developments, I am personally very optimistic about the future. Meanwhile, as you know, there is no way to be sure when or if these developments might lead to a treatment, but there are others things that can be done for you today such as prescribing optical devices that will allow you to use the vision that you do have more effectively. Let's start with that.

## COMMUNICATING WITH FAMILIES, FRIENDS, AND CARE GIVERS

Effective communication with the patient is not the only aspect of communication. It is also important that family members, care givers, and friends receive appropriate information, with the patient's permission, that will allow them to facilitate the rehabilitation process. General information about impaired vision can be made available on an information sheet similar to the sample below. Face-to-face conversations are important and effective. An information sheet or brochure should not be used to replace conversations but will serve to enhance information recall once patients have left the office.

---

### SAMPLE INFORMATION SHEET
### HINTS FOR FAMILY AND FRIENDS ABOUT VISION IMPAIRMENT

There are many ways in which friends and family members can be supportive of a person who is visually impaired. Part of being supportive is understanding some of the problems faced by those who are visually impaired and discovering appropriate ways to assist when necessary. The following thoughts may be helpful in this regard.

1. Sometimes it is hard to accept that a person is visually impaired if the eyes look perfectly normal. In fact, the eyes often look perfectly normal on the outside since many eye diseases affect only the structures inside the eye.
2. There is a certain folklore that suggests that people who lose some or all of their vision may compensate by developing extra sensory abilities such as a special sense of touch or hearing. This is not the case. They may learn to use their other senses more effectively, but their abilities are no different from anyone else in this regard. On the other hand, it is not unusual for some to assume that a person who is visually impaired is also hearing impaired, and they may speak to him or her in a loud tone of voice. This is not necessary unless there actually is a hearing impairment.
3. People who are visually impaired may not be able to recognize when someone is addressing them specifically if there are other people in the immediate area. It is therefore important to use their name first to indicate that you are speaking to them.
4. Don't walk away from people who are visually impaired without telling them that you are leaving. They may assume you are still there if they are not able to see well enough to find you.
5. You should not assume that people who are visually impaired are helpless. Offer assistance when appropriate but don't force it on them; for example, do not grab their arm to steer them into another room. Instead, ask, "Would you like some assistance moving to the dining room?" or, "Would you like to take my arm?"

6. People who are visually impaired may be hesitant to ask others to assist them with certain tasks for fear of seeming to be a burden. You can reduce their need to ask by volunteering; for example, if you are driving to the grocery store or downtown, ask if they would like to go with you.

7. It is not unusual for some people to assume that a person who is visually impaired will no longer enjoy activities that seem to require normal vision. This is not the case. A person who has become visually impaired will still enjoy many of the same activities he or she enjoyed in the past such as movies, television, museums, and browsing in stores. The experience may be different for him or her than in the past yet still provide pleasure.

8. You may be able to help your friend or family member by assisting him or her to learn to use optical aids or to make changes in the home or work environment such as improving lighting or using color and contrast to make things more visible. These and other techniques are discussed on other information sheets similar to this one.

9. Conditions such as glare, lighting, and surrounding colors may make a big difference in a person's ability to function visually from one moment to the next. There are also many causes of visual impairment that may allow a person to see better some days than other days. This is often confusing to friends and family members who may assume, falsely, that he or she ought to be able to see at the best level all day, every day.

10. It is not unusual for a person who becomes physically challenged to have periods of anxiety, depression, or denial. He or she will have to work through these changes, and one of the best forms of therapy is the continued support and acceptance by family and friends.

11. It may seem inappropriate to use words such as "see" or "look" when talking to someone who is visually impaired, but these are part of our everyday vocabulary and should not be avoided.

12. Most important of all, remember that your friend or family member is a person just like you who happens to be visually impaired. He or she has all the same emotions, feelings, concerns, needs, and aspirations that anyone else has but has some additional challenges to overcome. Be supportive.

## WHAT DO YOU TELL THE PATIENT WHO ISN'T HELPED?

Success is wonderfully invigorating when it occurs, but it is rarely easy to obtain; more often than most would like to admit, it just does not happen. Some people cannot be helped and some people simply will not be helped, but they all gain something from the experience. They all know that the clinician has tried to help them and, perhaps more importantly, that someone cares enough to try. This is therapeutic. They all gain information about what types of assistance are available and to what extent they may or may not be helpful. That is also therapeutic. At the conclusion of an apparently unproductive clinical encounter it is important to end on a positive note. The patient and family can be told something similar to the following:

> Ms. Smith, you have certainly learned a lot today, and I feel as if we accomplished a lot today. You now have a better understanding of your eye condition and what types of assistance are available to you. Even though you are not interested in pursuing any of them at this time, I hope you will think about what you have seen and will feel free to return, next week or next month, if you would like for me to demonstrate any of them again or if you would like to discuss anything else. Many people have the same reaction when they are examined for the first time, perhaps because they were expecting something different. A number of them return later, after thinking about it for a period of time, and find that some of these magnifiers are helpful in ways they didn't imagine at first. I hope you will do the same because I know from what you accomplished today that magnification could be helpful to you in some circumstances. I hope you will take advantage of it.

## SUMMARY

"Every patient needs mouth-to-mouth resuscitation for talk is the kiss of life."[10]

"There must come a time when diagnostic curiosity is satisfied and attention is turned to learning what it means to become therapeutic. Most of this learning comes by way of genuine conversations."[11]

## REFERENCES

1. Meyerscough PR: *Talking With Patients: A Basic Clinical Skill.* Oxford, Oxford University Press, 1989.

2. Lester GW, Smith SG: Listening and talking to patients. A remedy for malpractice suits? *West J Med* 158(3):268–272, 1993.
3. Husserl F: Effective communication: A powerful risk management tool. *J Lou State Med Soc* 145(1):29–31, 1993.
4. Johnson IA, Adelstein DJ: The use of recorded interviews to enhance physician-patient communication. *J Cancer Ed* 6(2):99–102, 1991.
5. Street RL Jr: Information-giving in medical consultations: The influence of patients' communicative styles and personal characteristics. *Social Sci Med* 32(5):541–548, 1991.
6. D'Eramo-Melkus GA, Demas P: Patient perceptions of diabetes treatment goals. *Diab Ed* 15(5):440–443, 1989.
7. Thompson SC, Nanni C, Schwankovsky L: Patient-oriented interventions to improve communication in a medical office visit. *J Health Psychol* 9(4):390–404, 1990.
8. Beisecker AE, Beisecker TD: Patient information-seeking behaviors when communicating with doctors. *J Med Care* 28(1):19–28, 1990.
9. Street RL Jr: Analyzing communication in medical consultations. Do behavioral measures correspond to patients' perceptions? *J Med Care* 30(11):976–988, 1992.
10. Broyard A: *Intoxicated by My Illness.* New York, Clarkson Potter, 1992, p 53.
11. Stephens GG: Acts of endearment. Attending to the affectional bonds between physicians and patients. *Can Fam Phys* 38:2842–2846, 1992.

## ADDITIONAL READING

Buckman R: *How To Break Bad News.* Baltimore, Johns Hopkins University Press, 1992.
Cassell EJ: *Talking With Patients, Volume I: The Theory of Doctor-Patient Communication.* Cambridge, MA, The MIT Press, 1985.
Cassell EJ: *Talking With Patients, Volume II: Clinical Technique.* Cambridge, MA, The MIT Press, 1985.
Cousins N: *Head First—The Biology of Hope.* New York, Dutton, 1989.
Fallowfield L: The ideal consultation. *Br J Hosp Med* 47(5):364–367, 1992.
Frank A: *At the Will of the Body.* Boston, Houghton-Mifflin, 1991.
Riccardi VM, Kurtz SM: *Communication and Counseling in Health Care.* Springfield, IL, Charles C. Thomas, 1983.
Stephens GG: Patients on patienthood: New voices from the high-tech arena. *JABFP* 6(2):517–522, 1993.

# MAGNIFICATION

*The most common therapeutic approach to assisting persons with low vision is to provide them with sufficient magnification to achieve their visual goals. There are several types of magnification that are utilized alone or in combination to help people use their remaining vision more effectively. Magnification must always be compared to some original reference in order to be meaningful; for example, the expression "two times bigger" is relative and not absolute—two times bigger than what? (Two times bigger than the reference size.)*

## TYPES OF MAGNIFICATION

*Relative distance magnification (RDM):* If an object is moved closer to the eye, it appears relatively larger. That is an example of RDM. A practical example is to have a student who is visually impaired sit closer to the blackboard. The concept of relative distance magnification is often applicable to adults who complain of difficulty seeing their television set. The television could be magnified by a spectacle-mounted telescope, but it would be easier and less expensive just to sit closer to the set. It seems intuitively obvious that an object might appear twice as large if it is moved twice as close (that is, to one-half the original distance). This can be shown to be true, and, in general, an object that is moved in to "1/k" of the reference (original) distance will appear "k" times larger. This relationship can be expressed as

$$RDM = r/d$$

where RDM is relative distance magnification, r is the reference (original) distance, and d is the new distance.

■ **Example 9–1.** A patient is just able to read 3M print at 40 cm. If the print is moved in to 20 cm, how much relative distance magnification will be achieved?

RDM = Reference distance/New distance
RDM = 40 cm/20 cm
RDM = 2X

*Relative size magnification (RSM):* An object that is difficult to distinguish may be enlarged to a sufficient size in order that the patient can see it. This is accomplished for students who are visually impaired by having their textbooks made available in large print. There are also many other large print books available in libraries and bookstores. Other examples of relative size magnification are large screen televisions, large print checks, and wrist watches with large numerals. Relative size magnification can be determined by measuring the new size and dividing that value by the reference (original) size.

■ **Example 9–2.** A teacher wants to enlarge a student's written test questions from their original size of 2M print. How much relative size magnification would be provided if he or she used 8M print in place of the 2M print?

RSM = New size/Reference size
RSM = 8M/2M
RSM = 4X

■ **Example 9–3.** If a reference acuity is established using letters that are 10 mm tall, how much relative size magnification would be achieved by using 35 mm tall letters held at the same distance?

RSM = New size/Reference size
RSM = 35 mm/10 mm
RSM = 3.5X

*Angular magnification:* Some optical devices are prescribed to provide angular magnification. These will be discussed in detail later, but an example for now would be binoculars or a hand-held monocular telescope used for spotting distant objects.

*Electronic magnification:* The image of an object can be enlarged electronically in a manner different from the other types of magnification. The closed circuit television (CCTV) is an example. This device consists of a television camera and monitor. The user places material beneath the camera, and an enlarged image is created on the monitor. Magnification can be altered with the camera lens. Contrast and brightness can be adjusted electronically for maximum visibility.

*Projection magnification:* An image can be enlarged by projecting it through an optical system such as an overhead projector, a slide projector, or an opaque projector. Such systems are used less often since the advent of the CCTV.

## MAGNIFICATION FROM MULTIPLE SOURCES

When magnification is derived from more than one source, the total magnification is determined by the product of the individual sources, not their sum. The general formula for "n" sources of magnification (M) is:

$$MAG_{total} = M_1 \times M_2 \times \ldots \times M_n$$

■ **Example 9–4.** A person is barely able to read 3M print when held at 40 cm. The examiner now shows her 9M print at 20 cm, and she reads it easily. What is the total magnification achieved?

The relative size magnification is 9M/3M = 3X. The relative distance magnification is 40 cm/20 cm = 2X. The total magnification is therefore:

$$MAG_{total} = (3X) \times (2X)$$
$$MAG_{total} = 6X$$

## DETERMINATION OF REQUIRED MAGNIFICATION

The approach used in this text to determine the amount of magnification the patient needs is first to establish a goal and then calculate the magnification required to achieve that goal. The magnification needed is calculated relative to a reference acuity that, in all cases, is determined *after* the patient's refractive error is corrected. Predictions of required magnification and the optical power needed to provide it are meaningless if they are determined before the patient's refractive error is corrected. (Have I made this point perfectly clear?)

By convention, magnification units are designated by an X; for example, three "times larger" is 3X. The general formula to determine required magnification is:

Magnification required = Reference size/Goal size

■ **Example 9–5.** If the patient reads 40-foot letters at 20 feet through the best correction and the goal is to read 20-foot letters at the same distance, then the required magnification is:

Magnification required = Reference size/Goal size
$$M = 40/20$$
$$M = 2X$$

The numerator of the acuity was ignored in the calculation. This is allowable only if the reference acuity and the goal acuity are expressed as equivalent acuities for the same distance. If not, they must be converted as in the example below.

■ **Example 9–6.** If the best corrected distance acuity is 10/40 and the goal is to read the equivalent of 20/20, the reference acuity is first converted to have the same numerator as the goal acuity. Then the required magnification is calculated:

$$10/40 = 20/80$$
$$\text{Magnification required} = \text{Reference size/Goal size}$$
$$M = 80/20$$
$$M = 4X$$

■ **Example 9–7.** The patient has a near acuity of 6M, and the goal is to read 2M print. The required magnification is:

$$\text{Magnification required} = \text{Reference size/Goal size}$$
$$M = 6M/2M$$
$$M = 3X$$

## MAGNIFICATION IS NOT CLARIFICATION

It is important for the clinician and the patient to realize that magnification does not provide the patient with a clearer image. It only provides a larger image. If patients have hazy vision from corneal clouding, they will still have hazy vision when looking through an optical device; however, they should distinguish more detail because the image is larger. If this is not emphasized to patients repeatedly, they will expect their prescription to render clear vision when it is finally dispensed. Their disappointment may result in rejection of a device that otherwise would have been very useful.

## THE MAGNIFICATION LABELING CONTROVERSY

Once the required magnification is known, the next step is to determine the optical device that will provide it. Manufacturers often label their devices with a magnification amount, but that is not necessarily the magnification that the patient will receive when using that device. The reason is obvious—the manufacturer has used an arbitrary reference distance that does not necessarily correspond to the reference distance for the patient.

For telescopes it is easy to select the appropriately powered aid since they are labeled, relatively accurately but not perfectly, in terms of the magnification they provide. This is not the case for other optical devices. For hand magnifiers, stand magnifiers, and microscopes it is necessary to determine what *dioptric strength* will provide the patient with the required magnification. This is discussed in detail in subsequent chapters.

## READING AS A MEASURE OF PREDICTED MAGNIFICATION

Reading is a very common everyday activity. When the clinician attempts to determine the magnification needed for near, a logical goal is to achieve the ability to read print of a given size. However, reading is not the only activity people want to perform at near, and acuity is not the sole criterion for determining functional reading ability. Legge et al.[1] investigated reading speed in 141 persons with low vision and found that acuity accounted for only 10% of the variance in reading speed and that age was a better predictor of reading speed. In fact, they found that all clinical predictors, such as central visual fields and clarity of the ocular media, even when combined, could account for only 30% of the variance in reading speed. Other factors that one might expect to influence reading function are eye movements, the degree and location of extrafoveal fixation, reading ability before vision loss, lighting, posture, print size, and quality of the printed material. Only a few of these can be manipulated clinically, and the major form of therapy—optical devices—can only affect the image size. The best measure of functional reading ability is to actually measure reading ability, preferably with the same materials the patient will use when an optical device has been prescribed. Visual acuity, measured with isolated letters, may serve as a convenient starting point for predicting the required magnification to achieve some functional goal, but since it is not the best predictor of functional reading ability, an acuity card with continuous text might serve as a better target to predict the required amount of magnification. When isolated letters are used, it should be anticipated that the patient will require more magnification than predicted, since reading continuous text is a more demanding task. The clinician also should not expect an acuity card and a newspaper or book with print of the same size to represent equivalent tasks since differences in paper, ink, and print fonts will influence reading performance.

Some people do not care to read, and it is therefore unrealistic to pursue this as a goal although the temptation is hard to resist since near function is typically determined by one's ability to distinguish print on an acuity card. But what about the patient who simply wants to distinguish food on his or her plate or enjoy photographs of his or her family? These activities cannot be adequately correlated with a specific acuity. One might assume that if the patient can distinguish newspaper-sized print, this might indicate adequate acuity for virtually all common near activities, but that remains an unproven assumption. Again, the best tests of functional ability involve performing the actual activity. This can be accomplished in the office by simulating or creating the activity that the patient wishes to pursue. For reading, it is easy to have many types of print available such as books, magazines, bills, menus, medication bottles, price tags, and newspapers. For those who seek assistance performing near tasks other than reading, it is also possible to have items available such as electronic components, silverware, sewing needles, insulin syringes, photographs, small tools, cosmetic products, and keys. Many similar objects are already present in the office; for those that are not, a small collection can be created. When it is not possible to make a reasonable simulation, the patient should be asked to bring his or her own material to the examination so the exact task can be recreated. Of course, the office setting may be quite different than the home or work place with respect to lighting and other factors, and this must be considered when the patient leaves with the prescribed device(s). Environmental adaptations for the home and work place are described in Chapter 24.

## SUMMARY

To reiterate—the purpose of determining a goal, the required magnification, and the optical aid that provides that magnification is to have an organized and systematic approach to the diagnostic evaluation of the patient. The aid that is demonstrated should give the desired result or one very close to it. The power can then be refined until the goal is achieved. When the result is not as expected, it indicates inconsistent data, the source of which must be determined. Some possibilities are an uncorrected refractive error, an improperly labeled device, or perhaps the patient's acuity is better or worse than measured because of lucky guessing, memorizing eye charts, or not having been "pushed" enough to get the best possible acuity measurement.

When the process is applied correctly, it avoids spending time prescribing or demonstrating devices that clearly are not appropriate, the demonstration of which would result in failure and hence loss of confidence in the examiner.

## REFERENCES

1. Legge GE, Ross JA, Isenberg JM, LaMay JM: Psychophysics of reading: Clinical predictors of low-vision reading speed. *Invest Ophthalmol Vis Sci* 33:677-687, 1992.

## ADDITIONAL READING

Bailey IL: Magnification for near vision. *Optom Monthly* 71:119-122, 1980.
Bailey IL: Equivalent viewing power or magnification? Which is fundamental? *Optician* 188(4970):32-35, 1984.

Brazelton FA: Magnification in microscopic lenses. *Am J Optom Arch Am Acad Optom* 46(4):304-308, 1969.

Brilliant R: Magnification in low vision aids made simple. *J Vis Impair Blind* 77(4): 169-171, 1983.

Ellerbrock VJ: Magnification for near vision. *Am J Opt* 31(2):67-77, 1954.

Elmstrom GP: Specifications of relative magnification for subnormal vision. *J Indiana Optom Assoc* 21(6):6, 1949.

Gordon DM, Ritter C: Magnification: Practical applications of the principles of magnification to the problems of subnormal vision. *Arch Ophthalmol* 54(5):704-716, 1955.

Gordon DM, Ritter C: Principles of magnification in subnormal vision problems. *Arch Ophthalmol* 54(2),301-302, 1955.

Sloan LL: Optical magnification for subnormal vision: Historical survey. *J Opt Soc Am* 62(2):162-168, 1972.

Thouless R: Apparent size and distance in vision through a magnifying system. *Brit J Psych* 59(2):111-118, 1968.

# Basic Optical Principles of Low Vision Devices

It is not necessary to have a complete grasp of complex optics in order to provide low vision care. However, it is important for the clinician to understand the basic optical principles of the devices that are demonstrated to the patient. This allows the clinician to evaluate and prescribe appropriate devices and to sort out problems when the devices do not work as expected. The approach taken in this and following chapters is to provide an overview of fundamental optical principles with clinically applicable examples. Some additional details are included that will be of interest to readers who want a more complete understanding of how the formulas are derived or how optical devices may function in unique situations. Because this chapter is lengthy and somewhat involved, it might be helpful to read the summary first in order to see where the information is leading. The reader who prefers to minimize his or her exposure to formulas and their derivation may simply study the examples in order to learn how they are applied.

## TELESCOPES

Telescopes are used to view distant objects but may be used for near with auxiliary lenses or if they have a wide range of focus. When used for near, they are referred to as telemicroscopes, reading telescopes, near point telescopes, or near vision telescopes. Telescopes for near are considered in a separate section.

Only two of the many different types of telescopes are used in low vision care: the Galilean (also called terrestrial) and the Keplerian (also called astronomical). The two types of telescopes differ in several important characteristics that will influence the choice for the final prescription. Either of these two types may be used as a hand-held device for occasional spotting of distant objects or may be mounted in spectacles, which leaves the hands free and is useful for continuous viewing or frequent spotting.

*The Galilean telescope.* In its simplest form, a Galilean telescope consists of two lenses. The objective ($F_1$) is a positive lens and is closest to the object, whereas the ocular ($F_2$) is a minus lens and is closest to the eye. The lenses are separated such that the posterior focal point of the objective coincides with the posterior focal point of the ocular (Figure 10-1). The image formed is erect. The separation (d) of the two lenses, considered as thin lenses, can be determined from the formula:

$$d = f_1 + f_2$$

For convenience, sign convention is ignored in that no stipulation is made about the direction of measurement from either lens, as demonstrated in Examples 10-1 and 10-2.

■ **Example 10-1.** What would be the lens separation (d) in centimeters for a Galilean telescope consisting of a +10 objective ($F_1$) and −20 ocular ($F_2$)?

$$f_1 = 100/F_1$$
$$f_1 = 100/10$$
$$f_1 = 10 \text{ cm}$$
$$f_2 = 100/F_2$$
$$f_2 = 100/-20$$
$$f_2 = -5 \text{ cm}$$
$$d = f_1 + f_2$$
$$d = 10 + (-5)$$
$$d = 10 - 5$$
$$d = 5 \text{ cm}$$

*The Keplerian telescope.* A Keplerian telescope, in its simplest form, consists of two convex lenses, separated such that the posterior focal point of the objective coincides with the anterior focal point of the ocular (Figure 10-1). In this case, the image formed is inverted, which necessitates that an image-erecting system of prisms and/or mirrors be included in order for the telescope to be useful to the patient. The separation, d, again considering the objective and ocular to be thin lenses, may be found by simply adding the focal lengths of the two lenses.

$$d = f_1 + f_2$$

■ **Example 10–2.** What would be the lens separation (d) in centimeters for a Keplerian telescope consisting of a +10 objective $(F_1)$ and +20 ocular $(F_2)$?

$$f_1 = 100/F_1$$
$$f_1 = 100/10$$
$$f_1 = 10 \text{ cm}$$
$$f_2 = 100/F_2$$
$$f_2 = 100/20$$
$$f_2 = 5 \text{ cm}$$
$$d = f_1 + f_2$$
$$d = 10 + 5$$
$$d = 15 \text{ cm}$$

The telescopes in Figure 10-1 are shown in their simplest form as a combination of two lenses with the appropriate separation. Less expensive telescopes may actually consist of only two lenses, or two lenses with an erecting system for the Keplerian design, but better quality telescopes are multielement lens systems designed to minimize aberrations and produce the sharpest possi-

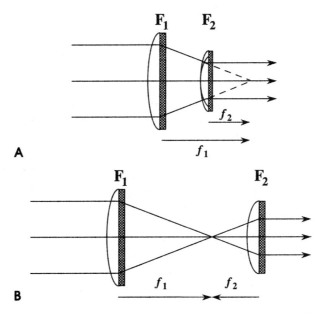

**Figure 10–1. (A)** A Galilean telescope, in its simplest form, consists of two lenses. The ocular is a concave lens, and the objective is a convex lens. The separation is such that the posterior focal point of the objective coincides with the posterior focal point of the ocular. **(B)** A Keplerian telescope, in its simplest form, consists of two convex lenses separated such that the posterior focal point of the objective coincides with the anterior focal point of the ocular.

ble image. The latter are similar to good quality camera lenses, and the cost is usually commensurate with the optical quality. A comparison of Examples 10-1 and 10-2 shows that a Keplerian telescope is longer than the equivalent Galilean telescope unless the path length is folded optically.

## Magnification by Telescopes

For either type of telescope the angular magnification it provides is the negative of the power of the ocular ($F_2$) divided by the power of the objective ($F_1$):

$$M = -F_2 / F_1$$

■ **Example 10-3.** Calculate the magnifying power of the telescope described in Example 10-1.

$$M = -F_2 / F_1$$
$$M = -(20/-10)$$
$$M = 2X$$

■ **Example 10-4.** Calculate the magnifying power of the telescope described in Example 10-2.

$$M = -F_2 / F_1$$
$$M = -20/10$$
$$M = -2X$$

Calculated in this manner, the magnification is negative for the Keplerian, which indicates that the image is inverted. Since there is going to be an erecting system, usually a prism, for the Keplerian telescopes used in vision rehabilitation, one may ignore the signs of the lenses and simply divide the two powers.

In the clinical situation, it is not usually necessary to calculate the magnification of telescopes because they are labeled, almost accurately, by the manufacturer, and no one is going to take them apart to see what the powers of the objective and ocular are. However, it is necessary to be able to calculate the lens separation and magnification provided by alternative telescope systems. These are covered elsewhere and include the contact lens telescope system (Chapter 17), the IOL telescope system (Chapter 12), and one in which an uncorrected aphakic eye serves as the ocular of a telescopic system (Chapter 12). There are other techniques that may be used to determine or verify the magnification of any telescope. These techniques are covered in Chapter 16.

By convention, telescopes are usually referred to as having some "power" as opposed to providing some magnification. Since a telescope is, by definition, an afocal system, the system has a dioptric power of zero. Although the use of the word "power" for "magnification" is technically inaccurate, it is well ingrained. The term "magnifying power" is used by some as a compromise.

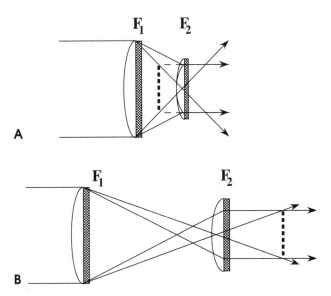

**Figure 10–2.** The exit pupil (dotted line) for a Galilean telescope (**A**) is within the telescope, whereas the exit pupil for a Keplerian telescope (**B**) is outside of the unit. The ray trace for each telescope type shows how the ocular forms an image of the objective, which creates the exit pupil of the telescope (see also Figures 16–1 and 16–2).

Two telescopes, one of each type, with the same power objective and the same total magnification differ as follows: the Galilean telescope is shorter (compare Examples 10-1 and 10-2), and, because there is no need for an erecting prism, it is lighter and less expensive to manufacture. One might therefore wonder why a Keplerian telescope is ever prescribed if the Galilean telescope has such advantages. There is one good reason—the Keplerian has a larger field of view due to the fact that the exit pupil is formed outside of the telescope and can therefore be placed close to or at the entrance pupil of the eye (Figure 10-2). A Galilean telescope has an exit pupil that is located within the telescope and therefore cannot be located at the entrance pupil of the eye (Figure 10-2). By definition, the exit pupil is the image of the objective lens as formed by the ocular. Figure 10-2 is a ray trace that localizes the position of the exit pupil for each of the two types of telescope. The generalizations given above about field of view, cost, size, and weight hold true for two telescopes that are virtually equivalent in design with the exception of telescope type (Keplerian versus Galilean).

## Diagnostic Trial of Telescopes

A telescope is first demonstrated, and then prescribed, with a particular goal in mind for the patient. In Chapter 9 it was shown that the examiner must determine the acuity level necessary to achieve the goal and then calculate the magnification that will provide it. The following two examples demonstrate how this might be accomplished with telescopes.

■ **Example 10–5.** A patient seeks improved distance vision for an on-the-job application of seeing a large meter located 20 feet across the room from his work station. His best corrected acuity is 5/40, and the numerals on the meter are the equivalent of a 40-foot letter. What telescope will allow him to distinguish these numerals?

The reference acuity is the best corrected acuity (5/40), which is equivalent to 20/160. The goal acuity is 20/40. As before, the magnification needed is determined by dividing the reference size by the goal size:

$$\text{Magnification needed} = \text{Reference size/Goal size}$$
$$M = 160/40$$
$$M = 4X$$

In this manner, it is determined that a 4X telescope, of either type, will achieve the goal.

■ **Example 10–6.** For general spotting purposes, when a specific goal is not identified, a telescope should be selected that allows the user to read the equivalent of approximately 20/50. If a patient has a best corrected acuity of 5/70, what telescope would theoretically allow him or her to read the equivalent of 20/50?

$$5/70 = 20/280$$
$$\text{Magnification needed} = \text{Reference size/Goal size}$$
$$M = 280/50$$
$$M = 5.6X$$

It is a simple matter to select a 4X telescope as needed in Example 10-5 because this is a common magnification; however, telescopes are not available with every desired magnification. When the predicted magnification required is not available, such as the 5.6X telescope in Example 10–6, the closest available power is selected. In this case the two closest choices would most likely be 4.0X and 6.0X, with the latter being the closest available option. As a general rule, the lower the magnification that achieves the goal, the better for the patient. A lower power telescope is easier to use because it has a wider field of view than a stronger but otherwise equivalent telescope, and because small hand tremors have a less noticeable effect on the image.

Telescopes can be prescribed for monocular or binocular use and can be hand-held or mounted in spectacles. The various considerations for each of these forms are presented in Chapter 12.

## CONVEX LENSES

A convex "lens" may be a single lens or a compound lens system, such as an achromatic doublet, designed to minimize selected aberrations. Convex lenses may be as powerful as +80.00 D or more but are usually prescribed as low vision devices in the +6.00 to +40.00 range. Convex lenses are used in three basic forms: as "microscopes," as hand-held magnifiers, or as stand magnifiers.

A high plus lens or lens combination that is mounted in spectacles is referred to, by convention, as a microscope. A true microscope, as used in the biology laboratory, is optically different, but both are used for magnifying a near object; hence those involved in vision rehabilitation have adopted the term microscope for a spectacle-mounted high plus lens. The lens design for a microscope may be full-diameter, lenticular, multifocal, or half-eye (see Chapter 13). A microscope is intended to be used with the material held at or near the focal point of the lens. Therefore, a very near working distance is necessitated with the higher powers. Patient adaptation is discussed in Chapter 13. Because of the high powers that are used, and because most patients have a preferred eye, microscopes are usually prescribed for monocular use by the better eye. The limitations to binocular use of microscopes are also covered in Chapter 13.

A hand magnifier or hand-held magnifier is a plus lens that is literally held in the hand, usually by means of a handle attached to the lens housing, and is familiar to everyone who has ever seen Sherlock Holmes at work. A stand magnifier is similar to a hand-held magnifier except that the lens is supported by the stand, not the hand, and remains a fixed distance from the page or other object. Unlike a microscope, which is in the spectacle plane, a hand-held or stand magnifier may be held any distance from the eye, and this often makes these devices preferred. An example of each of these three devices is shown in Figure 10–3.

The reader will recall from basic optics that a convex lens forms an erect virtual image outside the focal plane of the lens if the object is placed anywhere between the front focal plane of the lens and the lens itself. As the object is moved closer to the focal point, the image becomes larger and is formed farther from the lens (Figure 10–4). Maximum angular magnification by the lens itself is achieved when the object is placed at the focal point of the lens, which theoretically forms an image at optical infinity. With a stand magnifier, the object location, and hence the image size, are fixed relative to the lens since the stand is meant to be placed and maintained on the page of print or other object. This is advantageous for people who have difficulty holding a lens steady. With a hand-held magnifier or a microscope, the patient may position the lens at any desired distance from the object; thus, the image size and its location are variable. If the image size and location are variable, then the magnification achieved by the patient will be variable since the magnification depends on the image size and location compared to the reference size and location. Even simple convex lenses

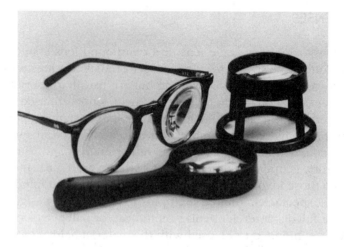

**Figure 10–3.** A convex lens may be prescribed in several forms, three of which are shown here: a hand-held magnifier, a stand magnifier, and a microscope (spectacle-mounted high plus lens).

cannot be prescribed effectively if the clinician does not understand how the outcome is affected by the manner in which the patient uses the device. Similarly, understanding basic optical principles enables the clinician to direct the patient's use of an optical device in order to accomplish the desired goal in the most effective manner.

If the object is located in the focal plane of the lens, the image is formed at "optical infinity," parallel light leaves the lens, and the image will be in focus when viewed through the best distance correction. If a convex lens is used to view an object that is inside the focal plane of the lens, the image is formed at a finite distance from the eye, and the patient must either accommodate or use an add in order to see it as clearly as possible. When an add or accommodation is used in combination with a convex lens, an optical system is created that has two lenses, and this will alter the amount of magnification compared to that of the magnifier alone. It might seem intuitively obvious that the magnification should be greater for the system as opposed to the magnifier alone, but this is not always true. Each of these situations is considered in subsequent sections.

## A Convex Lens with the Object Held at the Focal Point

This section develops a simple formula for clinical application. The derivation is given in some detail. Readers interested only in the "bottom line" may skip to Example 10–7.

The maximum angular magnification achievable by a convex lens is given by the formula $M = 1 + hF$, where M is magnification, h is the distance from the

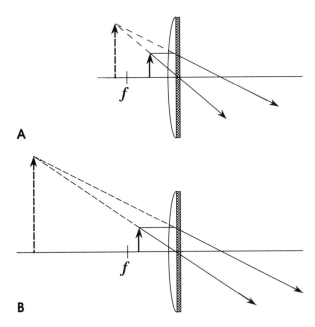

**Figure 10–4.** (**A**) A convex lens forms an erect virtual image of an object located between the lens and its anterior focal plane. (**B**) As the object is moved closer to the anterior focal plane of the lens, the image formed becomes larger and is located farther from the lens.

lens to the eye in meters, and F is the dioptric strength of the lens.[1] The magnification is relative to the object viewed without the lens compared to the image formed when the object is in the focal plane of the lens. In other words, the lens must be held at its focal length, $f$, from the page for this relationship to give the maximum angular magnification. If the print is maintained at the same distance at which the reference acuity was measured and the lens is inserted between the eye and the page, one focal length from the print, then the reference distance, r, is equal to the sum of h and $f$ as shown in Figure 10-5. This arrangement gives parallel light entering the eye, so the patient must have the best distance correction in place but does not have to accommodate or use an add.

If the print is moved after the reference acuity is measured and the lens is then inserted one focal length from the print at the new distance, the total magnification will be a combination of two separate types of magnification. The following sequence describes this situation. First, the near acuity is measured at the reference distance (r). Next, the patient moves the print to some other near distance (d), and, in order to put it in focus, a lens is inserted between the eye and the print, one focal length ($f$) from the print (Figure 10-6). The two types

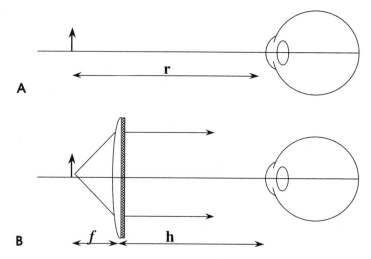

**Figure 10–5.** A convex lens held one focal length from the object of regard will create its maximum angular magnification, which is the total magnification to the viewer if the object remains at the reference distance. A clinical example would be as follows: (**A**) The patient reads an acuity card at some reference distance r, and then, (**B**) without moving the print, he or she places a convex lens one focal length in front of it. The distance of the lens from the eye is h; therefore, r = f + h, assuming the lens to be thin.

of magnification then are the relative distance magnification achieved by moving the print and the maximum angular magnification from the lens itself when it is inserted in front of the print at a distance of one focal length. (If the print had been moved sufficiently close to the eye, the lens might be approximately in the spectacle plane. This creates the situation described for a microscope, that is, a high plus lens mounted in a spectacle frame.)

The total magnification of a series of magnification steps is given by the product of the magnification from each step. For this example, the total magnification is the product of the relative distance magnification (RDM) and the maximum angular magnification (MAM) of the lens, inserted one focal length from the print.

$$M_{total} = RDM \times MAM$$

Since the RDM is r/d (reference distance over new distance) and the MAM is 1 + hF, we have:

$$M_{total} = r/d \times (1 + hF)$$

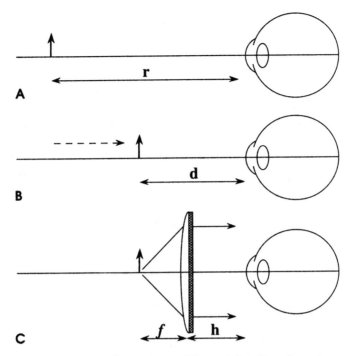

**Figure 10–6.** If an object is moved to a distance other than the reference distance, the viewer will receive the maximum angular magnification from the lens if it is held one focal length from the object, and relative distance magnification from the position change. A clinical situation would be as follows: (**A**) The patient reads an acuity card at some reference distance r, moves the print (**B**) to some new distance d, and then places a convex lens one focal length in front of the print (**C**) at the new distance. The distance of the lens from the eye is h; therefore, d = *f* + h, if the lens is considered to be thin.

The formula above is rather cumbersome, and, as luck would have it, there is a nice simplification. With a little algebraic manipulation the formula for total magnification reduces to $M_{total}$ = rF, as follows:

$$M_{total} = r/d \times (1 + hF)$$
$$M_{total} = r/(f + h) \times (1 + hF)$$
$$M_{total} = r/(f + h) \times (f/f + hF)$$
$$M_{total} = r/(f + h) \times (f/f + h/f)$$
$$M_{total} = r/(f + h) \times (f + h)/f$$
$$M_{total} = r/f$$
$$M_{total} = rF$$

This result shows that the magnification provided by a hand magnifier or a microscope, when the object is in the focal plane of the lens, can be determined from the formula M = rF, where r is the reference distance expressed in meters and F is the dioptric strength of the lens. Inspection of this formula reveals that the magnification depends only on the reference distance and the power of the lens used. Since there is no stipulation about the position of the lens relative to the eye, this formula holds true for a lens used as a hand magnifier as well as a lens mounted in spectacles and used as a microscope. It may seem intuitively wrong that a given lens provides the same magnification regardless of how far it is held from the eye as long as the object is maintained at the focal point of the lens. However, this is correct, although the intuitive notion is also partially correct since separate components of the total magnification do change with lens position; for example, while the total magnification remains constant, the relative proportions of the RDM and the MAM change, depending on the distance of the lens-print unit from the eye. The closer the lens-print unit is to the eye, the greater the contribution of the RDM and the less the contribution of the MAM from the lens. The closer it stays to the reference distance, the greater the contribution of MAM and the less the contribution of RDM. The magnification achieved with a microscope therefore is primarily relative distance magnification, *not* angular magnification.

■ **Example 10–7.** A patient reads 4M print at a distance of 40 cm through a +2.50 add over the best correction. What size print could she read with a +5.00 D hand-held lens held 20 cm from the print?

$$M = rF$$
$$M = (0.4)(5)$$
$$M = 2X$$

Since the lens provides 2X, she should now be able to read 2M letters through the distance correction, with the print held 20 cm from the lens:

$$Magnification = Reference\ size/Goal\ size$$
$$2X = 4M/Goal\ size$$
$$4/2 = Goal\ size$$
$$2 = Goal\ size$$

The reader should note that this calculated result is true only if the patient has the best distance correction in place and the near reference acuity is measured with the appropriate add if the patient cannot accommodate. In the example above, the patient was tested at 40 cm with a +2.50 add over the best distance correction; however, when the magnifier is used with the print at its focal point, the patient views the image through the distance portion of the glasses, not the add. The distance at which the magnifier is held from the eye does not alter the magnification as long as the print is maintained at the focal point of the lens.

■ **Example 10–8.** A patient reads 6M print at 33 cm with a +3.00 add over the best correction. What microscope would be required to read 1M print?

$$\text{Magnification required} = \text{Reference size/Goal size}$$
$$M = 6M/1M$$
$$M = 6X$$

Once the required magnification is known, the lens power that will provide it is calculated as follows:

$$M = rF$$
$$6 = (0.33)F$$
$$6/0.33 = F$$
$$+18.18 = F$$

With a +18.25 lens, the closest trial lens power, the patient should read 1M print when it is held about 5.5 cm ($f = 100/18.25 = 5.48$ cm) from the lens. The calculated dioptric power is the total power that the patient needs over the distance correction. The power of the add used to measure the reference acuity is *not* added on to the calculated value.

The formula $M = rF$ shows that, for a given power F, the magnification depends on the reference distance (r). Any given lens will therefore provide a different amount of magnification for a different reference distance. The low vision literature is, unfortunately, sprinkled rather liberally with the notion that the magnification of a lens is always determined by dividing its dioptric power by 4 or conversely that each 4 D of lens power gives 1X magnification. This is true only for the situation in which the reference distance is 25 cm. Since this is often the reference distance used by lens manufacturers, it is not hard to see how that notion has become ingrained and why manufacturers label some optical devices in terms of the magnification they would provide based on their reference distance. *The problem for the clinician is that the device will not provide that magnification for any patient unless the reference distance for the patient is the same as the reference distance used by the manufacturer.* The following two examples illustrate why it is not appropriate to accept unquestioningly the manufacturer's labeled magnification and why it is usually not appropriate to use the generalization that every four diopters provides 1X.

■ **Example 10–9.** A patient has a reference acuity of 0.4/10M through best correction and the appropriate add. The goal is to read 1M print. It requires 10X (10M/1M = 10X) to achieve that goal. The lens needed is determined as follows:

$$M = rF$$
$$10 = (0.4)F$$
$$+25 = F$$

If this patient wears a +25.00 D add over best distance correction and moves the print to 4 cm from the lens, he should read 1M print. In other words, the +25.00 diopter lens provides him with 10X magnification. Yet a manufacturer who used a reference distance of 25 cm would have labeled that +25.00 lens as a 6.25X microscope:

$$M = rF$$
$$M = (0.25)25$$
$$M = 6.25X$$

■ **Example 10–10.** Another patient has a reference acuity of 0.25/10M. (She can read the same size print as the first but must hold it almost twice as close in order to do so.) How much magnification this patient would get from that same +25.00 D microscope and the size print she would be able to read is determined as follows:

*Magnification*

$$M = rF$$
$$M = 0.25(25)$$
$$M = 6.25X$$

*Print size*

Magnification = Reference size/Goal size
Goal size = Reference size/Magnification
Goal size = 10M/6.25X
Goal size = 1.6M

In this case, only 6.25X is received from a +25.00 D lens, and she will only read 1.6M print. In order to read 1M print, this patient also needs 10X, just as in Example 10-9, but needs a +40.00 D lens to achieve it. That is determined as follows:

$$M = rF$$
$$10 = (0.25)F$$
$$+40 = F$$

This patient does get 1X for each 4 D of lens power (40 D/10X = 4 diopters per X), but only because the reference distance was 25 cm. However, in Example 10-9, where +25 D provided 10X, the patient received 1X for every 2.5 diopters, not for every 4 diopters.

In these two examples the same dioptric strength provided different amounts of magnification for the two patients because the reference distances were different. Both patients required 10X magnification to read 1M print, but in each case a different dioptric strength was needed. Why? Because the refer-

**TABLE 10–1. Dioptic power, determined by M = rF, needed to provide a given magnification for selected reference distances.**

| Mag | Reference Distance (Meters) | | | | | | | | |
|---|---|---|---|---|---|---|---|---|---|
| | 0.10 | 0.15 | 0.20 | 0.25 | 0.30 | 0.35 | 0.40 | 0.45 | 0.50 |
| 2X | **20.00** | 13.33 | 10.00 | 8.00 | 6.67 | 5.71 | 5.00 | 4.44 | 4.00 |
| 3X | 30.00 | **20.00** | 15.00 | 12.00 | 10.00 | 8.57 | 7.50 | 6.67 | 6.00 |
| 4X | 40.00 | 26.67 | **20.00** | 16.00 | 13.33 | 11.43 | 10.00 | 8.89 | 8.00 |
| 5X | 50.00 | 33.33 | 25.00 | **20.00** | 16.67 | 14.29 | 12.50 | 11.11 | 10.00 |
| 6X | 60.00 | 40.00 | 30.00 | 24.00 | **20.00** | 17.14 | 15.00 | 13.33 | 12.00 |
| 7X | 70.00 | 46.67 | 35.00 | 28.00 | 23.33 | **20.00** | 17.50 | 15.56 | 14.00 |
| 8X | 80.00 | 53.33 | 40.00 | 32.00 | 26.67 | 22.86 | **20.00** | 17.78 | 16.00 |
| 9X | 90.00 | 60.00 | 45.00 | 36.00 | 30.00 | 25.71 | 22.50 | **20.00** | 18.00 |
| 10X | 100.00 | 66.67 | 50.00 | 40.00 | 33.33 | 28.57 | 25.00 | 22.22 | **20.00** |

Example: A +20 lens provides 3X for a reference distance of 15 cm and 10X for a reference distance of 50 cm.

ence distances were different. This should make sense intuitively since they had very different acuities as evidenced by the fact that when the reference acuities were measured, the second had to have 10M print almost twice as close in order to distinguish it. It is therefore better not to use rules of thumb about magnification, but rather to calculate the needs for each patient based on the reference distance used when the best corrected acuity is measured. Similarly, lenses must be prescribed based on their dioptric strength, not a designated "X" value given by the manufacturer, since the reference distance used by the manufacturer may differ from that used by the clinician. Table 10-1 gives the lens power in diopters, from M = rF, necessary to provide given amounts of magnification relative to specific reference distances.

## A Convex Lens with the Object Not Held at the Focal Point

Most patients do not actually hold the material at the focal point of the lens because they quickly discover that more of the object can be seen if it is held within the focal point of the lens where the magnification is somewhat less. When the object is held very close to the focal point, the formula M = rF gives a good clinical approximation of the magnification that is achieved. When the object is further inside the focal point (that is, closer to the lens), the lens is used in a manner similar to a stand magnifier. Two things must then be considered: the image is located a finite distance from the eye, and the patient must accommodate or use an add to see as clearly as possible. This is covered in detail in the sections on stand magnifiers and magnifiers combined with an add or accommodation.

## A GENERAL FORMULA FOR MAGNIFICATION

The formula M = rF applies under the restriction that the object is held at the focal point, but since this is not always what happens clinically, the resultant magnification can be quite different. If the object of regard is held beyond the anterior focal point of the lens, the image is inverted. Patients quickly discover that this does not work for reading. When the object of regard is inside the anterior focal point, the lens forms an erect, virtual image some finite distance from the eye, and, if it is close enough, the patient must accommodate or have an add in order to see it as clearly as possible. How close is "close enough"? There is no clear answer because the effect of the resultant blur when the image is not in perfect focus depends on the residual visual acuity and the detail that the person is trying to resolve; for example, one diopter of blur is certainly more significant for a person with 20/50 residual acuity than for someone with 20/400.

The formula M = rF will be used for most of the clinical examples, but for readers who wish to have a general formula for magnification[2] the following is given:

$$M = \frac{rF}{1 - [xF(1 - hF)]}$$

where r is the reference distance, F is the power of the lens, $x$ is the distance of the object from the anterior focal point of the lens, and h is the distance of the lens from the eye. All distances are expressed in meters, and, for the clinical situations considered here, all distances are positive. While this formula appears cumbersome, the numerator should look familiar. It is possible to see that the formula simplifies to M = rF if the denominator is equal to 1, which happens in two unique situations. The first is when the object is at the focal point of the lens and therefore $x = 0$. In this case, the denominator becomes 1, and the formula reduces to M = rF. The second situation is that in which h = $f$. In this case, the term $1 - hF$ equals zero ($[1 - f(1/f) = 1 - 1 = 0]$), the denominator is therefore equal to 1, and the formula again reduces to M = rF.

These two situations may be summarized as follows. First, the magnification is constant and is equal to rF, regardless of where the lens is held, provided that the object is maintained at the focal point of the lens. That is precisely what was stated when the formula M = rF was derived earlier. Second, the magnification is constant and is equal to rF, regardless of the object location, provided that the lens is maintained one focal length from the eye. This is known as Badal's principle.[3] Badal's principle actually refers to the lens-eye separation being equal to the posterior (secondary) focal length, but the general term "focal length" has been used here in keeping with thin lens theory, in which the anterior and posterior focal lengths of a thin lens are equal.

If neither of these two special cases applies (that is, the object is not at the focal point of the lens and the lens is not held one focal length from the eye), the general formula given above applies. It is a simple matter to program it into a computer spreadsheet to cover any situation encountered clinically.

## EQUIVALENT LENS POWER

Prior to this point there has been no discussion of what measure of lens power is used. The correct lens power to use for predicting magnification is its equivalent power as opposed to, for example, front or back vertex power.[4] The equivalent power ($F_e$) for a lens or lens system is the power of the thin lens that has the property that, if positioned at the second principal plane of the system, its posterior focal point coincides with the posterior focal point of the system. By using equivalent powers, the clinician can predict performance with any other optical system since the patient should achieve the same magnification from equivalent systems; for example, if a person received 6X magnification from a convex lens with an equivalent power of +20.00 D, he or she would receive 6X magnification from any other system (stand magnifier, telemicroscope, convex lens used with an add, and so forth) provided its equivalent power was also +20.00 D. Furthermore, it is possible to predict performance in a linear manner; for example, if a patient can read 4M print with an equivalent power of +10.00 D, he or she should read 2M print with any system that has an equivalent power of +20.00 D and 1M print with any system that has an equivalent power of +40.00 D. These properties of equivalent power do not hold true for other measures of lens power, which is why equivalent power is an important parameter of optical devices used in vision rehabilitation.

Unfortunately, the use of equivalent power usually precludes using one's lensometer to determine lens power since the lensometer measures vertex power and not equivalent power. There can be considerable disparity between the equivalent power, the front vertex power, and the back vertex power for the same lens depending on the front and back surface curvatures and the lens thickness. There is an exception, however, for lenses that are plano-convex, in which case the front vertex power (curved surface) and the equivalent power are the same. The potential for disparity between vertex power and equivalent power is shown in Table 10-2.

Manufacturers of optical devices typically do not provide the equivalent power, although some have begun to recently. When a dioptric power is specified by a manufacturer, it is not necessarily the equivalent power, nor should one assume that it is. Distributors' catalogues may indicate an equivalent power, determined independently, for some optical devices. When the equiva-

TABLE 10–2. A comparison of equivalent power and front vertex power for selected theoretical thick lenses.

| | $F_1$ | $F_2$ | $t$ | $n$ | $F_e$ | $F_{fvp}$ | $F_{fvp} - F_e$ |
|---|---|---|---|---|---|---|---|
| 1 | 5.00 | 0.00 | 0.009 | 1.50 | 5.00 | 5.00 | 0.00 |
| 2 | 10.00 | 0.00 | 0.010 | 1.50 | 10.00 | 10.00 | 0.00 |
| 3 | 15.00 | 0.00 | 0.012 | 1.50 | 15.00 | 15.00 | 0.00 |
| 4 | 20.00 | 0.00 | 0.013 | 1.50 | 20.00 | 20.00 | 0.00 |
| 5 | 25.00 | 0.00 | 0.014 | 1.50 | 25.00 | 25.00 | 0.00 |
| 6 | 30.00 | 0.00 | 0.015 | 1.50 | 30.00 | 30.00 | 0.00 |
| 7 | 5.00 | 5.00 | 0.009 | 1.50 | 9.85 | 10.15 | 0.30 |
| 8 | 10.00 | 6.00 | 0.010 | 1.50 | 15.60 | 16.25 | 0.65 |
| 9 | 15.00 | 7.00 | 0.011 | 1.50 | 21.23 | 22.38 | 1.15 |
| 10 | 20.00 | 8.00 | 0.012 | 1.50 | 26.72 | 28.55 | 1.83 |
| 11 | 25.00 | 9.00 | 0.013 | 1.50 | 32.05 | 34.76 | 2.71 |
| 12 | 30.00 | 10.00 | 0.014 | 1.50 | 37.20 | 41.03 | 3.83 |
| 13 | 5.00 | 5.00 | 0.009 | 1.50 | 9.85 | 10.15 | 0.30 |
| 14 | 10.00 | 10.00 | 0.010 | 1.50 | 19.33 | 20.71 | 1.38 |
| 15 | 15.00 | 15.00 | 0.011 | 1.50 | 28.35 | 31.85 | 3.50 |
| 16 | 20.00 | 20.00 | 0.012 | 1.50 | 36.80 | 43.81 | 7.01 |
| 17 | 25.00 | 25.00 | 0.013 | 1.50 | 44.58 | 56.91 | 12.33 |
| 18 | 30.00 | 30.00 | 0.014 | 1.50 | 51.60 | 71.67 | 20.07 |

$F_1$ = front surface power, $F_2$ = back surface power, t = thickness in meters, n = index of refraction, $F_e$ = equivalent power, $F_{fvp}$ = front vertex power. The front vertex power and the equivalent power are the same for lenses that are plano-convex (rows 1–6) and are similar if the back surface has relatively little curvature (rows 7–10, 13–14); however, the difference may be large for biconvex lenses with a steeper $F_2$ (rows 11–12, 15–18).

lent power is not provided, it can be determined relatively easily for any lens or lens system, as will be shown in the section on stand magnifiers.

## ALTERNATIVE METHODS FOR DETERMINING NEAR ADDS

Kestenbaum proposed a formula to predict the near lens needed for achieving a given reading level, based on the patient's distance acuity.[5] Kestenbaum suggested that the quotient of the reciprocal of the best corrected distance acuity would equal the dioptric value of the add needed to read normal sized text at near; for example, a patient whose best corrected distance acuity was 20/100 should be able to read 1M print with a +5.00 D add (100/20 = 5). For this to be true, the test circumstances such as illumination, contrast, and target type would have to be precisely the same. This is not typically the case in clinical practice. Although distance and near acuities should correlate very closely for people with normal vision, this may not be the case for those who are visually impaired. There are many variables that allow people to perform better or worse at near than might be predicted from their distance acuity. Some examples include uncorrected refractive error, a difference in illumination, and the effect of pupillary constriction. Near lenses are best selected based on a measurement of near performance, not distance acuity, and the reciprocal of vision procedure can be used in this manner if the near acuity was, in fact, the reduced equivalent of the distance acuity.

The Lighthouse, Inc., and others produce near acuity cards such as The Lighthouse Near Acuity Test, which have an add printed next to each row of letters. For any row, if that is the best the patient can read with a +2.50 add at 40 cm, the printed add is the add considered necessary to read 1M print. The printed add is usually based on the reciprocal of vision described above.

## INTERIM SUMMARY

The formula M = rF can be used for prescribing microscopes and hand-held magnifiers. The only stipulation is that the user holds the object of regard at or near the focal plane of the lens and views through the distance correction of his or her spectacles. The power (F) refers to the equivalent power of the lens. While this may not be given by the manufacturer, it can be determined in the office by a procedure that is explained in the section on stand magnifiers. Telescopes provide distance magnification, and a specific magnifying power is prescribed by determining the goal and selecting the appropriate telescope.

## EQUIVALENT POWER AND MAGNIFICATION FOR COMBINATIONS OF MAGNIFIERS, ACCOMMODATION, AND ADDS

If the patient accommodates with an add or uses an add or accommodation in conjunction with a simple magnifier, a new optical system is created that is composed of two plus lenses separated by a finite distance. The equivalent power of two lenses separated (in air) by a distance of t meters is:

$$F_e = F_1 + F_2 - (t)(F_1)(F_2)$$

Once the equivalent power of the system is determined, magnification may be calculated from the formula M = rF, assuming that the object of regard is located at the anterior focal point ($f_e$) of the system and F is actually $F_e$ for the system.

### Accommodation with an Add

For the case of an add combined with accommodation, $F_1$ is the power of the add and $F_2$ is the amount of accommodation. If accommodation is considered to be approximately equivalent to a thin lens at the corneal surface, t is the vertex distance, which is typically small (10 to 15 mm). Therefore, the difference between $F_e$ and simply adding the two lenses together is relatively small, and the algebraic sum is a reasonable approximation to use clinically.[6] A similar situation exists for accommodation with a simple magnifier held close to the eye. Table 10–3 compares the $F_e$ with the algebraic sum for a series of adds ($F_1$) at a vertex distance of 10 mm from an eye that is accommodating +2.50 D ($F_2$). This table shows that the algebraic sum is a reasonable approximation to $F_e$ since the separation is small. This general rule holds true even for much larger amounts of accommodation on the order of +8 or +10 D (Table 10–4).

The clinician never really knows how much the patient is accommodating in conjunction with an add, but it can be estimated by measuring the distance that the object is held from the add and determining the approximate total power of the system as in Example 10–11.

■ **Example 10–11.** A young boy reads 3M print with a +8.00 add by holding the print 5 cm from the lens. How much accommodation is he using?

If it is assumed that the print is being held in the focal plane of the system, it must be a +20.00 D system (100/5 = +20), and the extra +12.00 D must come from accommodation.

The accuracy of this solution depends on the assumption that the system is actually in focus (that is, he is not simply accommodating +8.0 D and living with +4.00 of blur) and that 5 cm is the distance to the front focal plane of the system from the anterior principal plane of the system. Since neither of these is known clinically, the solution should be considered an approximation only.

■ **Example 10–12.** For the same person in Example 10–11, what add would be necessary to allow him to read 1M print while using only +5.00 D of accommodation?

**TABLE 10–3.** A comparison of equivalent power ($F_e$) versus the algebraic sum of powers for a series of adds ($F_1$) in combination with +2.50 D of accommodation ($F_2$) and a 10 mm vertex distance (t).

| $F_1$ | $F_2$ | t (meters) | $F_e$ | $F_1 + F_2$ | %* |
|-------|-------|------------|-------|-------------|------|
| 2 | 2.5 | 0.01 | 4.45 | 4.5 | 1.12 |
| 4 | 2.5 | 0.01 | 6.40 | 6.5 | 1.56 |
| 6 | 2.5 | 0.01 | 8.35 | 8.5 | 1.80 |
| 8 | 2.5 | 0.01 | 10.30 | 10.5 | 1.94 |
| 10 | 2.5 | 0.01 | 12.25 | 12.5 | 2.04 |
| 12 | 2.5 | 0.01 | 14.20 | 14.5 | 2.11 |
| 14 | 2.5 | 0.01 | 16.15 | 16.5 | 2.17 |
| 16 | 2.5 | 0.01 | 18.10 | 18.5 | 2.21 |
| 18 | 2.5 | 0.01 | 20.05 | 20.5 | 2.24 |
| 20 | 2.5 | 0.01 | 22.00 | 22.5 | 2.27 |

*Percentage difference between the algebraic sum, $F_1 + F_2$, and $F_e$

TABLE 10–4. A comparison of equivalent power ($F_e$) versus the algebraic sum of powers for a series of adds ($F_1$) in combination with +10.0 D of accommodation ($F_2$) and a 10 mm vertex distance (t).

| $F_1$ | $F_2$ | t (meters) | $F_e$ | $F_1 + F_2$ | %* |
|---|---|---|---|---|---|
| 2 | 10 | 0.01 | 11.80 | 12 | 1.69 |
| 4 | 10 | 0.01 | 13.60 | 14 | 2.94 |
| 6 | 10 | 0.01 | 15.40 | 16 | 3.90 |
| 8 | 10 | 0.01 | 17.20 | 18 | 4.65 |
| 10 | 10 | 0.01 | 19.00 | 20 | 5.26 |
| 12 | 10 | 0.01 | 20.80 | 22 | 5.77 |
| 14 | 10 | 0.01 | 22.60 | 24 | 6.19 |
| 16 | 10 | 0.01 | 24.40 | 26 | 6.56 |
| 18 | 10 | 0.01 | 26.20 | 28 | 6.87 |
| 20 | 10 | 0.01 | 28.00 | 30 | 7.14 |

*Percentage difference between $F_e$ and $F_1 + F_2$

■ **Solution.** The reference acuity is 3M, the goal acuity is 1M, and the reference distance at which he reads 3M print is 5 cm. Since it is assumed that the print is held at the focal plane of the system, the formula M = rF applies.

Magnification required = Reference size/Goal size
Magnification required = 3M/1M
Magnification required = 3X

$$M = rF$$
$$3 = (0.05)F$$
$$F = +60.00$$

Since he will accommodate +5.00 D, the lens has to be +55.00 D to give the total of +60.00.

## Magnifier Combined with an Add

A simple magnifier used with an add also comprises a two-element system with an equivalent power given by the equation $F_e = F_1 + F_2 - (t)(F_1)(F_2)$. If the patient holds a simple hand magnifier against his or her add or very close to it, t will be equal to zero and the equivalent power will simply be the sum of the two lenses. It might therefore seem logical that $F_e$ will always be greater than $F_1$ or $F_2$ but this is not the case, an important point to consider clinically. In fact, this point is worth emphasizing from another perspective. A person who uses an add with a magnifier may actually create a system that has less equivalent power than the power of the magnifier itself. It all depends on how far the magnifier is held from the add. The previous section considered a similar situation, accommodation with an add, but the distance between the two lenses was considered fixed and small. With a hand-held magnifier, the user may hold it any reasonable distance within arm's length from the add, which changes the situation substantially. The three theoretical possibilities that will be considered are those in which the equivalent power of the combination is equal to, greater than, or less than the power of the magnifier itself (yes, *less* than).

If it is assumed that the equivalent power of the combination ($F_e$) of a hand-held magnifier ($F_1$) with an add ($F_2$) is equal to the power of the magnifier itself, then the following relationships must be true:

$$F_e = F_1$$
$$F_1 + F_2 - (t)(F_1)(F_2) = F_1$$
$$F_2 - (t)(F_1)(F_2) = 0$$
$$F_2 = (t)(F_1)(F_2)$$
$$1 = (t)(F_1)$$
$$1/(F_1) = t$$
$$f_1 = t$$

This shows that if the magnifier is held one focal length from the add, the system will have an equivalent power equal to the power of the magnifier alone.

The same relationship can be expressed as an inequality to determine when $F_e$ might be greater than (>) or less than (<) $F_1$. The algebraic manipulations in each case never reverse the inequality since no step involves division or multiplication of each side by a negative number.

$$F_e > F_1$$
$$F_1 + F_2 - (t)(F_1)(F_2) > F_1$$
$$F_2 - (t)(F_1)(F_2) > 0$$
$$F_2 > (t)(F_1)(F_2)$$
$$1 > (t)(F_1)$$
$$1/(F_1) > t$$
$$f_1 > t$$

Finally,

$$F_e < F_1$$
$$F_1 + F_2 - (t)(F_1)(F_2) < F_1$$
$$F_2 - (t)(F_1)(F_2) < 0$$
$$F_2 < (t)(F_1)(F_2)$$
$$1 < (t)(F_1)$$
$$1/(F_1) < t$$
$$f_1 < t$$

The three possibilities can now be summarized as follows:

1. $F_e$ will be equal to $F_1$ if the magnifier is held one focal length from the add ($t = f_1$).
2. $F_e$ will be greater than $F_1$ if the magnifier is held less than one focal length from the add (i.e., $f_1 > t$).

**TABLE 10–5.** Equivalent power of a simple magnifier ($F_1$) separated (t) from an add ($F_2$) by increasing multiples of the focal length of the magnifier ($xf_e$).

| $F_1$ | $F_2$ | t (meters) | $F_e$ | $t = xf_e$ |
|---|---|---|---|---|
| 20 | 2.5 | 0.00 | 22.50 | 0f |
| 20 | 2.5 | 0.05 | 20.00 | 1f |
| 20 | 2.5 | 0.10 | 17.50 | 2f |
| 20 | 2.5 | 0.15 | 15.00 | 3f |
| 20 | 2.5 | 0.20 | 12.50 | 4f |
| 20 | 2.5 | 0.25 | 10.00 | 5f |
| 20 | 2.5 | 0.30 | 7.50 | 6f |
| 20 | 2.5 | 0.35 | 5.00 | 7f |
| 20 | 2.5 | 0.40 | 2.50 | 8f |
| 20 | 2.5 | 0.45 | 0.00 | 9f |

3. $F_e$ will be less than $F_1$ if the magnifier is held more than one focal length from the add (i.e., $f_1 < t$).

Table 10-5 gives the equivalent power of a system of two lenses: a magnifier ($F_1$) and an add ($F_2$) at different separations, which are multiples of the focal length of the magnifier ($F_1$). Table 10-5 should be compared with Tables 10-3 and 10-4, which showed that the algebraic sum is a reasonable approximation to $F_e$ if the separation is small.

The relationships just established can be used to assist in determining whether or not a presbyopic person should use his or her bifocal when using a simple magnifier and whether or not a nonpresbyopic person should use accommodation in combination with a simple magnifier[7]; for example, if the magnifier is held greater than one focal length from the add, the user will achieve the greatest magnification by viewing through the distance correction, not the add.

Once the equivalent power of the system is determined, magnification may be calculated from the formula M = rF, under the assumption that the object of regard is located at the anterior focal point ($f_e$) of the system and F is actually $F_e$ for the system.

## STAND MAGNIFIERS

A stand magnifier is a plus lens, or lens combination, mounted in a housing, the base of which sits on the material to be viewed. Most stand magnifiers are fixed focus, and therefore the lens is kept a fixed distance from the page. The stability of such an arrangement is advantageous for someone with a hand tremor or poor muscle control, or for a child who has trouble holding a hand magnifier the correct distance from the page. At first glance it might seem that the stand magnifier would have the same optical performance as a hand magnifier held one focal length from the object; however, this is not usually the case because the manufacturers select a stand height that will place the print inside the focal point of the lens when the base is resting on the page. This forms an erect virtual image some finite distance behind the page, and, unless it is formed very far from the lens, it becomes necessary for the patient to have the appropriate add or to be able to accommodate sufficiently to have as clear an image as possible (Figure 10-7). It also necessitates that the presbyopic patient hold the page and magnifier at a fixed distance so it remains in focus through the add. This situation is decidedly different from the hand-held magnifier in which the lens can be held at, or close to, one focal length from the page and the image is formed at "infinity," giving parallel light, and is in clear focus through the patient's distance prescription. In fact, it is identical to the situation discussed previously in which a simple magnifier is combined with an add. This creates a two-lens system in which the equivalent power of the system determines how much magnification the user actually gets.

The total magnification provided by a stand magnifier is a combination of two events. The lens provides an enlarged image of the object and relocates the

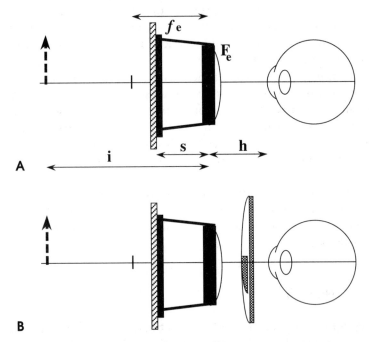

**Figure 10-7. (A)** A stand magnifier is placed on an object such as an acuity card. The stand height, $s$, is less than the focal length of the lens, $f_e$, and therefore the lens forms an erect virtual image (dashed arrow) some finite distance away. **(B)** Because the image is a finite distance from the eye, a presbyopic person will need an add over best distance correction in order to see it as clearly as possible. The exception to this rule is if the image is actually far enough away that it would be in focus through the distance portion.

object of regard (that is, the image) behind the page. This involves a change in distance, so there is relative distance magnification (or minification) as well as enlargement by the lens itself. The term enlargement is used instead of magnification to avoid confusion with the total magnification, which is a result of both enlargement by the lens and relative distance magnification (RDM). Because the RDM is determined by comparing the reference distance to the distance of the image, it is necessary to know where the image is located. This is also necessary in order to provide the patient with the appropriate add or to position the magnifier so the image is clear for an add that the patient already has. The enlargement of an object by the lens itself depends on the equivalent power of the magnifier lens and the emerging vergence. These are both discussed below, but first three examples are given to demonstrate the basic idea of how a stand magnifier works.

■ **Example 10–13.** A stand magnifier enlarges an object 5X, and the image is positioned 20 cm behind the lens. The patient has a +2.50 add and a reference acuity of 0.4/5M. Where must he hold the magnifier, and what size print should he be able to read?

Since the patient is in focus at 40 cm through his bifocal, the image must be located that distance from the spectacle plane. The magnifier lens must therefore be placed 20 cm from the spectacle plane since the image is 20 cm behind it (20 + 20 = 40). The image will be at 40 cm and 5X larger. The total magnification is the product of the RDM and the enlargement, E, by the lens:

$$M_{total} = RDM \times E$$
$$M_{total} = (40/40) \times 5X$$
$$M_{total} = 5X$$
$$\text{Magnification} = \text{Reference size/Goal size}$$
$$5X = 5M/\text{Goal size}$$
$$\text{Goal size} = 5M/5X$$
$$\text{Goal size} = 1M$$

■ **Example 10–14.** A stand magnifier enlarges 3X and has an image location 30 cm behind the lens. The patient is totally presbyopic and has a reference acuity of 0.25/8M through a +4.00 add. She prefers to hold the magnifier 14.5 cm from the spectacle plane. What size print should she read with this stand magnifier, and what add would be needed?

The image will be 44.5 cm from the eye (30 + 14.5 = 44.5), so a +2.25 add is needed (100/44.5 = 2.25).

$$M_{total} = RDM \times E$$
$$M_{total} = (25/44.5) \times 3$$
$$M_{total} = 0.56 \times 3$$
$$M_{total} = 1.68X$$

$$\text{Magnification} = \text{Reference size/Goal size}$$
$$1.68X = 8M/\text{Goal size}$$
$$\text{Goal size} = 8M/1.68X$$
$$\text{Goal size} = 4.76M$$

■ **Example 10-15.** The patient is totally presbyopic and has a best corrected near acuity of 0.4/4M through a +2.50 add. She tries a stand magnifier that has an enlargement of 2.5X and an image location (i) of 20 cm from the lens. How can she use this stand magnifier to read 1M print?

$$\text{Magnification required} = \text{Reference size/Goal size}$$
$$\text{Magnification required} = 4M/1M$$
$$\text{Magnification required} = 4X$$

Since the enlargement of the magnifier is only 2.5X, the relative distance magnification must provide 1.6X:

$$M_{total} = E \times RDM$$
$$4 = 2.5 \times RDM$$
$$1.6 = RDM$$

The RDM is found by dividing the reference distance, 40 cm, by the distance of the image from the eye. This latter distance is equal to the image location for the magnifier plus the distance of the magnifier from the eye (h).

$$RDM = 40/(20 + h)$$
$$1.6 = 40/(20 + h)$$
$$h = 5 \text{ cm}$$

Since the final image distance from the eye is equal to 25 cm (5 + 20), she will require a +4.00 D add to see the image as clearly as possible. A nonpresbyopic patient would have to accommodate +4 diopters. However, since the patient in this example is presbyopic, she needs to have bifocals or a reading lens prescribed with the stand magnifier in order to have the correct add. In these examples it appears that any magnification contributed by the add itself is ignored, but that is not the case, as will be seen when the appropriate formulas are derived.

The somewhat cumbersome calculations demonstrated above can be avoided by using a computer spreadsheet. There are many ways in which the spreadsheet can be formatted and used, but one suggestion is have input cells for the reference distance and acuity and a series of output cells that give the calculated magnification for different eye-lens distances along with the required add. The program can be repeated in several portions of the spreadsheet for the different stand magnifiers available in the office. This avoids the necessity of inputting the magnifier properties repeatedly.

The examples above demonstrate how the RDM and the enlargement by the lens interplay to provide the total magnification and also why the clinician must be sure that the patient either has the correct bifocal in place or holds the magnifier at the correct location to use the bifocal that he or she has. When stand magnifiers do not perform as expected, it is often because the clinician has failed to consider that the image and the focal plane of the add must coincide. This can be avoided if each stand magnifier in the diagnostic set is labeled with its enlargement factor and the position of the image.

As might be expected with respect to magnification, there is considerable difference between the labeling by the manufacturer and the magnification that the patient actually achieves because of the different reference distances and the difference between the labeled dioptric power versus the equivalent power of the lens. The following sections show how to determine these parameters for any stand magnifier in order to label it properly. The easiest technique, of course, is to find it in the literature if it has been published.[8-13] Published parameters for selected fixed-focus stand magnifiers are given in Table 10-6. Some companies have recently begun to provide this information, and, if others follow suit, this will eliminate the necessity of determining it in the office. Meanwhile, the following sections will show how to determine $F_e$, V, i, and, from these, E for any stand magnifier.

## How to Determine the Equivalent Power of a Convex Lens or Lens System

The equivalent power, $F_e$, of a convex lens or lens system may be determined by comparing an object of known size, at a known distance, with its image as formed by the lens.[8, 14] Once the image size is known, the image distance can be calculated and hence the focal length of the equivalent power. This can be done with similar triangles (see Figure 10-8 and Example 10-16). The image size can be measured by aligning a stand magnifier so an object of known size (O), at a known distance (d), forms an image (I) on the base of a contact lens reticle. The image height is measured with the reticle. Since d, O, and I are then known, it is possible to calculate $f_e$, the equivalent focal length. The reciprocal of that is the equivalent power.

$$\text{Image distance/Object distance} = \text{Image size/Object size}$$
$$f_e/d = I/O$$
$$f_e = dI/O$$
$$F_e = 1/f_e$$

These measurements are best accomplished with an optical bench, but they can also be done in the office with a little improvisation. The distance of the object should be measured from the anterior principal plane of the lens, but since its location is unknown, the distance is measured to the lens surface. The

**TABLE 10–6. Published parameters for selected fixed-focus stand magnifiers.**

| Magnifier | $F_e$ | E | V | i (cm) | Reference |
|---|---|---|---|---|---|
| Agfa-lupe AG-8 | 29.5 | 9.00 | −3.7 | 27.1 | 8 |
| COIL 5123 | 24.7 | 7.36 | −3.9 | 25.7 | 8 |
| COIL 5428 | 16.1 | 2.88 | −8.6 | 11.7 | 8 |
| Jupiter Standlupe #402 | 12.6 | 2.98 | −6.3 | 15.8 | 8 |

| Magnifier | $F_e$ | E | V | i (cm) | Reference |
|---|---|---|---|---|---|
| Eschenbach 1153 | 28.6 | 26.70 | −1.1 | 91.0 | 9 |
| Eschenbach 1550 | 29.8 | 8.50 | −3.7 | 27.0 | 9 |
| Eschenbach 1555 | 24.6 | 17.40 | −1.4 | 69.0 | 9 |
| Eschenbach 1558 | 16.7 | 4.80 | −4.2 | 24.0 | 9 |
| Eschenbach 1560 | 12.9 | 3.50 | −5.0 | 20.0 | 9 |
| Eschenbach 1565 | 7.3 | 1.80 | −9.1 | 11.0 | 9 |
| Eschenbach 1580 | 6.4 | 1.70 | −8.3 | 12.0 | 9 |
| Eschenbach 2020 | 7.7 | 1.70 | −10.0 | 10.0 | 9 |
| Eschenbach 2620 High | 11.2 | 2.80 | −5.6 | 18.0 | 9 |
| Eschenbach 2620 Low | 10.8 | 2.50 | −6.3 | 16.0 | 9 |
| Eschenbach 2623 | 6.8 | 2.10 | −6.3 | 16.0 | 9 |
| Eschenbach 2625 | 10.1 | 2.20 | −8.3 | 12.0 | 9 |
| Eschenbach 2627 | 13.4 | 3.20 | −5.6 | 18.0 | 9 |

| Magnifier | $F_e$ | E | V* | i (cm) | Reference |
|---|---|---|---|---|---|
| COIL 4206 | 18.2 | 7.70 | −2.7 | 37.0 | 10 |
| COIL 4208 | 22.6 | 12.50 | −2.0 | 51.0 | 10 |
| COIL 4210 | 29.8 | 10.00 | −3.3 | 30.0 | 10 |
| COIL 4212 | 34.6 | 9.20 | −4.2 | 24.0 | 10 |
| COIL 5123 | 23.8 | 7.00 | −4.0 | 25.0 | 10 |
| COIL 5226 | 18.4 | 8.80 | −2.4 | 42.0 | 10 |
| COIL 5228 | 23.2 | 14.50 | −1.7 | 58.0 | 10 |
| COIL 5210 | 29.3 | 7.20 | −4.8 | 21.0 | 10 |
| COIL 5212 | 34.5 | 7.70 | −5.0 | 20.0 | 10 |
| COIL 5472 | 6.6 | 2.00 | −7.1 | 14.0 | 10 |
| COIL 5474 | 8.6 | 2.50 | −5.6 | 18.0 | 10 |
| COIL 5428 | 17.4 | 3.60 | −6.7 | 15.0 | 10 |

| Magnifier | $F_e$ | E | V | i (cm)† | Reference |
|---|---|---|---|---|---|
| COIL 4206 | 16.8 | 7.10 | −2.8 | 36.4 | 11 |
| COIL 4208 | 23.0 | 12.50 | −2.0 | 50.0 | 11 |
| COIL 4210 | 27.7 | 8.80 | −3.6 | 28.2 | 11 |
| COIL 4212 | 31.8 | 8.50 | −4.3 | 23.5 | 11 |
| COIL 5210 | 29.2 | 8.30 | −4.0 | 25.0 | 11 |
| COIL 5212 | 34.5 | 7.90 | −5.0 | 20.0 | 11 |
| COIL 5213 | 6.7 | 2.30 | −5.3 | 19.0 | 11 |
| COIL 5214 | 9.7 | 5.30 | −2.3 | 44.4 | 11 |
| COIL 5226 | 16.7 | 6.60 | −3.0 | 33.3 | 11 |
| COIL 5228 | 22.2 | 11.10 | −2.2 | 45.5 | 11 |
| COIL 5855 | 2.3 | 1.42† | −5.5 | 18.2 | 11 |
| Peak 1960 | 13.9 | 6.60 | −2.5 | 40.0 | 11 |

**TABLE 10–6.** *(continued)*

| Magnifier | $F_e$‡ | E | V§ | i (cm) | Reference |
|---|---|---|---|---|---|
| Agfa loupe 8X | 28.9 | 7.80 | −4.3 | 23.5 | 12 |
| COIL 5123 | 21.7 | 6.80 | −3.7 | 26.7 | 12 |
| COIL 5428 | 15.5 | 3.30 | −6.8 | 14.8 | 12 |
| COIL 5472 | 5.0 | 2.00 | −5.0 | 20.0 | 12 |
| COIL 5474 | 6.8 | 2.70 | −4.0 | 25.0 | 12 |
| Eschenbach 1550 | 32.5 | 11.00 | −3.2 | 30.8 | 12 |
| Eschenbach 1555 | 20.5 | 17.40 | −1.3 | 80.0 | 12 |
| Eschenbach 1558 | 14.4 | 3.40 | −6.0 | 16.7 | 12 |
| Eschenbach 1560 | 11.6 | 3.20 | −5.3 | 19.0 | 12 |
| Eschenbach 1565 | 5.6 | 1.80 | −7.0 | 14.3 | 12 |
| Eschenbach 1580 | 5.2 | 1.80 | −6.5 | 15.4 | 12 |
| Jupiter loupe | 12.3 | 3.90 | −4.3 | 23.5 | 12 |
| Peak 10X illuminated | 22.1 | 6.9 | −3.7 | 26.7 | 12 |
| Peak 10X nonilluminated | 25.2 | 7.3 | −4.0 | 25.0 | 12 |
| Peak 15X illuminated | 35.0 | 8.0 | −5.0 | 20.0 | 12 |
| Peak 15X nonilluminated | 41.0 | 9.6 | −4.8 | 21.0 | 12 |
| Selsi Bar #377 | 25.0 | 1.50 | −50.0 | 2.0 | 12 |
| Selsi plano-convex #404 Chrome | 10.7 | 1.60 | −17.9 | 5.6 | 12 |
| Selsi plano-convex #404 Plastic | 10.7 | 1.80 | −13.3 | 7.5 | 12 |

*A value for V was not published and was calculated by the author from i. †A value for i was not published; these values were calculated from V. ‡Calculated from the investigators' data. §$F_e$ and V were not published and were calculated from i and E. Some values in this table may differ slightly from the actual published values due to rounding. It will be noted that the same magnifier may have different values published by different investigators. This is due to variations in measurement as well as variations in quality control by the manufacturers.

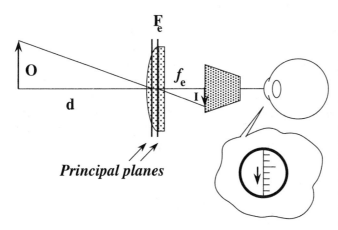

**Figure 10–8.** The equivalent power of a lens or lens system can be determined by measuring the height (I) of the image formed by an object of known size (O) placed at a known distance (d) from the lens. The image height is measured with a contact lens reticle or similar device. The equivalent focal length, $f_e$ is calculated from similar triangles ($f_e$ = dI/O), and the equivalent power ($F_e$) is then determined from the relationship $F_e = 1/f_e$.

111

TABLE 10–7. Equivalent power comparison for published values[8] and those calculated by measuring the base curves and center thickness.

| Magnifier | Published $F_e$ | Calculated $F_e$ | Difference |
|-----------|-----------------|------------------|------------|
| COIL #5123 | +23.8 | +24.98 | +1.18 D |
| COIL #5428 | +17.4 | +18.24 | +0.84 D |

difference will be relatively small provided the object is located several meters away.

It is also possible to determine the equivalent power by measuring the front ($F_1$) and back surface ($F_2$) powers and the center thickness (t) in meters, provided the index of refraction (n) is known.

$$F_e = F_1 + F_2 - (t/n)(F_1)(F_2)$$

These measurements may not be possible without disassembling the stand magnifier, in which case the first technique is preferred. Since aspheric surfaces cannot be measured accurately with the lens gauge, a small error may also be introduced. A comparison of equivalent powers measured by these two techniques is given in Table 10-7 for two commercially available lenses.

## Enlargement by the Magnifier Lens Alone

The enlargement (E) by the lens is dependent on the equivalent power of the lens ($F_e$) and the vergence (V) leaving the lens from the image formed by an object at the base of the stand. The system consists of the magnifier lens ($F_1$) and the patient's add or accommodation ($F_2$) separated by a distance t. The equivalent power of the system is therefore

$$F_e = F_1 + F_2 - (t)(F_1)(F_2)$$

The amount of accommodation ($F_2$) is determined by the distance of the image from the eye. This distance is h + i, as can be seen from Figure 10-7; therefore, $F_2 = 1/(i + h)$. (The distance h is measured to the eye for an eye that is accommodating or to the spectacle plane for an add.) This value can be substituted into the formula above for $F_2$. Some algebraic manipulation will give a value for the enlargement (E) by the magnifier. For this derivation, sign convention is ignored, which does not create a problem as long as it is remembered that V, the vergence emerging from the magnifier lens, is a negative number.

$$F_e = F_1 + F_2 - (t)(F_1)(F_2)$$
$$F_e = F_2[F_1/F_2 + 1 - (t)(F_1)]$$
$$F_e = F_2[F_1(i + h) + 1 - (t)(F_1)]$$
$$F_e = F_2[F_1(i + h) + 1 - (h)(F_1)]$$
$$F_e = F_2[F_1(i) + F_1(h) + 1 - (h)(F_1)]$$
$$F_e = F_2[F_1(i) + 1]$$

It is now possible to substitute $1/V$ for i, but since we have treated i as a positive number and V is a negative number (remember?), the absolute value of V will be used.

$$F_e = F_2[F_1/|V| + 1]$$
$$F_e = F_2[F_1/|V| + |V|/|V|]$$
$$F_e = F_2[(F_1 + |V|)/|V|]$$

The term $(F_1 + |V|)/|V|$ is substituted for the enlargement factor E, and this gives

$$F_e = F_2(E)$$

This form shows that the equivalent power of the system (magnifier plus add or accommodation) can be determined by multiplying the enlargement factor E by the add or accommodation. This is useful clinically since a person should achieve the same magnification from any two systems that have the same equivalent power; for example, if the patient can read 2M print with a microscope that has an equivalent power of +20 D, then he or she should also be able to read 2M print with a stand magnifier and bifocal combination that has a system equivalent power of +20 D. The system equivalent power can easily be determined by multiplying the enlargement factor of the stand magnifier by the patient's bifocal power or by the add that should be prescribed to create the appropriate system.

Bailey gives an equivalent alternative form for E,

$$E = (V - F)/V$$

and refers to it as the MULTACC factor.[15] This term should look familiar as an expression for transverse magnification[16] ($M_t$), where

$$M_t = (L' - F)/L'$$

and since $L' - F = L$ for a thin lens,

$$M_t = (L)/L' \text{ or } l'/l$$

The emerging vergence (V) can be estimated experimentally by placing the magnifier on a page of print and adding plus lenses on top of the magnifier lens until the image is first blurred. Since the emerging vergence is negative, the plus lenses neutralize it, and the largest power plus lens without blur will be equal to, but opposite in power to, the emerging vergence. If the emerging vergence is known, the position of the image behind the page is also known; for example, if $V = -4$, then i = 25 cm from the lens. Once V and $F_e$ are known, E can be calculated. It is now possible to determine exactly how a stand magnifier will perform, as is shown in the next example.

■ **Example 10–16.** A new stand magnifier arrives in the office mail. The label reads +24.00 D and, not surprisingly, 6X is in parentheses next to it. The clinician places it on a page of fine print, adds plus lenses just until the print appears blurred, and finds that a +5.00 D lens is the largest plus power that keeps a clear image. The emerging vergence is therefore −5.00 D, and the image must be located 20 cm behind the lens. The clinician now views an object that is 50 cm tall, and 3 meters away, through the lens. The image in sharp focus on the screen of the contact lens reticule is 8.5 mm tall. By similar triangles the equivalent focal length, $f_e$, in millimeters, is found as follows:

$$f_e = dI/O$$
$$f_e = (3,000)(8.5)/500$$
$$f_e = 25,500/500$$
$$f_e = 51 \text{ mm or } 5.1 \text{ cm}$$
$$F_e = 1,000/f_e$$
$$F_e = 1,000/51 \text{ or } 100/5.1 = +19.6 \text{ D}$$

The equivalent power of the magnifier is therefore +19.6 D. The enlargement that the lens will provide by itself is then determined.

$$E = (F_e + |V|)/|V|$$
$$E = (19.6 + 5)/5$$
$$E = +24.6/5$$
$$E = 4.92X$$

or alternatively,

$$E = (V − F_e)/V$$
$$E = (−5 − 19.6)/(−5) = (−24.6)/(−5) = 4.92X$$

The clinician now prepares a label for the box with the following information: image location = 20 cm, enlargement = 4.92X (or 5X), equivalent power = +19.6. This may seem like a lot of work, but it only has to be done once for a given type of stand magnifier if the information has not been published or is not provided by the manufacturer.

When properly labeled, it is easy to use the magnifier successfully since the clinician now knows how to determine the expected results and the correct positioning of the lens for the patient's add.

■ **Example 10–17.** A patient enters with a goal to read 1M print and a reference acuity of 0.4/4M through best correction and a +2.50 add. With the stand magnifier above, could that goal be achieved, and where should the lens be positioned for the image to be clear?

Because the patient is in focus at 40 cm, the lens must be 20 cm from his add, which will put the image at 40 cm. The total magnification will be:

$$M_{total} = RDM \times E$$
$$M_{total} = 40/40 \times 4.92X$$
$$M_{total} = 4.92X$$

Since 4M/4.92X = 0.81M, the patient should be able read 1M print, which is slightly larger than 0.81M print. The patient must be instructed to hold the magnifier 20 cm from the spectacle plane and to view through the bifocal segment.

***Hand Magnifiers Revisited.*** When hand-held magnifiers were discussed previously, the formula M = rF assumed that the object was held at, or very near to, the focal point of the lens. This is not always how patients use hand magnifiers. It should now be clear that if the object is held inside the focal length of the lens, a situation is created that is identical to that of a stand magnifier. The image will be erect, virtual, and located some finite distance from the patient's eye, and a presbyopic patient will need an add to see it as clearly as possible. The total magnification will be a combination of the enlargement by the lens and the relative distance magnification, just as with a stand magnifier.

## TELEMICROSCOPES

A telemicroscope, as the name implies, combines features of a telescope and a microscope. It is a telescope that has been made to focus at a near point either by adding an auxiliary lens or by having a focusing apparatus that allows sufficient separation between the ocular and the objective. A telescope without these alterations is useful only for distances close to optical infinity, perhaps 10 feet and further. If one looks through a telescope at a near object, it does not appear clear. This is easily shown by following the vergence of light from a point source located near the objective lens. Figure 10–9 illustrates a 2X telescope used to look at an object 40 cm away. The vergence entering the telescope is −2.50 D. As the light immediately leaves the objective, it has +7.50 D of convergence. When it meets the ocular, it has +12 D of convergence, which becomes −8 D of divergence as it exits from the telescope.

The divergence was −2.50 D entering but −8.00 D leaving. A telescope therefore is a "vergence amplifier" when used to view a near object. This should make it clear that a presbyopic patient cannot use a telescope to view near objects without some optical modification. If a patient can use the telescope in this example to view objects clearly at 40 cm, then he or she is either accommodating 8.00 D or has 8.00 D of uncorrected myopia. In order for a patient to be able to use a telescope for near, we must either add a plus lens, called a cap, to the objective or be able to separate the lenses enough to have parallel light exiting the telescope. In the example given, the cap would be a +2.50 D lens, placed over the objective, which makes the light entering parallel so the telescope behaves in the normal fashion of having parallel light entering and exiting. This gives the patient a clear image through his or her distance correction (Figure 10–9). The cap can also be added permanently by increasing the

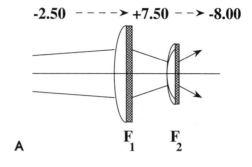

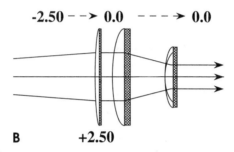

**Figure 10–9. (A)** A telescope, focused for distance, acts as a vergence amplifier when used to view a near object. In this example, 2.50 D of divergence from an object 40 cm away is amplified to 8.00 D of divergence by a 2.0X Galilean telescope, where $F_1$ = +10.00 D and $F_2$ = −20.00 D. **(B)** A telescope may be used to view near objects if the appropriate convex lens is used as a "cap" to produce parallel light from the object of regard.

power of the objective to +12.50. This is often done but sacrifices the potential use of the device as a telescope since there is no longer a cap that can be removed. (The astute reader may correctly observe that a −2.50 cap can be used in this case to allow the telescope to be used for distance.)

## Magnification by a Telemicroscope

The magnification provided by a telemicroscope is the product of that given by the telescope and that given by the cap, which can be considered to be a microscope. The formula is given below, where $M_{tms}$ is the total magnification provided by the telemicroscope (tms), $M_{cap}$ is the magnification of the cap, and $M_{ts}$ is the magnification of the telescope.

$$M_{tms} = M_{cap} \times M_{ts}$$
$$M_{tms} = rF \times M_{ts}$$

■ **Example 10–18.** What letter size should a patient be able to read if her best corrected near acuity with a +2.50 add over best correction is 0.4/5M and she uses a 2X telescope with a +5.00 D cap?

$$M_{tms} = rF \times M_{ts}$$
$$M_{tms} = (0.4)5 \times 2$$
$$M_{tms} = 2 \times 2$$
$$M_{tms} = 4X$$

Magnification = Reference size/Goal size

$$4X = 5M/Goal\ size$$

Goal size = 5M/4X

Goal size = 1.25M

■ **Example 10–19.** What cap would be necessary for this patient to read 2M print using the same telescope?

Magnification = Reference size/Goal size

Magnification = 5M/2M

Magnification = 2.5X

$$M_{tms} = M_{cap} \times M_{ts}$$
$$2.5 = (0.4)F \times 2$$
$$2.5 = (0.8)F$$
$$2.5/0.8 = F$$
$$+3.12 = F$$

■ **Example 10–20.** The same patient wants to read the equivalent of 1M print on an instrument at work and must do so at 25 cm. What telemicroscope would achieve this goal?

The requirement to read at 25 cm fixes the cap at +4.00 D. Therefore, the only variable is the telescope power.

Magnification needed = Reference size/Goal size

Magnification needed = 5M/1M

Magnification needed = 5X

$$M_{tms} = M_{cap} \times M_{ts}$$
$$5 = (0.4)4 \times M_{ts}$$
$$5 = 1.6 \times M_{ts}$$
$$5/1.6 = M_{ts}$$
$$3.12X = M_{ts}$$

A 3.12X telescope is needed. Since there is not one with that exact magnification, the one with the closest magnification, probably 3.0X, is demonstrated to the patient.

A telemicroscope has several disadvantages compared to a microscope in that it is heavier, longer, and more expensive and may have a smaller field of view. There is, however, one significant advantage that makes it the device of choice in some situations: a telemicroscope gives the patient a longer working distance than the equivalent microscope. Because many patients resist the near working distance of a microscope, the telemicroscope is the only other choice for a spectacle-mounted device. These two devices are compared in the next example.

■ **Example 10–21.** Determine the microscope and telemicroscope that will allow a patient whose near acuity is 0.4/8M to read 2M print. For this example use a telescope that is 2.2X. Compare the work distances for the two results.

$$\text{Magnification required} = \text{Reference size/Goal size}$$
$$\text{Magnification required} = 8M/2M$$
$$\text{Magnification required} = 4X$$

*Microscope*

$$M = rF$$
$$4X = (0.4)F$$
$$+10 = F$$

The *work distance* is defined as the required object distance from the most anterior part of the device.[17] For the microscope, the work distance is 10 cm from the lens.

*Telemicroscope*

$$4 = M_{cap} \times 2.2X$$
$$4/2.2 = M_{cap}$$
$$1.82 = M_{cap}$$
$$M_{cap} = rF$$
$$1.82 = (0.4)F$$
$$+4.5 = F$$

For the telemicroscope, the work distance is 22.22 cm (100/4.5) from the cap (the most anterior portion of the device).

The telemicroscope in this example gives a work distance that is more than twice as great as the microscope. One occupational application where this is a clear advantage is surgery. Thoracic surgeons require magnification to suture fine coronary vessels but must have a comfortable work distance. The surgical loupes they use are telemicroscopes with the appropriate cap power built into the system for their preferred work distance. Persons who are visually impaired may also have occupational demands that require a longer work distance, or they may simply prefer it.

■ **Example 10–22.** The patient prefers to read at 25 cm and needs to read 1M print. Her reference acuity is 0.4/6M through a +2.50 add. Design a telemicroscope that allows her to achieve the stated goal.

The magnification needed to achieve her goal is 6X (M = 6M/1M = 6). The need, or desire, to read at 25 cm fixes the cap power at +4.00 D. The magnification by the telescope is the remaining variable. The cap gives 1.6X ($0.4 \times 4 = 1.6$); therefore, the telescope must provide 3.75X. This is determined as follows:

$$M_{tms} = M_{cap} \times M_{ts}$$
$$6X = 1.6X \times M_{ts}$$
$$6X/1.6X = M_{ts}$$
$$3.75X = M_{ts}$$

■ **Example 10-23.** Consider the same patient as in Example 10-22. This time, suppose that the only telescope in the diagnostic kit is 2.5X. What cap would be needed to achieve the same goal?

The total magnification needed remains 6.0X. Since 2.5 of it comes from the telescope, 2.4X must come from the cap. In this case, the cap must be 6 diopters.

$$M_{tms} = M_{cap} \times M_{ts}$$
$$6.0X = M_{cap} \times 2.5X$$
$$6.0/2.5 = M_{cap}$$
$$2.4X = M_{cap}$$
$$2.4X = rF$$
$$2.4 = (0.4)F$$
$$2.4/0.4 = F$$
$$+6\,D = F$$

When comparing a microscope with a telemicroscope, the clinician should understand that there is not just one telemicroscope, but many, that will provide the equivalent magnification to the microscope. Other equivalent telemicroscopes are found by adjusting the cap power and telescope magnification accordingly. A lower magnification telescope requires a higher power cap and hence a shorter working distance. A higher magnification from the telescope allows a lower power cap and a greater working distance. In fact, there is a nice relationship that is very useful in determining a series of telemicroscopes that all have the same total magnification. The product of the cap, expressed in diopters, and the telescope's magnification is constant for all equivalent telemicroscopes and is equal to the equivalent power of the microscope ($F_e$) that gives the patient the same magnification. The relationship is:

$$F_{cap} \times M_{ts} = \text{Equivalent microscope (in diopters)} = F_e$$

This relationship is established as follows: If the magnification of the microscope ($M_{ms}$) is equal to the magnification of telemicroscope ($M_{tms}$), then the following statements must be true:

$$M_{ms} = M_{tms}$$
$$M_{ms} = M_{cap} \times M_{ts}$$
$$M_{ms} = rF_{cap} \times M_{ts}$$
$$rF = rF_{cap} \times M_{ts}$$
$$F_e = F_{cap} \times M_{ts}$$

**TABLE 10–8. Four telemicroscopes equivalent to a +20.00 D microscope.**

| $F_{cap}$ (diopters) | $M_{ts}$ | $F_e$ System |
|---|---|---|
| +2.00 | 10X | +20.00 |
| +4.00 | 5X | +20.00 |
| +5.00 | 4X | +20.00 |
| +10.00 | 2X | +20.00 |

Example: A telemicroscope composed of a 5X telescope and a +4.00 cap has an equivalent power of +20.00 D (4 × 5 = 20). $F_{cap}$ is the power of the cap, $M_{ts}$ is the magnifying power of the telescope, and $F_e$ is the equivalent power of the system ($F_e = F_{cap} \times M_{ts}$).

The telemicroscopes given in Table 10–8 all provide the same total magnification. The numerical value of the magnification is equal to the equivalent power of the microscope that also gives the patient that same magnification.

■ **Example 10–24.** If a patient achieves a goal with a +20.00 D microscope, he can also achieve the same goal with any of the four telemicroscope combinations in Table 10–8. One might be selected over another depending on the preferred work distance or the desired use of the telescope when the cap is removed.

## SUMMARY

An understanding of the basic optical principles of low vision devices is central to prescribing them rationally. If the clinician understands how these devices provide magnification and what results the patient should achieve, then it becomes possible to predict which devices should be tried and, specifically, what optical strength is required to achieve the patient's goal.

In order to keep the preceding sections basic yet clinically relevant, certain optical considerations have been ignored; for example, other components of the total eye-lens system such as refractive correction, axial length of the eye, and lens design all contribute to the total magnification. Similarly, the patient typically does not hold the object precisely at the focal point of the lens, so the maximum angular magnification, as determined by any calculation using M = rF, may not be achieved. Nevertheless, this formula is appropriate for the clinical setting, and the clinician is prepared for any deviation from the expected results by accepting that the calculated values, similar to retinoscopy, serve only as a logical starting point. The final lens power is refined by subjective testing.

Hand-held magnifiers and microscopes can be prescribed with the use of M = rF, provided that the patient is instructed to hold the material at the focal point of the lens. If he or she does not, then the magnification achieved will be different but can be determined from the general magnification formula. Stand magnifiers are somewhat more complex to prescribe rationally. The magnification that the patient receives is determined by the enlargement and the position of the image relative to the reference size and distance. At the very least, the clinician should know the image location in order to be sure that the image is in the best possible focus. The magnification can be determined easily if the parameters of the magnifier are known and a spreadsheet or other computer program is used to perform the calculation. Stand magnifiers can be prescribed easily if the enlargement factor is known by remembering that the enlargement factor multiplied by the add (or accommodation) determines the equivalent power of the system. The magnification should be equivalent to that provided by any other device with the same equivalent power (see Example 10–25).

The two types of telescopes used in vision rehabilitation are the Galilean and the Keplerian. The main advantage of the Keplerian is the fact that it has a wider field of view than the equivalent Galilean. Telescopes are used for viewing distant objects unless they have a sufficient range of focus to be used for near or unless the appropriate cap is used. When used for near, they are called telemicroscopes. The main advantage of a telemicroscope compared to a microscope that provides the same magnification is that the telemicroscope allows the object to be held farther away; this may be a significant and desirable advantage for some. The following example illustrates the main points and should convince the reader that some low vision care can be provided with a very small inventory and that the optics are not insurmountable.

■ **Example 10–25.** Suppose your inventory of optical devices consists only of a 2.5X telescope, a trial lens set, and a stand magnifier with an enlargement factor of 3.0X and an image location of 15 cm from the lens. The first person who presents as a patient with a visual impairment has best corrected acuity of 20/250 at distance and 0.4/5M at near with a +2.50 add over best correction. What size letters should he be able to read with the telescope at distance? What microscope would allow him to read 1M print? What hand magnifier would allow him to read 1M print? What add would be required for the stand magnifier to allow him to read 1M print? What cap would be required for the telescope to create a telemicroscope that allows him to read 1M print?

*Telescope:* In previous examples a goal was set and the required telescope was determined. Since you only have one telescope, the same formula is used, but it is the goal that is calculated, not the telescope power.

$$\text{Magnification} = \text{Reference size/Goal size}$$
$$2.5X = 250/\text{Goal size}$$
$$\text{Goal size} = 100$$

The patient should read the equivalent of 20/100 through his best distance correction with the telescope.

*Microscope:* Your inventory doesn't include any microscopes, but you have trial lenses that serve the same purpose.

$$\text{Magnification needed} = \text{Reference size/Goal size}$$
$$M = 5M/1M$$
$$M = 5X$$
$$M = rF$$
$$5 = (0.4)F$$
$$+12.5 = F$$

With a +12.5 trial lens over best distance correction the person should read 1M print if he holds it at the focal point of the lens (100/12.5 = 8 cm). A tape measure is used to make sure that the correct distance is maintained.

*Hand-held magnifier:* The same lens that was used as a microscope can be used as a hand-held magnifier, and 1M print should be readable as long as it is maintained at the focal point of the lens and the patient views through his distance correction. Trial lenses have a little handle and can be used to demonstrate a hand-held magnifier even though their apertures are too small.

*Stand magnifier:* It has already been determined that he should be able to read 1M print with a lens that has an equivalent power of +12.5 D. This part of the problem therefore reduces to determining what add, combined with the stand magnifier, gives a system with that same equivalent power of +12.5 D. If E is multiplied by the add $(F_2)$, the product is the equivalent power $(F_e)$ of the system.

$$F_e = F_2(E)$$
$$12.5 = F_2(3)$$
$$+4.17 = F_2$$

Since there is no +4.17 D trial lens, the next best choice would be +4.25 D, which should give a small measure of reserve (very small). Since the image is 15 cm from the lens, the magnifier must be held 8.5 cm from the add in order for the image to be in its focal plane (23.5 cm = 100/4.25). He should be able to read 1M print with this stand magnifier and a +4.25 add over best correction. Unlike the hand-held magnifier, this time he must view through the add.

*Telemicroscope:* Once again, since he can read 1M print with a +12.5 add, he should read 1M print with a telemicroscope that has a equivalent power of +12.5 D. This is an application of the formula for equivalent power of a telemicroscope.

$$F_e = F_{cap} \times M_{ts}$$
$$12.5 = F_{cap} \times 2.5$$
$$+5 = F_{cap}$$

If a +5.00 D trial lens is held against the objective of the telescope, he should read 1M print held 20 cm (100/5 = 20) from the cap. The advantage of this system over a microscope is the large increase in work distance (20 cm compared to 8 cm).

## REFERENCES

1. Ogle, KN: *Optics,* 2 ed. Springfield, IL, Charles C. Thomas, 1971, p 98.
2. Keating MP: *Geometric, Physical, and Visual Optics.* Boston, Butterworths, 1988, pp 247-266.
3. Keating MP: *Geometric, Physical, and Visual Optics.* Boston, Butterworths, 1988, p 256.
4. Bailey IL: Verifying near vision magnifiers. Part 1. *Optom Monthly* 72(1):42-43, 1981.
5. Kestenbaum A, Sturman R: Reading glasses for patients with very poor vision. *Arch Ophthalmol* 3:451, 1956.
6. Bailey IL: Combining accommodation with spectacle additions. *Optom Monthly* 71:397-399, 1980.
7. Bailey IL: Combining hand magnifiers with spectacle additions. *Optom Monthly* 71:458-461, 1980.
8. Bailey I, Loshin DS: Standardization: Stand magnifiers. *J Vis Rehab* 2(3):25-27, 1984.
9. Raasch TW, Bailey IL, Loshin, DS: Standardization: Eschenbach magnifiers. *J Vis Rehab* 3(1):26-28, 1985.
10. Bullimore MA, Bailey IL: Stand magnifiers: An evaluation of new optical aids from Coil. *Opt Vis Sci* 66(11):766-773, 1989.
11. Chung STL, Johnston AW: New stand magnifiers do not meet rated levels of performance. *Clin Exp Optom* 73(6):194-199, 1990.
12. Freed B: A new method for the measurement of transverse magnification; initial results in 21 elected stand magnifiers. *J Vis Rehab* 1(2):47-50, 1987.
13. Dillehay SM, Pennsyl CD: Low vision aids and the presbyope. *J Amer Optom Assoc* 62(9):704-710, 1991.
14. Bailey IL: Verifying near vision magnifiers. Part 2. *Optom Monthly* 72(2):34-38, 1981.
15. Bailey IL: The use of fixed focus stand magnifiers. *Optom Monthly* 72(8):37-39, 1981.
16. Fannin TE, Grosvenor T: *Clinical Optics.* Boston, Butterworths, 1987, p 411.
17. *American National Standard for Ophthalmics—Low Vision Aids Requirements.* Merrifield, VA, Optical Laboratories Association, 1993, p 4.

## ADDITIONAL READING

### General Optics

Bailey IL: Magnification for near vision. *Optom Monthly* 71:119-122, 1980.
Cole RG: A unified approach to the optics of low vision aids—Part 1. *J Vis Rehab* 2(1)23-36, 1988.

Cole RG: A unified approach to the optics of low vision aids—Part 2. *J Vis Rehab* 2(2):45-53, 1988.

Cole RG: A unified approach to the optics of low vision aids—Part 3. *J Vis Rehab* 2(4):69-79, 1988.

Cole RG: Predicting the low vision reading add. *J Am Optom Assoc* 64:19-27, 1993.

Jalie M: *The Principles of Ophthalmic Lenses,* 2 ed. London, C. F. Hodgson & Son, Limited, 1972.

## Hand Magnifiers

Lederer J: The design of single-lens ophthalmic magnifiers. *Australian J Optom* 40:445, 1957.

Loshin DS, Bailey IL: Standardization: Hand-held magnifiers. *J Rehab Optom* 1(2):29-32, 1984.

## Loupes

Linksz A: Optical principles of loupe magnification. *Am J Ophthalmol* 40(6):831-840, 1955.

Blommaert FJJ, Neve JJ: Reading fields of magnifying loupes. *J Opt Soc Am* A, 4:1820-1830, 1987.

## Stand Magnifiers

Bailey IL: Locating the image in stand magnifiers. *Optom Monthly* 72(6):22-24, 1981.

Bailey IL: Locating the image in stand magnifiers—an alternative method. *Optom Monthly* 74:487-488, 1983.

Bailey IL, Raasch TW, Loshin D: Stand magnifiers. *J Rehab Optom* 1(2):29-32, 1985.

Bailey IL, Loshin DS: Hand held magnifiers. *Rehab Optom* 1:29-32, 1984.

Bailey IL, Loshin DS: Eschenbach magnifiers. *J Vis Rehab* 3(1):26-28, 1985.

Fonda G, Livingston NJ: Visolett magnifier. Evaluation and optics. *Arch Ophthalmol* 94(9):1614-1615, 1976.

Freed B: Clinical categories of stand magnifiers: Measurements and applications. *J Vis Rehab* 4(1):49-52, 1990.

Loshin DS, Bailey IL: Standardization: Stand magnifiers. *J Vis Rehab* 2:235-250, 1984.

Sloan LL: New focusable stand magnifiers. *Am J Ophthalmol* 58:604-608, 1964.

Spitzberg LA, Kuether CL, Jose RT: The new writing magnifier. *J Vis Rehab* 1(2):23-27, 1987.

## Telescopes

Bailey IL: Distance telescopes and ametropia. *Optom Monthly,* 72(12):22-26, 1981.

Bailey IL: Afocal telescopes. *Optom Monthly* 72(11):17-20, 1981.

Bailey IL: Image brightness and telescopes. *Optom Monthly* 73:391-400, 1982.

Berliner ML: A new type of telescopic lens. *Arch Ophthalmol* 16:649-654, 1936.

Browning RA: Charting the field of view through telescopic low vision aids. *Rehab Optom* 1(1):7-8, 1983.

Eggers M: Optical principles of telescopic lenses. *Transac Am Ophthalmol Soc* 27:410, 1939.

Katz M, Citek K, Arditi A: An instrument for measuring the modulation transfer functions of low power telescopes and telemicroscopes. *Am J Optom Physiol Optics* 65(3):190-197, 1988.

Katz M, Citek K, Price I: Optical properties of low vision telescopes. *J Am Optom Assoc* 58:320-331, 1987.

Katz M, Yager D, Lewis A, Citek K, Sanchez N, Arditi A: Modulation transfer and contrast sensitivity through low vision telescopes. *Applied Optics* 28:1103-1109, 1989.

Margach CB: Optical characteristics of focusable ophthalmic telescopes. *Opt J Rev Optom* 111(8):12-16, 1974.

Morgan M, Peters H: Telescopic lenses, in *The Optics of Ophthalmic Lenses*. Millbrae, CA, The National Press, 1948.

Otto D, Woo GC: Notes on the use of low magnification telescopes in low vision care. *Clin Exp Optom* 73(2):37-42, 1990.

## Telemicroscopes

Bailey IL, Loshin DS: Keeler near vision telescopes. *J Vis Rehab* 3(2):19-21, 1985.

Jose RT, Morse SE: Telescopes: To cap or not to cap. *Rehab Optom J* 1(3):9-11, 1983.

Kleinstein RN: Reading with a 10X telescope. *Am J Optom and Physiological Optics* 55(10):732-734, 1978.

Krefman RA: Working distance comparison of plus lenses and reading telescopes. *Am J Optom Physiol Optics* 57(11):835-838, 1980.

Margach CB: Optical characteristics of focusable ophthalmic telescopes. *Opt J Rev Optom* 111(8):12-16, 1974.

Margach CB: Telescopic microscopes. *Opt J Rev Optom* 113(2):56-59, 1976.

Smith G: Magnification of afocal telescopes when used focally. *Austr J Optom* 64: 202-205, 1981.

Williams DR: Magnification in telescopic loupes. *J Am Optom Assoc* 45(9):1068-1071, 1974.

# GENERAL GUIDELINES FOR PRESCRIBING OPTICAL DEVICES

*The prescription of optical devices is somewhat different from the prescription of pharmaceuticals or other medical treatments. The patient does not usually have an in-office demonstration of how each of several pills or ointments work so he or she can choose the one that seems most desirable, yet this is exactly how optical devices are most often prescribed. The sense of a device being "prescribed" is maintained by not allowing the patient to randomly try each and every device in the office until some satisfactory subset is selected. The clinician must present the diagnostic trial to the patient as a planned sequence of tests, each of which leads to the next. The use of a logical sequence and systematic approach is the central theme of this text. The diagnostic trial should always be under the control of the clinician, and it should be clear to the patient that the clinician knows where the process is headed. This cannot happen if devices are tried randomly.*

*The next several chapters give specific recommendations for prescribing each of the main categories of optical devices. There is a certain planned redundancy in the format that hopefully will reinforce guidelines that are helpful in practice. Before specific devices are considered, however, some general guidelines are presented in this chapter.*

## A BASIC PHILOSOPHY FOR PRESCRIBING OPTICAL DEVICES

Low vision devices should be prescribed in a systematic manner in order to achieve the best outcome. This approach requires that the practitioner understand how each device works and be able to predict an expected result when it is demonstrated to the patient. If the patient does not achieve the expected result, then some data are inconsistent, the source of which can be uncovered. Such an approach also allows the practitioner to select the most appropriate device(s) to demonstrate and prescribe, and spares the patient all of the disadvantages and disappointments associated with multiple trials of devices that are too strong or too weak for the desired goals. By way of example, suppose that a patient requires an add of +40.00 D to read newsprint. The practitioner, not knowing how to determine this in advance, proceeds to try a number of adds such as +4, +6, +8, +10, +12, +14, and so forth. None of these is even close to what the patient needs, and with each hapless trial another failure is realized. Clearly, this is not conducive to developing patient confidence in the practitioner's expertise. The following is the recommended process:

- Determine the best distance correction
- Measure the best corrected acuity (the reference acuity)
- Determine the goal acuity
- Calculate the magnification needed
- Demonstrate the appropriate device to the patient

There are so many excellent devices and options available that it is often difficult to know where to start once the goal and required magnification have been determined. A good general rule is to prescribe the most conventional device possible when there is a choice; for example, glasses, because they are a familiar appliance, are preferred over hand-held and stand magnifiers or other obvious assisting devices. Similarly, bifocals or prism-compensated half eyes are more natural appearing and hence better received than a full-diameter microscope. Because telescopes and telemicroscopes are cosmetically conspicuous, they are often rejected early in the rehabilitative course but may be better received at a later point. It may be unreasonable to expect to achieve the patient's goal initially because of the difficulties involved in learning to use optical appliances and residual vision effectively. When this is the case, a sequential approach to prescribing is helpful in which lower power devices are used initially for less demanding tasks. As facility in the use of the device improves, stronger powers may be prescribed until maximum efficiency is reached. This may take a long time, so communication is the key to maintaining the patient's motivation.

In the author's experience the sequence in which optical devices are considered is: high adds, full-diameter microscopes, hand magnifiers, stand magnifiers, telescopes, and finally telemicroscopes. This sequence is based on the types of devices that patients seem to accept most readily.

There is no one device that can compensate for all the functions of the human eye. It is therefore unreasonable to assume that patients must be tested until *the* right device is found for them. When the clinician engages in a pursuit of "the right device," it can soon seem like a "quest for the Holy Grail." It is the rule, not the exception, that multiple devices are eventually prescribed to meet the many needs of each patient. It is just as important not to investigate too many devices as this can also be counterproductive. When there are numerous similar devices that might be useful to the patient, the clinician must be directive in order to avoid an unnecessarily lengthy and potentially confusing demonstration session.

One way to get locked into an unnatural "quest" is to invite the patient into a demonstration area where all of the optical devices are openly displayed. This invites unreasonable comparisons for the sake of courtesy when the patient expresses an interest in "that one over there." Once the appropriate lens power has been determined, it should be only a matter of demonstrating some of the forms in which it can be prescribed, not every available magnifier in the office. This keeps the process under the control and direction of the provider.

## AVOIDING FALSE EXPECTATIONS

In spite of the clinician's best efforts, patients often expect their device(s) to appear different from those they were shown during the examination because this is what has happened in the past. For example, they may expect a telescope to look like a conventional spectacle lens because in previous eye examinations, before the loss of vision, the best correction was demonstrated as a collection of trial lenses in a heavy, ugly trial frame, yet the glasses received at dispensing had light lenses in a fashionable frame.

Patients also often expect to have a larger field of view, greater ease of use, and perhaps even better vision than the actual device offers. These false expectations can be reduced by repeated emphasis that the device they are shown is exactly what they would get if it were prescribed for them. It is helpful to have examples of spectacle-mounted devices available for demonstration and to reiterate several times that *"Your glasses will look just like these."* Also, as the patient prepares to leave, it is a good idea to mention that *"Your glasses will look just like these."*

## WHEN TO BE DIRECTIVE

Patients can easily become confused over the many choices they are presented with. When this is the case, it is up to the practitioner to make a professional judgment and to prescribe the appropriate devices based on clinical experience; for example, when it is obvious that a less cosmetically pleasing device is the better choice, it is the role of the practitioner to help the patient accept that fact and use the prescribed device effectively. If the device required to achieve the patient's goal is too strong to be used effectively at first, then it is reasonable to prescribe a lower power initially, followed by progressively stronger devices as performance improves. This is more expensive for the patient but is more likely to result in a satisfactory outcome.

## TRAINING IN THE PROPER USE OF THE DEVICE

Spectacle-mounted devices require practice to use as effectively as possible. The patient must be educated about the care and use of the device. This can require several sessions during which the correct focal distance and adjustment are demonstrated along with the use of proper lighting, reading stands, or other environmental adaptations that will provide the optimum circumstances for successful utilization. No matter how well a patient uses the device initially, he or she will probably use it even more effectively following a course of programmed instruction.

## LOANING DEVICES

It is convenient for patients to borrow a device for home trial prior to investing in it for permanent use. In-office training and home trials with loaned devices serve to assist patients in adapting to the limitations imposed by any optical device before they actually commit to obtaining their own; however, there are several pitfalls that can make loaning devices a poor idea. When a device is loaned, there may be a tendency by patients to regard it less seriously. If patients purchase the device initially, they have a vested interest in making it work for them. From an economic point of view, it is expensive for the clinician not only to purchase a large inventory of devices for loaning to patients but also to maintain it when devices are lost, broken, and worn out. When a person uses the device without supervision, he or she may not use it effectively and may not appreciate how useful it could be under the right circumstances. This latter concern is reduced by in-office training before the device is actually loaned.

## FRAME SELECTION FOR SPECTACLE-MOUNTED DEVICES

A spectacle-mounted telemicroscope, telescope, or multielement microscope is heavy and requires precise adjustment with respect to the line of sight. This necessitates careful attention to the selection of an appropriate frame. The ideal frame is sturdy and has large, adjustable nose pads and spring-loaded temples. Temples that are slightly longer than would be selected for conventional spectacles should be chosen in order to give extra holding power around the ears. The bridge should be slightly larger than usual to allow for lateral adjustment. This can compensate for a minor laboratory error if the position of the device within the carrier lens is slightly off.

A small eye size is preferred to keep the weight of the lens and frame as low as possible. A small eye size is also preferred for microscopes that are manufactured in the lenticular form. The selection of an eye size that is circular and small enough to approximate the size of the bowl can mask the transition line from the power zone to the carrier portion of the lens.

The most important guideline for the selection of the frame, however, is whether or not the patient will wear it. It may seem surprising at first, but it is natural that some patients want a particular frame because it is cosmetically pleasing even though it has a telescope or telemicroscope protruding from the lens. If the patient will not wear the device, it does not really matter how carefully it was designed from an optical perspective.

## OPHTHALMIC OPTICS CONSIDERATIONS FOR THE CORRECTION OF HIGH REFRACTIVE ERRORS

Some visually impaired patients require complex spectacle prescriptions for correction of the refractive error. Careful attention to ophthalmic materials design can result in the optimum end result. Some examples are high plus and minus lenses in which a more cosmetically appealing and comfortable design may make the difference between whether or not a patient continues to use the prescription. These and other special design considerations are considered in the sections that follow. It often seems that the greatest problem is not designing the prescription but finding a laboratory that can fabricate it correctly.

### High Plus Lenses

High plus lenses for the correction of refractive error used to be prescribed most frequently for aphakic patients but are less common now with the widespread use of the intraocular lens. Nevertheless, there are still some patients who are aphakic and some who have unusually high hyperopia. Regardless of the etiology, the design considerations are the same.

A number of manufacturers have designed high plus lenses with aspheric surfaces that they believe offer the best optical result. While asphericity probably does not offer any advantage until the lens power is +8.00 D or higher, high plus lens with aspheric surfaces are available in lower powers. The ideal high plus lens has the following characteristics: minimum center thickness, minimum edge thickness, an aspheric front surface, and a relatively flat curve on the posterior surface. Minimum center thickness reduces spectacle magnification and gives a better cosmetic appearance since the patient's eyes appear less magnified to observers. Minimum edge thickness prevents an unsightly thick edge. The aspheric front surface reduces optical aberrations in the higher powers. The flat posterior surface keeps the front surface flatter and, again, reduces the amount of spectacle magnification. The edge thickness can be controlled to some extent by keeping decentration to a minimum, which in turn is accomplished by selecting a frame with the bridge size and eyewire size such that the geometrical center of the eyewire falls over the line of sight.

## High Minus Lenses

High minus lenses must be designed to minimize edge thickness. Edge thickness can be controlled by keeping the eye size to a minimum and by beveling the edge to remove excess material. A flat front surface curve keeps the posterior surface curve to a minimum; in fact, for lenses above $-10.00$ D, it is desirable to order a biconcave lens. Lens reflections are particularly bothersome with minus lenses. An antireflective coating and edge coating may reduce these reflections substantially. For patients who are particularly concerned about cosmesis, a light mirror coating on the front surface can mask some of the more noticeable effects. If the weight is a considerably greater concern than the optical quality, a Fresnel membrane can be used on a base lens to provide a portion of the total power.

High plus and high minus lenses can both be obtained in full-diameter and lenticular forms. The lenticular forms are less desirable from a cosmetic standpoint but offer the advantage of lighter weight. High index glass and plastic should be used to reduce thickness and weight.

## DISPENSING AND FOLLOW-UP

Patients should be rescheduled for follow-up to ensure that the devices prescribed are actually being used. If they are not being used effectively, then either additional training is indicated or perhaps an alternate device must be prescribed.

The environment in which the device will be used should be altered when necessary to enhance performance. For near devices of any type, proper lighting is always a consideration for achieving optimum use. Increased illumination may be provided through the use of illuminated magnifiers and/or auxiliary lamps. When lamps are used, some attention should be given to the bulb type and the wavelengths emitted in order to reduce glare and heat. Incandescent bulbs are bright but very hot. Fluorescent lamps have a discontinuous spectrum and increased UV emission but produce much less heat than tungsten bulbs. The advantages of each can be combined by using the two simultaneously, with the tungsten bulb located farther away when possible to reduce heat. Some lamps are available that have both bulbs in the same housing for separate or simultaneous use. There are also some new bulbs available that emit a more natural spectrum and may provide better functional ability for reading. The Chromalux® bulb is one example (see Chapter 19). Reading stands, reading guides, and correct posture can all contribute to success and should be demonstrated for each patient. Finally, the patient must know how to care for each of the devices. An expensive investment can be ruined on the first day by careless handling or by cleaning with inappropriate materials (see Chapter 30 for some of the author's experiences in this regard).

A written copy of the patient's prescription may be provided just as is done with glasses or medications. This adds to the patient's sense that optical devices are prescription items and thus enhances their therapeutic value.

## SUMMARY

Low vision devices should be prescribed in a systematic manner. The practitioner must understand how each device works and be able to determine an expected result when it is demonstrated to the patient. If the patient does not achieve the predicted result, then some data are inconsistent, the source of which can be uncovered. This approach allows the practitioner to select the most appropriate device(s) to demonstrate and prescribe.

The prescription of specific optical devices is considered in more detail in the following chapters. The general guidelines presented here are intended to serve as an introduction; hopefully, they will assist the reader in avoiding some of the mishaps involved in learning these lessons the hard way. Some of the author's experiences in prescribing optical devices (learned the hard way) are presented in Chapter 30.

## ADDITIONAL READING

*Protocols for choosing low vision devices—Consensus statement.* National Institute on Disability and Rehabilitation Research, 1(4), 1993.

Innes A: Prescribing spectacles for low vision patients, in Rosenthal BP, Cole RG (eds): A structured approach to low vision care. *Problems in Optometry* 3(3):462–483, 1991.

# CHAPTER XII

# HOW TO PRESCRIBE TELESCOPES

*The basic optical principles of telescopes were described in Chapter 10. Telescopes are prescribed for viewing distant objects. A distant object, by strict optical definition, is one that is located at optical infinity. From a practical point of view, 20 feet approximates optical infinity, and most telescopes have a sufficient range of focus to be used at least as near as 10 feet. When closer viewing is required, the patient must accommodate substantially, or the telescope must be modified in focusing ability by extending the range or adding an auxiliary lens referred to as a cap. Telescopes modified for near are called telemicroscopes. The diagnostic evaluation and prescription of telemicroscopes is the subject of Chapter 15. This chapter presents a procedure for prescribing telescopes that should not be considered the only approach but rather one that can be tried and modified by the individual clinician.*

## A DIAGNOSTIC SEQUENCE FOR PRESCRIBING TELESCOPES

There are many considerations in the determination of the final prescription of a telescope including cost, cosmesis, weight, frequency of use, purpose of use, age, physical abilities, and potential for binocularity. The basic choices are those that can be hand-held, spectacle-mounted, or clipped onto glasses temporarily. Hand-held telescopes are prescribed for occasional use such as spotting signs. More prolonged and/or frequent use requires a spectacle-mounted telescope. In general, hand-held telescopes are the least expensive option. Before considering the much more expensive option of a custom-designed spectacle-mounted device, it is a good idea to prescribe a hand-held or clip-on telescope first in order to make sure that the patient will utilize such a device. Any of these telescope types may be prescribed as a monocular or binocular system; however, most telescopes, and most low vision devices for that matter, are prescribed for monocular use with the better eye. Coincidentally, this is also the least expensive, lightest, and possibly least conspicuous option. These and other considerations are discussed below.

The diagnostic test sequence for prescribing telescopes must provide a systematic approach to determining the proper prescription for the patient. The following sequence provides such an approach:

- Determine the best distance correction
- Measure the best corrected acuity
- Determine the goal acuity
- Calculate the magnification needed
- Demonstrate the appropriate telescope magnification to the patient
- Explain the available options
- (Loan a device for home trial)
- Design the final prescription

The step of loaning a device is placed in parentheses since it has both advantages and disadvantages that make this an optional step that may be used for some patients but not for others. This is discussed in greater detail below.

## Determining the Appropriate Magnification

Determination of the goal acuity and calculation of the required magnification were discussed in the sections on magnification and optical principles of telescopes, but a few additional examples are given below. When someone seemingly could benefit from a telescope for general spotting but has no clear goal, it is reasonable to prescribe the power that would allow him or her to read the equivalent of approximately 20/50. The practical limits within which telescopes are prescribed are 2.0X to 8.0X in order to have enough magnification to be useful but not so much that the field of view is extremely limited or that it is not possible to maintain a steady image. Because telescopes are limited in the availability of powers, the exact power required often is not available, so the closest alternative must be selected. As a rule, it is best to prescribe the lowest power that will be adequate. This gives the patient the best field of view and the least noticeable effect on the image from small movements induced by hand tremors or movements.

■ **Example 12–1.** A patient wants a telescope that will give her the equivalent of 20/20 acuity. If her best corrected distance acuity is 10/80, what telescope would be expected to allow her to achieve that goal?

First, the acuities are converted to have the same reference distance (10/80 = 20/160). In order to go from 160 to 20 the patient needs 8X magnification (160/20 = 8). Therefore, an 8.0X telescope should allow this patient to achieve her goal.

■ **Example 12–2.** A patient desires a hand-held telescope for general daily activities such as spotting street signs and bus numbers. If her best corrected distance acuity is 20/200, what telescope would meet her needs?

A reasonable goal to strive for, when a specific need is not determined, is the equivalent of 20/50. Therefore, the patient needs a 4.0X telescope (200/50 = 4.0X).

■ **Example 12–3.** A patient desires to read an instrument dial 15 feet from his work station. The numerals on the dial are 44 mm tall. What telescope would allow him to achieve that goal if his best corrected distance acuity is 10/100?

A 20-foot letter is 8.7 mm tall; therefore, the numerals are approximately equivalent to a 100-foot letter (44/8.7 is approximately 5, and 5 × 20 = 100). Since this patient must read the equivalent of 15/100, the acuities are converted to have the same reference distance (10/100 = 20/200, and 15/100 ≈ 20/130). In order to go from 20/200 to 20/130 he needs about 1.5X. A 1.5X telescope should work, but most telescopes are stronger. The next closest available power, which is probably 2.0X or 2.5X, should be tried.

## Demonstration to the Patient

The ideal situation is to have exactly the desired telescope available for demonstration, but this is unrealistic unless an extensive diagnostic inventory is maintained. The next best choice is to have a reasonable diagnostic set and to prescribe, for the most part, only those telescopes. This avoids the problem of showing the patient one thing and ordering another. If the patient requires a relatively strong telescope, it is wise to demonstrate a lower power first since the larger field of view makes it easier to use. Larger targets should be used in conjunction with the lower powers. As patients become more comfortable using the device, stronger powers can be demonstrated. If the telescope is focusable, the practitioner can focus it for the test distance as long as patients use their distance correction with the telescope. If patients use the telescope without their glasses, then they must focus the telescope themselves to compensate for the spherical component of the uncorrected refractive error. As a general rule, the user gets a larger field of view without his or her glasses in place because the telescope can be held closer to the eye and the exit pupil of the device can therefore be located closer to the entrance pupil of the eye.

## Explaining the Available Options

Once the power has been determined and demonstrated satisfactorily to the patient, it is necessary to decide which telescope, from the available options, is prescribed and in what form it is dispensed to the patient. The age of the patient is certainly an important consideration when deciding which of the various options is most appropriate. Children may have trouble treating optical devices with the care necessary to keep them in good functioning order, so it is wise to provide them with devices that are less expensive and consequently more easily replaced when broken or lost. Spectacle-mounted devices may be hard to keep in adjustment when subjected to the strenuous physical activities of youngsters. Older patients, on the other hand, might prefer a spectacle-mounted device because of difficulty in holding a telescope steady; however, the weight is a concern if the frame causes excessive pressure on the thin skin of the bridge of the nose. This can be partially alleviated with larger nose pads and/or soft covers for the nose pad.

When it is clear that a child will benefit from distance magnification later in life, it is a good idea to start him or her with a telescope at a young age even though the benefits seem minimal at that time. The child will learn to use magnification and to adapt to the limitations of optical devices that will be prescribed later. This should make the transition easier when or if it becomes necessary to use a telescope for daily function.

### *Hand-held Versus Spectacle-mounted.*

Telescopes may be hand-held or spectacle-mounted. If the primary use is for occasional spotting, the hand-held device is preferred; for example, if the telescope is to be used only to spot bus numbers in order to commute to and from work, a hand-held device would suffice. It is conveniently carried in a pocket or a purse and removed when needed. Some telescopes come with a cord and can be worn around the neck for easy access. When the patient uses the telescope for extended periods of viewing, it is more convenient to have the telescope mounted in spectacles. Other considerations are weight, cosmesis, whether both hands must be free during use, and whether or not the telescope can be held steady enough by hand. A student might use the telescope for viewing the blackboard during school and prefer to have both hands free for writing or page turning. This would require a spectacle-mounted device.

### *Monocular Versus Binocular.*

If the patient has one eye that is significantly better than the other, a monocular device for the better eye is indicated. Monocular devices are also preferred if the telescope is to be hand-held so it is more convenient to carry, but hand-held binoculars are certainly another option and may actually be easier to manipulate. If the two eyes are relatively similar in ability, and if there is binocular potential, it is reasonable to consider prescribing two telescopes for simultaneous use. The patient might have some preference in this regard. As with microscopes, it is possible to prescribe two devices for *biocular* use if both eyes have similar ability but no binocular potential. The disadvantages associated with prescribing two telescopes are the increased weight and cost. Cosmesis is probably less of a concern since two telescopes are not a lot more conspicuous than one.

*Cost.* There is a reasonably large number of good quality, relatively inexpensive telescopes that can be mounted in spectacles or hand-held, so cost need not be a major factor in the prescription. If cost is of concern to the patient, a hand-held device avoids the cost of spectacles to support it, and, of course, one is cheaper than two of the same thing.

## Loaning a Device for Home Trial

Prior to determining the final prescription, a telescope may be loaned for a period of time in order to allow the patient to determine if it really will be useful. While this has certain advantages, there are also certain disadvantages; for example, the clinician must maintain an inventory of devices for loaning, which can be expensive, especially when some are lost or damaged. Financial loss can be circumvented, to some extent, by asking the patient to make a deposit on a loaned device. If this is done, there must be a clear understanding of what the deposit covers and under what circumstances it might not be returned.

Since it is not possible to maintain an inventory of every possible device, patients must often borrow something different from what would be prescribed for them. This negates an important aspect in their decision whether or not the device is something they want to own. Another important consideration is whether or not a home trial will actually be accomplished in an effective manner. If patients are unable to use the device correctly, no amount of home trial is going to allow them to decide whether or not it could be useful to them. No device should be loaned for use away from the office until the borrower demonstrates that he or she can use it effectively or until the clinician can arrange for someone to provide training in the home setting.

Each clinician must temper his or her willingness to allow patients a home trial with the disadvantages mentioned above. Loaning certainly has some significant advantages when the exact device to be prescribed can be loaned or when the patient can make a rational choice based on experience with a similar, but different, device. For the latter example, it is a good idea to loan a trial device before a patient is asked to purchase an expensive custom-designed spectacle-mounted system. Even though the trial device may be quite different from the prescribed device, the patient can decide about the potential usefulness.

## Design of the Final Telescope Prescription

Spectacle-mounted telescope systems must be carefully designed in order to work successfully. There are also several alternative telescope options that require special design considerations, and these are discussed in subsequent sections and in Chapter 17.

***Hand-held Telescopes.*** Hand-held telescopes are relatively easy to prescribe once the final power is determined. The main design criterion is the telescope type and optical quality. The selection of type is a trade-off between the improved field of view with the Keplerian and the more compact size of the equivalent Galilean. Also, telescopes of equivalent power are available in very different optical quality. Better optical quality is typically more costly and is not always appreciated by the patient with a significant visual impairment. When cost is a factor, it is appropriate to let the patient try the options in various settings and to offer a professional opinion, based on objective testing, about which telescope offers the best performance weighed against the other differences. Several hand-held telescopes are shown in Figure 12–1.

***Clip-on Telescopes.*** A number of hand-held telescopes can be converted to act as spectacle-mounted devices by inserting them into a clip that can be fastened temporarily to a frame (Figure 12–2). The device can be removed at will, thus offering the advantage of flexibility. The disadvantages of this approach are that the spectacle lens eventually becomes scratched, the field of view may be limited since the telescope is farther away from the eye, and most of the devices are heavier than a permanently mounted device due, in part, to the weight of the clip. However, if intermittent spectacle-mounted use is the main

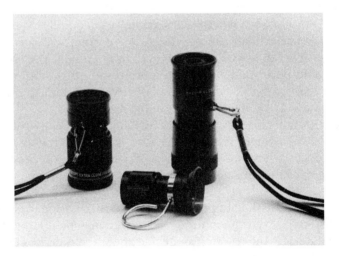

**Figure 12–1.** Hand-held telescopes are typically prescribed as monoculars. They may be worn around the neck with an attached cord as shown on the 4.0X (**left**) and 6.0X (**right**) models. The smaller telescope is 2.75X. The attached ring allows it to be held inconspicuously in the palm while secured around a finger.

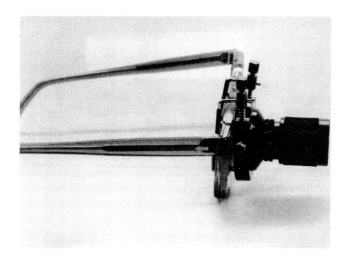

**Figure 12-2.** Many monoculars have an optional clip-on attachment that allows them to be fastened reversibly to spectacles. This is practical only for telescopes that are reasonably light, usually 4.0X or less. Two disadvantages are the smaller field of view caused by having the exit pupil further from the eye than if the telescope was used without spectacles, and the fact that the spectacle lens is likely to become scratched.

consideration, this option allows the same telescope to be used both as a hand-held device and as a spectacle-mounted device. This is less expensive than having two devices for alternate use.

***Spectacle-mounted Telescopes Fabricated by the Manufacturer.*** Telescopes can be permanently mounted in glasses (Figure 12-3) by some specialized optical companies or by the private practitioner. Spectacle-mounted telescopes are relatively expensive, so it is reasonable, prior to prescribing this option, to let the person try a hand-held telescope for a period of time to ascertain that a telescope will actually be of benefit to him or her.

Telescopes designed for mounting in spectacles are available in trial rings (Figure 12-4) that allow them to be demonstrated in the trial frame or in a clip attached to the patient's spectacles.

Some manufacturers prefer that a particular frame be used. If that frame is not used, or if the practitioner mounts the telescope personally, the frame selected should be sturdy with large adjustable nose pads and spring-loaded temples to keep the telescope properly positioned. If the device tends to slide down the patient's nose, a retaining strap just as athletes wear may be of help.

Spectacle-mounted telescopes must be placed precisely within the frame. Each unit is located horizontally at the patient's *monocular* pupillary distance. If the patient views eccentrically, the location must be altered to take this dif-

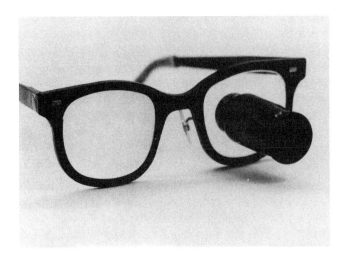

**Figure 12–3.** A telescope may be permanently mounted in spectacles. This one from Designs for Vision, Inc., is focusable and has the patient's prescription incorporated in the ocular of the telescope. It was mounted in the center of the frame for continuous use as opposed to the "bioptic" position (above the line of sight) for intermittent spotting.

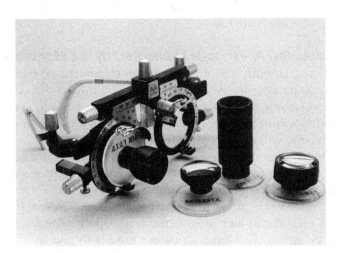

**Figure 12–4.** Telescopes that are intended to be permanently mounted in spectacles can be obtained in trial rings for demonstration. These telescopes, from Designs for Vision, Inc., are a 4.0X (in the trial frame) and (from left to right) a 2.2X Bioptic Model I, a 3.0X Expanded Field Spiral, and a 2.2X F.D.T.S. (full-diameter telescope).

ference into account. The vertical placement depends on the manner in which it is to be used. For continuous use, the telescope is centered before the line of sight. For spotting, the telescope must be above the line of sight such that it does not interfere with the patient's straight-ahead gaze and such that the telescope can be used with as small a head tilt as possible to allow rapid spotting. The best way to determine telescope placement is to have the *exact* frame that the patient will use and adjust it for proper fit prior to making the measurements. The measurements should be repeated and specified exactly, preferably with a drawing, for the laboratory.

If the telescope is placed above the line of sight, it must be angled slightly upward so that it will be aligned straight ahead when the patient tilts the head to view through it. A company that manufactures such devices will determine the angle but will also provide custom angles at the practitioner's request. The maximum placement above the line of sight is limited by the edge of the lens, and, as a general rule, the upper edge of the telescope housing must be ≈3 or more millimeters from the lens edge to prevent cracking. Given that restraint, the maximum superior placement of the unit from the top of the carrier lens is equal to 3 mm plus one-half of the diameter of the telescope housing that surrounds the ocular (Figure 12–5). Since the patient lowers the chin in order to spot through the telescope, the unit must be angled up so it is horizontal when the head is tilted down (Figure 12–6). As a general rule,[1] for each one millimeter above the line of sight, the telescope must be angled up 2°. Note that the angle is relative to the spectacle plane, not a true vertical line, since there is customarily some pantascopic tilt. The angle of inclination can be measured with a protractor and plumb line[2, 3] as illustrated in Figure 12–7. Telescopes (and telemicroscopes) that are designed to be mounted by the practitioner can

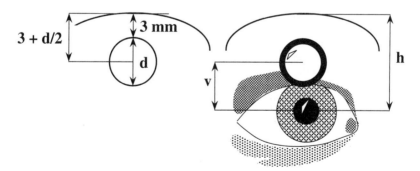

**Figure 12–5.** The maximum superior placement of a telescope from the top of a spectacle lens is equal to 3 mm plus one-half of the diameter (d) of the portion that is inserted in the lens. V is the maximum placement of the center of the telescope above the line of sight and is calculated as follows: v = h − (3 + d/2), where h and d are expressed in millimeters.

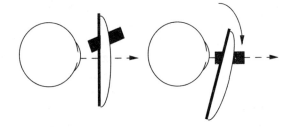

**Figure 12–6.** A telescope mounted in the "bioptic" position must be angled upwards in order to be aligned straight ahead when the head is tilted downward to view through the device.

be angled by the use of mounting rings that are thicker on one side than the other (see below). Custom-made spectacle-mounted telescopes manufactured by Designs for Vision, Inc., have standard angles for each telescope unless the practitioner specifies something different. If the practitioner uses the standard angle and it doesn't work for the patient, alterations are made very reasonably by the company.

When a binocular system is prescribed, it is not sufficient to measure the interpupillary separation and divide by two. Each unit must be placed horizontally at a position corresponding to the monocular pupillary distance. A pupilometer may work fine for measuring the monocular distance pupillary separations but often does not measure accurately for the near distances required for telemicroscopes. An alternative method for measuring the monocular pupillary distance is the Englemann technique, which is covered in Chapter 15.

**Figure 12–7. (A)** The angle of inclination for a spectacle-mounted telescope can be verified with a protractor and a plumb line. If the base of the protractor is aligned parallel to the lens with the telescope horizontal, angle ø will be equal to the angle of inclination as shown in B and C. **(B)** The vertical arrow represents the lens, and the angled arrow represents the telescope at an angle of inclination ø. **(C)** The lens is rotated ø° until the telescope is horizontal. The angle below, a vertical angle, must also be equal to ø. A line (p) parallel to the lens serves as the base of the protractor, and the vertical arrow pointing downward is the plumb line. The plumb line and line p form an angle that must also equal ø.

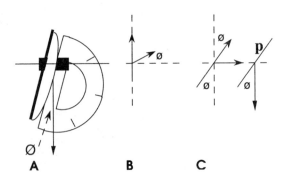

Designs for Vision, Inc. (DVI), the company founded by Dr. William Fein-bloom, has developed a number of spectacle-mounted telescopes that they have called bioptic telescopes. This name has come into general use now, similar to Kleenex and Xerox, and it is not unusual to see references to placing any telescope in the "bioptic" position, meaning above the line of sight. There are also full-diameter telescopes that are so named because they occupy virtually the full diameter of the spectacle lens. These are meant to be used constantly, as opposed to the bioptic type, which can be used alternately with the conventional spectacle correction for distance. A permanently mounted telescope is usually inserted through a hole drilled in the spectacle lens. This means that the distance correction is lost and must therefore be incorporated in the ocular of the telescope. This accounts for some of the increased expense. If the spectacle correction does not enhance vision through the telescope, it can be omitted from the system.

There has been a recent increase in the number of very small spectacle-mounted telescopes.[4, 5, 6, 7] Most of these take additional advantage of a special mounting technique in which the telescopes are mounted entirely or partially behind the spectacle lens to make them less conspicuous and hence more cosmetically acceptable. The fact that they pose some increased threat to the patient's eye in the event of trauma causes concern about the liability involved with their use. It is recommended that patients sign a waiver or statement of intended use that excludes sports or other vigorous activities, but the effectiveness of such waivers still awaits litigation. Selected examples of miniature telescopes are shown in Figures 12–8 and 12–9. It should be clear from the discussion of optical principles of telescopes in Chapter 10 that shorter telescopes will probably be Galilean in design since this type has a shorter separation of the two lenses than the equivalent Keplerian. This design, along with the small lens diameter, limits the field of view since the exit pupil for a Galilean telescope is located within the telescope. The clinician must be able to assist the patient in selecting a smaller system for cosmesis versus a larger one for the field of view. It is very helpful, and perhaps mandatory, to have examples for demonstration in the office.

***Spectacle-mounted Telescopes Fabricated by the Practitioner.*** Special double eyewire frames exist that have plano lenses in front with holes already in them. These are somewhat adjustable for the patient's pupillary separation and have the additional advantage that the lenses flip up so that the telescope(s) can be completely out of the line of sight while the patient views through the distance prescription. There are also plano lenses that have a predrilled slot for a telescope (Figure 12–10) or telemicroscope. The slot allows for horizontal adjustment to match the patient's monocular pupillary distance. These lenses can be placed in the Polysnap frame. Both lenses and frames are available from the New York Lighthouse (see Resources, Chapter 31).

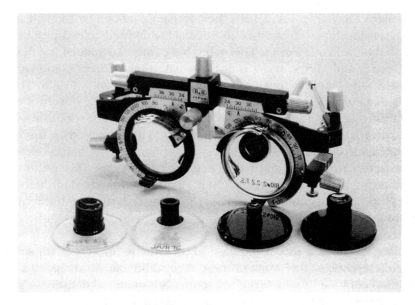

**Figure 12–8.** These telescopes, designed to be mounted permanently in spectacles, are very small and may be more cosmetically acceptable because they are less conspicuous. Three of these are from Designs for Vision, Inc.: Bioptic #2 2.2X Model II (trial frame), Eagle-eye 2.2X (left), and a 2.2X Micro Spiral (second from left). The remaining two, from Edwards Optical, are a 4.0X BITA 5/16″ (second from right) and a 3.0X BITA 1/2″ (right).

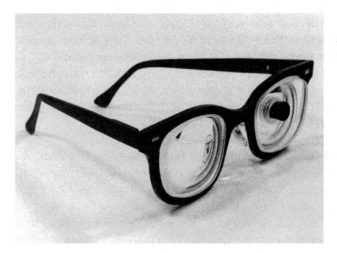

**Figure 12–9.** A 2.2X Micro Spiral Galilean focusable telescope (Designs for Vision, Inc.) is permanently mounted in a −11.50 D.S. carrier. The patient's spectacle prescription is also incorporated in the ocular of the telescope.

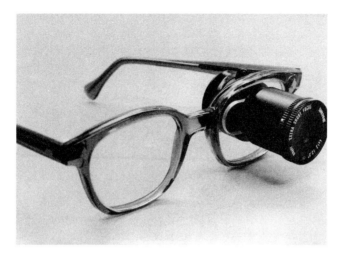

**Figure 12–10.** A monocular may be spectacle-mounted inexpensively using slotted lenses and a Polysnap frame available from the New York Light House. The slot allows the telescope(s) to be adjusted to the patient's monocular pupillary separation.

There are telescopes that can be hand-held or mounted by the practitioner in a manner similar to those discussed above by drilling a hole in the patient's spectacle lens to receive the telescope. Since the spectacle correction is literally drilled out, the telescope must be sufficiently focusable to correct the spherical refractive error. If a large astigmatic correction is required, a different approach, discussed below, must be taken.

A spectacle lens can be drilled with a drill press or even a hand-held drill using a "hole saw" of the appropriate diameter (Figure 12–11). The hole saw (the type of bit used to drill holes for mounting locks or door knobs) is the best drill bit in the author's experience. It does not require drilling a pilot hole first since the hole saw has a central pilot bit. Polycarbonate lenses should be used, and an rpm of about 500 works well for this material. This is a simple procedure and can be accomplished easily after practicing on two or three lenses.

The following procedure is suggested for mounting telescopes in the office:

1. Order the patient's glasses with polycarbonate lenses, and order two lenses for the side that will be drilled. (The astute reader will immediately see the value of doing this!)
2. Place the spectacles on the patient's face, and adjust them for a precise fit. Mark the location for the placement of the telescope with a felt-tip pen.

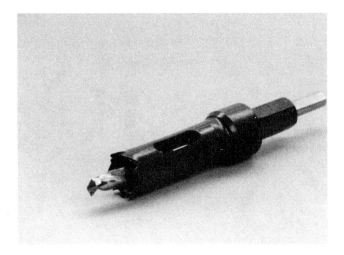

**Figure 12–11.** A hole saw works well for drilling polycarbonate lenses. A variety of diameters should be available in a good hardware store.

3. Remove the frame, and then replace it to make sure the mark remains in the same relative location with respect to the patient's eye. If not, check the frame adjustment.

4. The hole can be drilled from the front without removing the lens from the frame, and, in fact, it is much easier to hold steady if it remains in the frame. If there is concern about bending the frame, the lens can be removed for drilling. The temples will have to be removed in most cases. The lens can be protected from scratches by plastic debris if a thin transparent plastic film is pressed over it. It is at this point, when the hole is drilled, that the spare lens becomes most appreciated. It can avoid a lengthy delay if a second lens is required.

5. As the telescope is mounted, the angle can be adjusted by the use of spacers that are thicker on one side than on the other (Figure 12-12).

Keeler Optical makes telescopes that can be mounted by the practitioner without the necessity of drilling a hole in the lens. Their approach is to glue a plastic threaded ring onto the front surface of the spectacle lens and then screw the telescope into the ring as shown in Figure 12-13. This allows the system to have the patient's best correction preserved in the spectacle lens, which is particularly advantageous for those with significant astigmatism. The threaded mounting ring is attached to the spectacle lens with a cyanoacrylate glue. Since

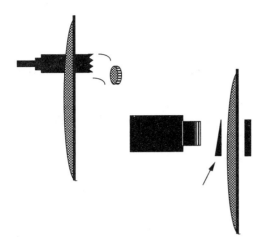

**Figure 12–12.** Some telescopes that can be mounted in polycarbonate lenses have spacer rings available that are thicker on one side than the other. The use of one or more of these rings allows the telescope to be angled or may simply serve to make the fit approximately flush with the curved surface of the lens. The telescope is secured in place by a threaded ring on the posterior side of the lens.

rings are available that are higher on one side, the telescope can be angled if desired. It takes some practice to glue the ring to the lens without making a mess. Cyanoacrylate glue is an excellent lubricant until it dries, and it is easy to smear glue across the surface of the lens when pressing the ring into place. The same procedure as outlined for drilling lenses should be followed, except that no hole is required. After step three, the dot is transferred to the back surface of the lens with a felt-tip pen, and the front surface is cleaned. The ring is glued in place and allowed to dry. If a different power is required at a later time, it is a simple matter to unscrew one and insert another.

***Complex Telescope Combinations.*** A spectacle-mounted telescope, mounted by the practitioner or a manufacturer, can be combined with a bifocal

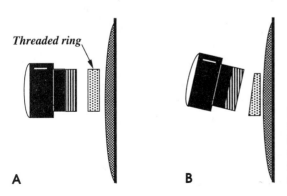

*Threaded ring*

A                    B

**Figure 12–13. (A)** Keeler Optical uses a threaded ring that is glued to the spectacle lens. **(B)** Rings are available that are taller on one side. This allows the device to be angled in any desired direction.

or trifocal to give the patient several viewing options. This combination is referred to as a "trioptic," again borrowing DVI's term. The combination of a telescope with a bifocal or bifocal-type microscope limits the portion of the spectacle lens available for the distance correction but is still an option that many patients find satisfactory.

It is also possible to have two different telescopes, one before each eye, for alternate use and to have a telemicroscope mounted in the bottom of the lens. Almost any combination of lenses can be fabricated if time and money are not an issue.

***Other Telescope Options.***  The Ocutech Vision Enhancing System[8, 9, 10, 11] is a spectacle-mounted Keplerian telescope developed as the "horizontal lightpath" telescope. It is a monocular system that is mounted transversely on the top of a frame. This clever design allows for the longer optical path length required by a Keplerian design without having the telescope protrude in front of the patient's spectacles (Figures 12–14 and 12–15). It is currently available in magnifications of 3.0X, 4.0X, and 6.0X. It has an adjustable horizontal position for centering before the patient's eye and an adjustable angle of inclination, and can be focused for near work distances. The telescope can be reversed by the practitioner, left to right, for use by either eye. The frame to which the telescope is attached is essentially a half-eye frame in terms of style and shape. The patient's distance and/or near prescription is placed in the frame. The telescope is suffi-

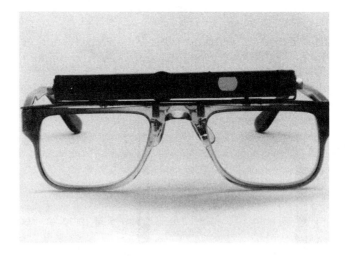

**Figure 12–14.** The Ocutech Vision Enhancing System is a Keplerian telescope mounted horizontally across the eyewire. Light is deflected in a manner similar to a periscope (Figure 12–15), which allows the system to be used in the horizontal position.

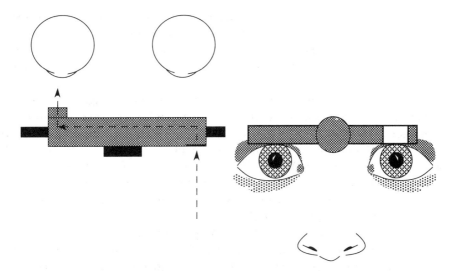

**Figure 12–15.** The objective of the Ocutech Vision Enhancing System is in front of the left eye, as illustrated here, and the ocular is in front of the right eye. The telescope can be reversed, right for left, by the clinician to allow the patient to view with the preferred eye.

ciently focusable to adjust for most patients' spherical refractive error and to be used for near viewing distances.

Aphakia has become less common with the success of intraocular lens implants; however, when a person who is aphakic and visually impaired is encountered, there is a unique possibility for creating a telescopic system.[12] If the patient removes his or her glasses, the uncorrected eye acts as a negative lens, of about −12.50 D on the average, and can become the ocular of a Galilean telescope. The person holds a low plus lens at the appropriate distance from the eye, and the system is completed. For example, with an eye that requires a +12.50 correction, if the correction is removed and a +5.00 hand-held lens located about 12 cm from the eye, a 2.5X system is created ($-(-12.5)/5 = 2.5$X). Compared to other Galilean systems, this system has the advantage of having the exit pupil much closer to the entrance pupil of the eye and hence a greater field of view. Although rarely encountered, high hyperopia, not secondary to aphakia, is amenable to the same approach.

It is possible to create a Galilean system using a contact lens as the ocular and a spectacle lens as the objective. While some clinicians have claimed great success with such a system, it has not been widely utilized. When first attempting to design such a system, the clinician quickly realizes that, unless the patient is Pinocchio, both the spectacle lens and the contact lens have to be rather high in power to achieve a reasonable vertex distance. The high minus contact lens (−30 to −50 D) required is often difficult to obtain as a soft lens or is too uncomfortable as a hard lens due to edge thickness. Nevertheless, it is possible to prescribe such a system. It requires a spectacle frame with extendible nose pads to achieve the longer than usual vertex distance. This system is described in greater detail in the chapter entitled Contact Lenses in Vision Rehabilitation (Chapter 17).

Intraocular lens (IOL) telescope systems have been designed for patients who have both cataracts and macular disease and who are potential candidates for cataract extraction.[13, 14, 15, 16] The system creates a Galilean telescope consisting of a high minus IOL and a high plus spectacle lens. It is therefore similar to a contact lens telescope but should provide a better field of view since the exit pupil is closer to the entrance pupil of the eye. One style of IOL designed to serve as the ocular of a telescope has a small diameter high minus "myodisc" in the central zone of approximately −60.00 D.[15] The carrier portion serves as the distance correction (Figure 12-16). A spectacle lens of up to +20.00 D is used, and therefore the magnification is equal to 3.0X or more. Higher magnification requires a lower power spectacle lens and greater vertex distance.

There are several inherent problems in this system. The spectacle lens is very difficult to fit since the positioning must be exact. There is currently no satisfactory frame that allows adjustment of the vertex distance. The position of the IOL is also critical since the central portion must be centered precisely within the pupil. Four iridotomies may be located at the 3, 6, 9, and 12 o'clock positions around the pupil border to limit pupil constriction. The magnification is limited by virtue of the high spectacle lens power needed. The ideal candidate would therefore have relatively mild macular disease that was stable. Lower power spectacle lenses will create greater magnification but require such long vertex distances that they are not practical. The system reportedly has poorer contrast than standard telescopes and has not worked well for reading. Because the central zone is small, this IOL seems to function as well as a conventional IOL if the telescope system is abandoned.

Another clever spectacle-mounted design was the Behind-the-Lens telescope.[7] This design had the body of the telescope mounted behind the spectacle lens but off-center. It incorporated a bent design similar to a periscope in

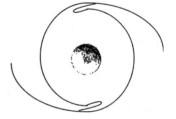

**Figure 12-16.** The high minus center portion of the IOL serves as the ocular for a Galilean telescope, while the carrier portion corrects the distance ametropia.[15]

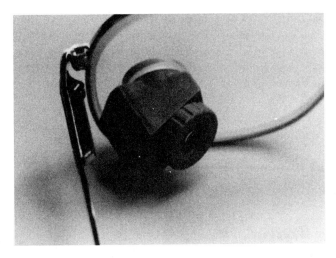

**Figure 12–17.** The Behind-the-Lens telescope was designed with a bent light path to allow the telescope to be placed off-center yet allow the user to view straight ahead. The major portion of the body is behind the spectacle lens, which make the device less conspicuous, especially if clip-on tinted sun lenses are worn in front of the spectacles.

order to have it off-center yet allow the user to view straight ahead (Figure 12-17). The user viewed straight ahead by rotating the eye to view through the telescope. At the time of writing, the company was no longer manufacturing this telescope, but a number were prescribed and may still be encountered by the low vision practitioner.

Autofocusing telescopes have future potential if effective and affordable designs can be developed.[17] Several investigators have reported on prototypes.[18] Autofocusing is advantageous for those with impaired vision who may have difficulty judging the best focus and for those with physical limitations that make focusing difficult.

## AVOIDING FALSE EXPECTATIONS

The various options must be carefully and completely explained to the patient. Some patients expect a spectacle-mounted telescope to look just like ordinary glasses when it is finally dispensed, even after a careful explanation. For this reason it is very helpful to have, and show, an example of the device as it will appear in its final form, emphasizing to the patient, *"Your glasses will look just like these."* This should be done several times to make sure there is no misunderstanding. It should also be emphasized that the vision through the dispensed device will be just the same as it was through the demonstrated device. It is natural for patients to want restoration of the vision that they enjoyed previously, and it is natural for them to think that the new "glasses" will give them clear vision just as new prescriptions did in the past. Careful presentation of the treatment plan avoids the disappointment associated with false expectations.

Prior to ordering an expensive custom-designed spectacle-mounted telescope, patients should be clearly informed that this device cannot be returned because it is designed specifically for them and is of no use to anyone else. This helps to ensure that they will make a commitment to successful use and that the clinician does not develop a large inventory of "demonstrators."

## ADAPTATION TO TELESCOPES

It is not safe to assume that a patient will adapt to telescope use even though he or she can demonstrate satisfactory manipulation of the device with respect to focusing, target location, and other user skills. Demer et al.[19] found that about 20% of normal subjects wearing telescopic spectacles initially had symptoms of oscillopsia and motion discomfort. They measured the vestibulo-ocular reflex (VOR), a mechanism for producing rapid compensatory eye movements during head movements, to investigate adaptation in normal subjects of this reflex to spectacle magnifiers. They found considerable interindividual variability in adaptation to telescopic spectacles, unrelated to spectacle power, as measured by VOR gain adaptation. Adaptation was associated with amelioration of symptoms of oscillopsia and motion discomfort.

Adaptation also requires acceptance of the physical constraints such as inconvenience of use, weight, difficulty in locating objects, difficulty in focusing, and cosmesis. Each of these might become more significant after a more lengthy trial than was experienced during early practice with a loaned device. The most effective means of ensuring adaptation for those who experience difficulty is to provide a comprehensive training program[20, 21] similar to those used for learning to drive with bioptic telescopes (Chapters 22 and 23).

## DISPENSING AND FOLLOW-UP

Patients should never be allowed to take home any device until they have learned to use it correctly. To do otherwise almost guarantees failure. This is not to imply that use must be mastered in the office but rather that the patient should at least be able to demonstrate proper technique in order to practice successfully at home. The proper care and handling should be demonstrated at dispensing, and a follow-up appointment should be made for two weeks later to assess progress and reinforce proper use. If a follow-up appointment is not made automatically, the patient is likely to call at the first hint of unsuccessful use and not give the device an adequate trial.

A spectacle-mounted telescope requires careful attention to frame adjustment in order to have the most comfortable fit. These devices are notably heavier than glasses and require large nose pads adjusted to spread the weight evenly over as large an area as possible. Vertex distance has a significant effect on the field of view and, in general, should be as short as possible.

## SUMMARY

There are many options for patients who might benefit from a telescope. Because of their variety and complexity, professional guidance is important. Patients should not choose designs on their own, but rather the telescope should be prescribed for them. For the clinician who is just beginning to provide low vision services, it is reasonable to start with hand-held telescopes and add other designs as confidence is gained. The prescription of spectacle-mounted telescopes may seem intimidating at first but should not be. They can be incorporated into one's clinical armamentarium systematically by first working with predrilled lenses, followed by drilling lenses in the office, and then by ordering custom designs from manufacturers.

## REFERENCES

1. Bailey IL: A scientific angle on bioptic telescopes. *Optom Monthly* 70:131–138, 1979.
2. Bailey IL: Determining the angle for bioptic telescopes. *J Vis Rehab* 2(2):5–19, 1988.
3. Freed B: A method for measurement of the vertical drilling angle of headborne telescopes. *J Vis Rehab* 3(2):4–5, 1985.
4. Harkins T, Maino JH: The BITA telescope: A first impression. *J Amer Optom Assoc* 62(1):28–31, 1991.
5. Williams DR: The bi-level telemicroscopic apparatus—(BITA), in Rosenthal BP, Cole RG (eds): A structured approach to low vision care. *Problems in Optometry* 3(3):495–503, 1991.
6. Hoeft WW: The microspiral Galilean telescope, in Rosenthal BP, Cole RG (eds): A Structured approach to low vision care. *Problems in Optometry* 3(3):490–494, 1991.
7. Spitzberg LA, Jose RT, Kuether CL: Behind the lens telescope: A new concept in bioptics. *Optom Vis Sci* 66(9):616–620, 1989.
8. Siwoff R: Patient preference between new cosmetically appealing spectacle telescope systems. *J Vis Rehab* 4(3):7–14, 1990.

9. Greene HA, Pekar J, Brilliant R, Freeman PB, Lewis HT, Siwoff R, Paton C, Madden DJ, Westlund R: The Ocutech Vision Enhancing System (VES): Utilization and preference study. *J Amer Optom Assoc* 62(1):19-26, 1991.

10. Greene HA, Pekar J, Brilliant R, Freeman PB, Lewis HT, Siwoff R, Madden DJ, Westlund RE: Use of spectacle mounted telescope systems by the visually impaired. *J Amer Optom Assoc* 64(7):507-513, 1993.

11. Greene HA: The Ocutech Vision Enhancing System (VES): A new low vision spectacle telescope system, in Rosenthal BP, Cole RG (eds): A structured approach to low vision care. *Problems in Optometry* 3(3):484-489, 1991.

12. Nowakowski RW, Pierce S: A simple Galilean telescope system for an aphakic patient with retinochoroidal coloboma. *So J Optom* 6:27-29, 1988.

13. Donn A, Koester CJ: An ocular telephoto system designed to improve vision in macular disease. *CLAO* 12:81-85, 1986.

14. Bailey IL: Critical view of an ocular telephoto system. *CLAO* 13:217-221, 1987.

15. Peyman GA, Koziol J: Age related macular degeneration and its management. *J Cataract Refract Surg* 14:421-430, 1988.

16. Jacobi KW, Nowak MR, Strobel J: Special intra-ocular lenses. *Fortschritte Der Ophthalmologie* 87 Suppl:S29-32, 1990.

17. Greene HA, Beadles R, Pekar J: Challenges in applying autofocus technology to low vision telescopes. *Optom Vis Sci* 69(1):25-31, 1992.

18. Kuyk T, James J: A pilot study of a telescopic low vision aid with motorized focus. *J Vis Rehab* 4(4):21-29, 1990.

19. Demer JL, Porter FI, Goldberg J, Jenkins HA, Schmidt K: Adaptation to telescopic spectacles: Vestibulo-ocular reflex plasticity. *Invest Ophthalmol Vis Sci* 30(1): 159-170, 1989.

20. Walls MAK, Molenda MM: Training procedures for more cosmetically appealing miniaturized telescopes. *J Vis Rehab* 5(1):11-15, 1991.

21. Hoeft W: Bioptic telescopes: Training and adaptation. *Optom Monthly* Sept:71-74, 1980.

## ADDITIONAL READING

Abbot AN: A discussion of telescopic spectacles and their use. *Am J Optom* 51(5): 321-324, 1938.

Bailey IL: New expanded field bioptic systems. *Optom Monthly* 69:981-984, 1978.

Bailey IL: Telescopes—their use in low vision. *Optom Monthly* 69(9):143-147, 1978.

Biessels WJ: Binocular low vision telescopic spectacles. *J Am Optom Assoc* 44(12): 1239-1243, 1973.

Brady HR, Hecke D, Culliton P: Spectacle-mounted telescopic lenses for children. *Annals Ophthalmol* 15(3):286-289, 1983.

Bruner AB: Telescopic lenses as an aid to poor vision. *Am J Ophthalmol* 13(8):667-674, 1930.

Choyce DP: A Galilean telescope using an anterior-chamber implant as eyepiece. *Lancet* 1:794, 1960.

Demer JL, Porter FI, Goldberg J, Jenkins HA, Schmidt K, Ulrich I: Predictors of functional success in telescopic spectacle use by low vision patients. *Invest Ophthalmol Vis Sci* 30(7):1652–1665, 1989.

Demer JL, Goldberg J, Porter FI, Schmidt K: Validation of physiologic predictors of successful telescopic spectacle use in low vision. *Invest Ophthalmol Vis Sci* 32(10): 2826–2834, 1991. (Published erratum appears in *Invest Ophthalmol Vis Sci* 33(3): 691, 1992.)

Eggers M: An inexpensive telescopic spectacle. *Arch Ophthalmol* (Chicago) 10:515, 1933.

Faye EE: Guide to selecting reading spectacles, hand magnifiers, stand magnifiers, telescopes, electronic aids, and absorptive lenses, in Faye EE (ed): *Clinical Low Vision,* 2 ed. Boston, Little, Brown and Company, 1984.

Fonda G: Evaluation of telescopic spectacles (thirty-nine cases changed to simpler lenses). *Am J Ophthalmol* 51(3):433–441, 1961.

Fonda G, Fonda A: Distant magnification for low vision patients with aphakia. *Transac Am Acad Ophthalmol* 66:790–794, 1962.

Freedman B: A method for measurement of the vertical drilling angle of headborne telescopes. *J Vis Rehab* 3(2):4–5, 1985.

Friedenberg HL: Notes on the application of telescopic spectacles with reports of three cases. *Am J Optom* 26(1):3–8, 1949.

Friedman G: Distance low-vision aids for primary level school children. *New Outlook for the Blind* 70(9):376–379, 1976.

Gerstman DR, Levene JR: Galilean telescopic system for the partially sighted. New application of the Fresnel lens. *Brit J Ophthalmol* 58(8):766–769, 1974.

Gradle HS, Stein J: Telescopic spectacles and magnifiers as aids to poor vision. *Trans Am Acad Ophthalmol Otolaryngol* 77(3):229–253, 1973.

Gruber E: A modified telescopic aid for the low vision patient. *EENT Monthly* 54(12): 468–470, 1975.

Hoeft W: Bioptic telescopes: Training and adaptation. *Optom Monthly* Sept:71–74, 1980.

Hoff HJ: Application of telescopic and microscopic spectacles in subnormal vision. Part 1. *Opt J Rev Optom* 83(11):36, 1946.

Hoff HJ: Application of telescopic and microscopic spectacles in subnormal vision. Part 2. *Opt J Rev Optom* 83(12):41, 1946.

Hoff HJ: Application of telescopic and microscopic spectacles in subnormal vision. Part 3. *Opt J Rev Optom* 83(13):29, 1946.

Kelleher DK: A pilot study to determine the effect of the bioptic telescope on young low vision patients' attitude and achievement. *Am J Optom and Physiological Optics* 51(3):198–205, 1974.

Kestenbaum A: New kinds of application of telescopic systems. *Am J Ophthalmol* 53(3):443–444, 1962.

Lauber H: Telescopic spectacles. *Arch Ophthalmol* (Chicago) 89:401, 1915.

Levy AH: Telescopic spectacles. *Brit J Ophthalmol* 13:593, 1929.

Lewis H: Considerations of telescopic field of view in prescribing of low vision lenses. *Am J Optom Arch Am Acad Optom* 48(11):953–960, 1971.

Lloyd JH: Use of telescopic aids for vocational purposes. *J Vis Impair Blind* 78:216–220, 1984.

Marks R: Factors concerning the prescription and use of telescopic spectacles. *Am J Optom Arch Am Acad Optom* 25(6):262–274, 1948.

Mayer LL: Visual results with telescopic spectacles. *Am J Ophthalmol* 10:256–260, 1927.

Mayer LL: Further visual results with telescopic glasses. *Arch Ophthalmol* 2:315–321, 1929.

Newman JD: Telescopic systems, in Faye EE, Hood CM: *Low Vision.* Springfield, IL, Charles C. Thomas, 1975.

Pascal JI: Telescopic spectacles in ophthalmological practice. *Eye, Ear, Nose and Throat Monthly* 28:171, 1949.

Scott K: Telescopic eyeglasses. *Ophthalmol* 7:445, 1911.

Scott K: Telescopic spectacles. Ophthalmol 9:444, 1913.

Spitzberg LA, Jose RT, Kuether C: Behind the lens telescope: A new concept in bioptics. *Optom Vis Sci* 66(9):616–620, 1989.

Stoll KL: Telescopic spectacles: Their history, practicability and future. *Lancet-Clin* 108:120, 1912.

Waiss B, Cohen JM: Modification of common low vision devices for uncommon needs. *J Amer Optom Assoc* 62(1):65–68, 1991.

Walters GB: A bioptic telescope clip. *Rev Optom* 117:52–54, 1980.

Woo GC: An overview on the use of a low magnification telescope, in Woo GC (ed): *Low Vision: Principles and Applications.* New York, Springer-Verlag, 1987, pp 262–271.

# CHAPTER XIII

# HOW TO PRESCRIBE MICROSCOPES

*A microscope, when defined as a low vision device, is a high plus lens mounted in glasses. The main consideration for near is whether to prescribe a hand-held magnifier or a spectacle-mounted microscope. The major consideration in the choice between a microscope and a hand-held magnifier is the work distance. Other considerations are the weight of spectacles, cosmesis, whether both hands must be free during use, whether or not the hand-held magnifier can be held steady enough, and field of view. In general, a microscope has a larger field of view than a hand-held magnifier of equal equivalent power, since it is closer to the eye. (Field of view for hand magnifiers is discussed in Chapter 14.) Many patients prefer a spectacle-mounted lens over a hand-held or stand magnifier because it is a more natural ocular appliance and somewhat less likely to draw attention. However, when the power is so high that the short working distance is a major drawback, the hand-held devices become more appealing. Hand-held devices are considered in more detail in Chapter 14.*

## A DIAGNOSTIC SEQUENCE FOR PRESCRIBING MICROSCOPES

Microscopes are prescribed in a logical sequence, similar to telescopes. The recommended test sequence is as follows:

- Determine the best distance correction
- Measure the best corrected near acuity through the appropriate add
- Determine the goal acuity
- Calculate the magnification and equivalent power needed

- Demonstrate the appropriate microscope power to the patient
- Demonstrate the different forms in which it can be prescribed
- (Loan a device for home trial)
- Design the final prescription

## Determination of the Goal Acuity

The dioptric power of the microscope is determined by the goal to be achieved. When patients seemingly could benefit from a microscope for general reading but have no clear goal, it is reasonable to prescribe the power that allows them to read 1M continuous text smoothly. This is approximately the size of newspaper print and the print found in typical books. As a rule, it is best to prescribe the lowest power that is adequate yet still leaves some measure of reserve. This gives the patient the best field of view, the least noticeable peripheral distortions, and the longest work distance.

## Calculation of the Magnification and Equivalent Power Needed

The magnification needed is that which allows the patient to achieve his or her goal based on the reference acuity. Several examples were given in Chapter 10, and two more are given below. These examples assume that the patient holds the material near enough to the focal plane that the formula M = rF will apply.

■ **Example 13–1.** A 60-year-old male has a reference acuity of 0.4/3M through a +2.50 add over best distance correction. What microscope will allow him to read 1M print?

Magnification required = Reference size/Goal size
Magnification required = 3M/1M
Magnification required = 3X

The dioptric strength required is found by substitution into M = rF.

$$M = rF$$
$$3 = (0.4)F$$
$$3/0.4 = F$$
$$+7.5 \text{ D} = F$$

The patient in this example requires +7.50 D over the best distance correction and must hold the print at or near the focal point (13.33 cm) in order to achieve the desired goal.

■ **Example 13–2.** A 55-year-old woman has an example of print that she must be able to read on her job. The letters are 4.35 mm tall. Her reference acuity is

0.33/8M. What microscope will allow her to read her material assuming she has no usable accommodation?

A 1M letter is 1.45 mm tall; therefore, her material is equivalent to 3M print (4.35 mm/1.45 mm = 3). In order to read 3M print she needs 2.67X (8M/3M). The lens power that provides that magnification is found from M = rF, where M = 2.67 and r = 0.33 meters. Solving for F, she needs a +8.10 D lens, which will allow her to read her print if it is held at, or very near, the focal point of the lens. This assumes that her reference acuity was determined with a task of similar difficulty with respect to font, letter spacing, and contrast. A +8.00 lens serves as a starting point and is refined using her specific print sample. The final power should allow her to accomplish the goal with a measure of reserve; in other words, she should read with some ease as opposed to being just able to discern the print.

## Demonstrating Microscopes to the Patient

Most people initially reject a microscope because of the near work distance that a high plus lens necessitates. The examination chair makes a good place for the initial demonstration of near adds. The head rest can be placed firmly against the back of the person's head to prevent a retreating eye as the print is advanced toward the microscope. Once the patient is more accepting of the near work distance, adds can be demonstrated in more appropriate surroundings, such as at a reading table, where it is also possible to demonstrate reading stands and adjustable lamps similar to those that might be used in the home or work place.

Because of the initial resistance to high adds, it is usually best to demonstrate lower adds with larger print and work sequentially toward the calculated power by decreasing the print size until it can no longer be read with a given lens and then increasing the lens power. Lower power lenses are easier to use initially, and this sequential approach eases the patient in the direction of the calculated lens power.

The clinician should prove that the lens makes the difference in the patient's ability to read by having him or her hold the print that he or she just read, without moving it, while the trial frame or microscope is lifted. The clinician asks, "How does it look without the lens?" (*"Can't see it at all."*) Next, the frame is lowered again, and the patient is asked, "Now, how does it look?" (*"I can read it again."*) "So this lens makes a big difference, doesn't it?"

Examples of everyday reading tasks—for example, labels from cans of food, price tags of various types, utilities bills, and a newspaper—should be available in the office for demonstration. No device should be prescribed for a specific task until the patient has been allowed to try it for that task. If a patient has a particular task in mind that cannot be simulated adequately with what is available in the office, he or she can be asked to bring actual examples to the next appointment in order that each device may be demonstrated for its intended task.

If the patient has a central scotoma and does not view eccentrically with some degree of consistency, it is better to postpone further evaluation until after the provision of some training in techniques of eccentric viewing.

***Binocularity with Microscopes.*** A microscope requires a very close working distance since the material to be viewed must be held at the focal point of the lens. This limits the ability to use microscopes binocularly because of the extreme demand on convergence. The practical limit on binocular use of microscopes is approximately +10 diopters. It is easy to see why this is true. The total convergence demand (c), in prism diopters, depends on the patient's distance interpupillary separation (DPS), the focal length ($f$) of the add, and the distance (d) from the center of rotation of the eye to the spectacle plane (Figure 13–1). Since the object is held at the focal point of the lens, the total distance to the point of convergence is $f$ plus the distance from the center of rotation of the eye to the microscope lens. The total convergence demand is determined as follows,[1] where the DPS is given in centimeters and the distances are in meters:

$$c = DPS \times 1/(f+d)$$

The distance of the object from the lens is known ($f$), but the location of the center of rotation of the eye is not; therefore, an approximation of 0.027 meters is used for the distance (d) from the spectacle plane to the center of rotation of the eye. It can also be seen in Figure 13–1 that base-out prism is in-

**Figure 13–1.** The convergence demand in prism diopters for a near viewing distance depends on the distance pupillary separation (DPS), the distance (d) from the center of rotation of the eye to the spectacle plane, and focal length (f) of the add. The exact location of the center of rotation of the eye is not known; 0.027 meters is used as an approximation of its distance from the spectacle plane.

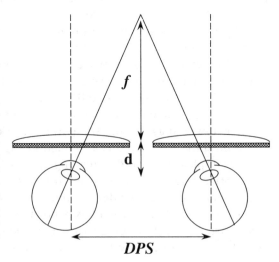

duced by a plus lens that has not been decentered for the near interpupillary separation. This adds to the overall convergence demand but has been ignored in the above formula, which specifies only the convergence demand with respect to the point of fixation.

■ **Example 13–3.** Determine the total demand on convergence for a patient using +10.00 O.U. who has a distance interpupillary separation of 62 mm (6.2 cm). (Ignore any prism induced by the lens itself.)

The lens has a focal length of 10 cm or 0.10 meters.

$$c = \text{DPS} \times 1/(f + 0.027)$$
$$c = 6.2 \times 1/(0.10 + 0.027)$$
$$c = 6.2 \times 1/0.127$$
$$c = 6.2 \times 7.87$$
$$c = 48.8^\Delta \ (24.4^\Delta \text{ base-in for each eye})$$

The above example shows why there is a practical limit of about +10.00 diopters for the binocular use of microscopes. The total convergence requirement induced by various adds for a patient with an interpupillary separation of 62 mm is shown in Table 13-1. The effect of various distance interpupillary separations on convergence demand for a given add is shown in Table 13-2.

Faye[2] has suggested that some special tests may indicate when a binocular system is preferred; for example, patients who have better contrast sensitivity under binocular conditions than under monocular conditions or who have a less noticeable central scotoma with the Amsler grid under binocular conditions than monocular conditions may benefit from a binocular system. Of course, this would only be a consideration when binocularity can actually be achieved physically.

**TABLE 13–1.** Total convergence demand (c) by high adds for a distance interpupillary separation (DPS) of 62 mm.

| DPS (mm) | Add | c* |
|---|---|---|
| 62 | 2.50 | 14.52$^\Delta$ |
| 62 | 3.00 | 17.21$^\Delta$ |
| 62 | 4.00 | 22.38$^\Delta$ |
| 62 | 5.00 | 27.31$^\Delta$ |
| 62 | 6.00 | 32.01$^\Delta$ |
| 62 | 7.00 | 36.50$^\Delta$ |
| 62 | 8.00 | 40.79$^\Delta$ |
| 62 | 9.00 | 44.89$^\Delta$ |
| 62 | 10.00 | 48.82$^\Delta$ |
| 62 | 11.00 | 52.58$^\Delta$ |
| 62 | 12.00 | 56.19$^\Delta$ |

*c = DPS × 1/(f + 0.027), where DPS is in cm and f is in meters

TABLE 13–2. Effect of increasing distance interpupillary separation (DPS) on total convergence demand for a given add of +8.00 D.

| DPS (mm) | Add | c* |
|---|---|---|
| 60 | 8.00 | 39.47△ |
| 61 | 8.00 | 40.13△ |
| 62 | 8.00 | 40.79△ |
| 63 | 8.00 | 41.45△ |
| 64 | 8.00 | 42.11△ |
| 65 | 8.00 | 42.76△ |
| 66 | 8.00 | 43.42△ |
| 67 | 8.00 | 44.08△ |
| 68 | 8.00 | 44.74△ |
| 69 | 8.00 | 45.39△ |
| 70 | 8.00 | 46.05△ |

*c = DPS × 1/(f + 0.027), where DPS is in cm and f is in meters

**Lens Decentration for Near.** If the optical center of the add is not decentered for near, the patient will receive base-out prism from the add, which increases the convergence demand. This may be compounded further by the distance correction if the patient is hyperopic or reduced if he is myopic. High plus adds may require considerable decentration to allow the optical center to be in alignment with the patient's line of sight when viewing at the focal point of the lens. This is an important optical consideration even if the patient is not binocular, since better optical quality is achieved when viewing through the optical center of the lens. The near pupillary separation (NPS) in the spectacle plane can be calculated, similar to the near convergence demand, based on the patient's distance pupillary separation (DPS) and the point of convergence when using the add to view material held at its focal point. If the distance from the center of rotation of the eye is considered to be 0.027 meters, and $f$ is the focal length of the add (assuming a thin lens), the near pupillary separation can be determined by similar triangles (Figure 13–2) as follows:

$$NPS/DPS = f/(f + d)$$
$$NPS = (DPS)(f/(f + d))$$

The decentration required for each lens individually, to be in line with the visual axis, can be approximated by subtracting the NPS from the DPS and dividing by two, or it can be calculated by using the patient's monocular DPS (MDPS) and calculating the lens decentration using similar triangles (Figure 13–2) in a manner similar to calculating the NPS:

$$Monocular\ lens\ decentration/MDPS = d/(f + d)$$
$$Monocular\ lens\ decentration = (MDPS)(d/(f + d))$$

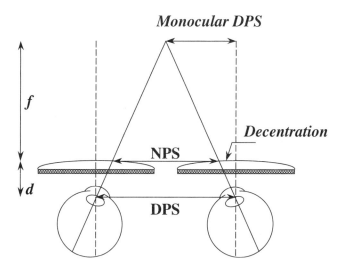

*Monocular DPS*

*Decentration*

NPS

DPS

*f*

*d*

**Figure 13–2.** The near pupillary separation (NPS) in the spectacle plane, when viewing at the focal point of an add, can be determined from the distance pupillary separation (DPS) and the focal length of the add (*f*) by similar triangles. The distance from the center of rotation of the eye to the spectacle plane (d) is estimated to be 0.027 meters. The lens decentration required to align the optical center of the add with the line of sight for the near viewing distance can also be determined by similar triangles from the monocular DPS, *f*, and d.

The calculated NPS and lens decentration for a series of adds used by patients with different distance pupillary separations are shown in Table 13-3 and Table 13-4 respectively. A rule of thumb proposed by Bailey is to decenter the near adds a total of 1.5 mm for each diopter of add and increase that value by one more millimeter if the DPS is more than 65 mm.[3]

It is easiest to use tables or rules of thumb when determining lens decentration, but, if desired, the values can be calculated directly as in Examples 13-4 and 13-5 below.

■ **Example 13–4.** For a patient whose distance pupillary separation (DPS) is 66 mm, calculate the near pupillary separation (NPS) when using a +10 add and reading print held at the focal point of the add.

$$\text{NPS} = (\text{DPS})(f/(f + \text{d}))$$
$$\text{NPS} = (66)(100/(100 + 27)$$
$$\text{NPS} = 51.96 \text{ mm}$$

The answer for this example from Table 13-3 is 52, the rounded value.

■ **Example 13–5.** For the patient in Example 13-4, determine the decentration required for each lens to place its optical center at the NPS. Assume that

**TABLE 13–3. Calculated near pupillary separation (NPS) (mm) in the spectacle plane, based on distance pupillary separation (DPS) and near add.**

| DPS (mm) | ADD | | | | |
|---|---|---|---|---|---|
| | +4 | +6 | +8 | +10 | +12 |
| 58 | 52.3 mm | 49.9 mm | 47.7 mm | 45.7 mm | 43.8 mm |
| 60 | 54.2 | 51.6 | 49.3 | 47.2 | 45.3 |
| 62 | 56.0 | 53.4 | 51.0 | 48.8 | 46.8 |
| 64 | 57.8 | 55.1 | 52.6 | 50.4 | 48.3 |
| 66 | 59.6 | 56.8 | 54.3 | 52.0 | 49.8 |
| 68 | 61.4 | 58.5 | 55.9 | 53.5 | 51.4 |

Example: A person with a distance pupillary separation of 64 mm would have a near pupillary separation of 52.6 mm, measured at the spectacle plane, when converging adequately to use a +8.00 add.

the monocular distance pupillary separation (MDPS) for each eye is exactly one-half of the total DPS.

$$\text{Monocular lens decentration} = (MDPS)(d/(f + \text{d}))$$
$$\text{Monocular lens decentration} = (33)(27/(100 + 27))$$
$$\text{Monocular lens decentration} = 7.02 \text{ mm}$$

If this value were obtained from Table 13-4, one would find 7.0 mm, which is rounded from 7.016.

The decentration can also be calculated using the alternative approach above:

$$\text{Monocular lens decentration} = (DPS - NPS)/2$$
$$\text{Monocular lens decentration} = (66 - 51.96)/2$$
$$\text{Monocular lens decentration} = 14.04/2$$
$$\text{Monocular lens decentration} = 7.02 \text{ mm}$$

**TABLE 13–4. Monocular decentration (mm) required for each add to align the optical center of the add with the calculated near pupillary separation based on distance pupillary separation (DPS) and near add strength.**

| DPS (mm) | ADD | | | | |
|---|---|---|---|---|---|
| | +4 | +6 | +8 | +10 | +12 |
| 58 | 2.8 mm | 4.0 mm | 5.2 mm | 6.2 mm | 7.1 mm |
| 60 | 2.9 | 4.2 | 5.3 | 6.4 | 7.3 |
| 62 | 3.0 | 4.3 | 5.5 | 6.6 | 7.6 |
| 64 | 3.1 | 4.5 | 5.7 | 6.8 | 7.8 |
| 66 | 3.2 | 4.6 | 5.9 | 7.0 | 8.1 |
| 68 | 3.3 | 4.7 | 6.0 | 7.2 | 8.3 |

Example: If the DPS was 64, a +8.00 add would have to be decentered 5.7 mm for each eye to place the optical center at the calculated near pupillary separation.

■ **Example 13–6.** For the patient in Example 13–4, determine the total lens decentration using the rule of thumb given above.

Total decentration = 10(1.5) + 1
Total decentration = 16 mm, or 8 mm per lens

The values determined in the examples above are for lens decentration to place the optical center of the add at the line of sight when viewing through the add. This eliminates base-out prism induced by the add but does not give the necessary base-in prism to achieve fusion. Decentration for base-in prism may be determined by Prentice's rule, which states that lens-induced prism is equal to the product of the lens power (F) in diopters and the distance (d) in centimeters from the optical center.

Prism = d(F)

■ **Example 13–7.** For Example 13–5, how much additional decentration would be required to achieve $5^\Delta$ base-in per lens?

Prism = d(F)
5 = d(10)
d = 5/10
d = 0.5 cm, or 5 mm

Therefore, each lens would have to be decentered nasally 12 mm (7 mm +5 mm) to achieve $5^\Delta$ base-in per lens, for a total of $10^\Delta$ base-in. The patient would have to provide $42^\Delta$ of additional convergence since the total calculated demand is $\approx 52^\Delta$ due to his large DPS and high add. Even if the laboratory could fabricate a +10 add with $12^\Delta$ base-in per lens, the remaining demand is quite large, and binocularity would not be a reasonable pursuit.

## Demonstration of Available Options

The major portion of the magnification provided by a microscope comes from moving the object closer (Chapter 10), and the lens serves primarily to put it into clear focus. Since accommodation does the same thing, age is an important consideration when prescribing microscopes. Children have sufficient accommodation that microscopes often are not necessary. If it seems that the accommodative effort is bothersome, an add can be prescribed that will alleviate all or some of that effort. It is also true that children may have trouble treating glasses with the care necessary to keep them in good functioning order, so it is wise to provide them with devices, such as a hand-held magnifier, that are less expensive and consequently more easily replaced when broken or lost. Spectacle-mounted devices may be hard to keep in adjustment when subjected to the strenuous physical activities of youngsters. Older people, on the other hand, may prefer a spectacle-mounted device because of difficulty holding a hand-held magnifier steady.

***Monocular Versus Binocular.*** In general, microscopes are prescribed for the better eye as a monocular device. If the two eyes are relatively similar in ability and if there is binocular potential, it is reasonable to consider prescribing two microscopes for simultaneous use; however, as shown previously, it is very difficult to achieve binocularity beyond +8.00 D.

If a monocular device is prescribed and the patient is bothered by interference from the other eye, that interference can be reduced by frosting the lens or using a clip-on occluder. The clip-on occluder is preferred over frosting the lens since many patients find that the interference from the other eye is less bothersome once they have adapted to the microscope. They may also prefer to have the glasses look as inconspicuous as possible. When this is the case, the occluder can easily be removed. A frosted lens would have to be replaced, which is more expensive. If, after a period of trial with the occluder, permanent occlusion is determined necessary, a clear lens can always be frosted later.

When binocular use is desired and the power is not too great, base-in prism can be prescribed to help with the convergence demand. This adds considerable thickness and weight to the lenses; $12^\Delta$ base-in is about the practical limit for each eye. The weight can be reduced by prescribing the microscopes in half-eye form with the appropriate prism. A full-diameter prism-compensated lens is available from Eschenbach Optik (see Resources, Chapter 31).

Microscopes can also be prescribed for "biocular" use in which a lens is prescribed for each eye to use alternately, but not binocularly. This can be advantageous for a person whose eyes have similar visual potential but no binocularity or for someone who simply prefers to use each eye some of the time. Two different strength microscopes, one for each eye, prescribed for a patient who is not binocular but whose eyes have a similar visual acuity allows more flexibility in sizes of print that can be read.

***Lens Form.*** A microscope can be prescribed as a full-diameter lens, a half-eye lens, or as a bifocal (Figure 13–3). Most optical suppliers can routinely provide adds of up to +10.00 D. Bifocal lens blanks with adds of +6.00, +9.00, +12.00, and +18.00 D are available from American Optical Corporation. When higher bifocal adds are desired, several companies have special designs (Figure 13–4), such as corrected doublets, or bifocals in the "Ben Franklin style" made by cementing together two lens halves, in the desired powers for distance and near, to give an executive-style bifocal. Designs for Vision, Inc., makes a series of microscopes that are compound lenses designed to reduce peripheral distortions. These are available in both full-diameter and bifocal form.

Full-diameter microscopes in a variety of strengths are available already mounted in a frame, which can be dispensed immediately to the patient. The term full-diameter refers to the fact that a single lens is centered before the eye as opposed to a multifocal design. These "stock" devices have acceptable optical quality and are very useful devices to have available provided that the fit is adequate and that the patient will accept the frame style and color. These pre-

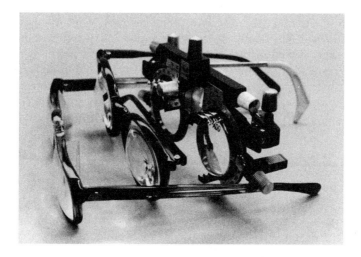

**Figure 13–3.** A convex lens, to be used as a microscope, may be prescribed in several forms, three of which are shown here: prism-compensated half-eyes (left), a full-diameter aspheric lenticular lens (middle), and a high add (right).

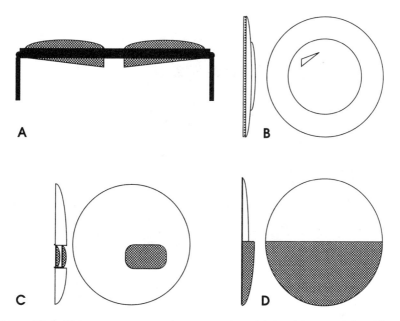

**Figure 13–4.** High power convex lenses can be obtained in a variety of lens forms: (**A**) prism-compensated half-eyes, (**B**) lenticular, (**C**) bifocal doublet, and (**D**) "Ben Franklin" style bifocal.

fabricated microscopes typically have good quality aspheric surfaces and a lenticular lens form. The higher powers are rather conspicuous since the actual lens is a relatively small button centered in the larger carrier.

Several optical companies make a series of prism-compensated half-eyes ranging in power from +4.00 D with 6△ base-in for each eye to +12.00 D with 14△ base-in for each eye; however, the stated prism amount is not always accurate for a given patient unless the major reference point of the lens corresponds with the patient's line of sight in straight-ahead gaze.[4] Patients often prefer this half-eye form because it looks more like normal glasses than a full-diameter high plus lens (Figure 13-3).

An inexpensive microscope can be produced quickly in either full-diameter or bifocal form by using Fresnel lenses. The major drawback is the poor optical quality of the Fresnel lens, but this may not be that noticeable to some patients. A Fresnel lens may be used to construct an inexpensive demonstration device for home trial.

At the time of publication, Unilens Corporation was test marketing a removable add designed to be placed on the patient's spectacle lens with an adhesive ring (UniVision™ low vision lens application system). This lens can serve as a temporary lens for home trial or be dispensed permanently with the option of removing it if the patient so desired or replacing it later with one of another power (Figure 13-5). This concept is more feasible if the person has single vision lenses rather than multifocals.

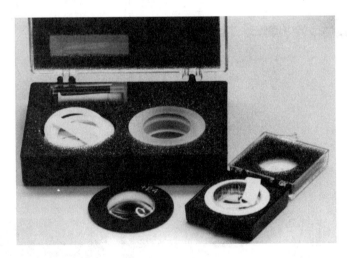

**Figure 13-5.** The UniVision application system, being introduced as this book goes to press, utilizes high plus lenses that can be reversibly mounted to a spectacle lens using an adhesive ring. This system works best on a single vision lens. Shown here are a +24.00 D lens in a trial ring and the same power lens with an adhesive mounting ring attached (right). In the background is the mounting kit.

*Cost.* There are a reasonably large number of good quality, inexpensive microscopes, so cost need not be a major factor in the prescription. If it is of concern to the patient, then a hand-held device avoids the cost of spectacles to support it. If cost is part of the decision in whether or not a binocular or biocular device is to be prescribed, the clinician should remember that one is cheaper than two of the same thing. Therefore, a monocular microscope may suffice.

## DESIGN OF THE FINAL PRESCRIPTION

As a general rule, single lenses over +8.00 D will offer improved optical quality if the surface is aspheric. Below this amount, asphericity is probably of little benefit to the patient. Full-diameter aspheric microscopes are available in a standard frame with plastic aspheric lenses. These are available in stock spherical powers ranging from +8.00 to +64.00 D. These work fine if the patient is satisfied with the frame and if it fits properly. The consideration of fit must include not only physical comfort but also the location of the optical center of the lens with respect to the line of sight. The lens blanks can also be ordered by a finishing laboratory if a different frame is desired. The disadvantages of the prefabricated microscopes are that the lens decentration is fixed and the frame is plastic without nose pads, so it cannot be adjusted as precisely as some other frames. A good alternative is to use lenses designed to correct aphakia. They are readily available in full-diameter and lenticular designs with spherical and cylindrical powers on aspheric surfaces, and they can be edged to fit almost any desired frame.

New aspheric full diameter designs have been announced recently by Tech-Optics and Designs for Vision, Inc. The former introduced the HI-45 lens, and the latter, the ClearImage II®. The ClearImage II® is a compound lens made of high index glass. It can be dispensed as a stock lens or can include the patient's refractive correction. There are several considerations to be made when comparing new designs to available lenses. For example, the clinician must weigh the cost against the value of better optics for a patient whose media and acuity level may preclude noticing any advantage offered by better optical designs; however, visual performance is not the only consideration. The clinician should also consider improved cosmesis and the lighter weight offered by designs that reduce lens thickness and curvature.

If a prefabricated microscope is prescribed, it must be remembered that the patient's refractive correction is not incorporated in the lens and is lost when he or she she removes his or her glasses and puts on the microscope. This affects the power of the add, as shown in the following three examples.

■ **Example 13–8.** A prefabricated microscope of +24.00 D is dispensed to a patient who has a refractive error of +6.50 DS. What is the actual power of the add for this patient?

Some of the microscope power goes to correct the patient's refractive error, and the remainder is the actual add:

$$\text{Microscope} - \text{Refractive error} = \text{Add}$$
$$+24.00 \text{ DS} - (+6.50) = \text{Add}$$
$$+17.50 \text{ D} = \text{Add}$$

■ **Example 13-9.** A prefabricated microscope of +24.00 D is dispensed to a patient who has a refractive error of −8.00 DS. What is the actual power of the add for this patient?

In this example, the patient's refractive error increases the total add since uncorrected myopia acts as an add:

$$\text{Microscope} - \text{Refractive error} = \text{Add}$$
$$+24.00 \text{ DS} - (-8.00) = \text{Add}$$
$$+24.00 \text{ DS} + 8.00 = \text{Add}$$
$$+32.00 = \text{Add}$$

■ **Example 13-10.** A prefabricated microscope is to be used for a patient whose reference acuity is 0.4/6M. If his refractive correction is +4.00 DS, what power microscope would be necessary to allow him to read 1M print?

$$\text{Magnification needed} = \text{Reference size/Goal size}$$
$$\text{Magnification needed} = 6M/1M$$
$$\text{Magnification needed} = 6X$$
$$M = rF$$
$$6 = (0.4)F$$
$$+15.00 \text{ D} = F$$

He needs a total of +15.00 D, but +4.00 of the microscope is needed to correct his refractive error. He therefore needs a +19.00 microscope. Since prefabricated microscopes do not come in all possible powers, the closest available is probably a +16.00 or a +20.00.

If a binocular system is to be prescribed, base-in prism will be required for most adds beyond +4.00 D or +5.00 D to assist the patient in achieving sustained fusion. The total convergence demand can be calculated as shown previously, and prism may be provided through the use of stock prism-compensated devices or by custom design.

When a custom microscope is designed for monocular use, the lens is decentered. Therefore, the optical center of the lens corresponds with the line of sight for the near viewing distance required by that lens, not the near pupillary separation as is usually measured clinically for adds up to +2.50 D.

## Frame Selection

The best frames to use have small eye sizes to keep lens weight minimal and are selected with a bridge and eyewire size that do not require decentration to match the optical centers with the patient's line of sight. This avoids an unsightly thick edge on one side unless prism is incorporated, in which case some increased edge thickness is unavoidable. When a lenticular lens is prescribed, the eyewire should be as close to spherical as possible and should approximate the bowl size in order to minimize the appearance of the transition zone.

## OTHER MICROSCOPE OPTIONS

Bifocals and even trifocals with each lens designed for near offer some flexibility; for example, a patient who is emmetropic might use bifocals with +4.00 in the "distance" portion and a +4.00 D "add" in the segment. This gives +4.00 D for intermediate tasks and a total of +8.00 for the maximum add. Similarly, a patient with a refractive error of −2.00 D sphere might use a bifocal with +2.00 D in the "distance" portion and a +4.00 D "add" in the segment for two different near tasks. This also gives +4.00 D for intermediate sized print and a total of +8.00 D for the maximum add. Two diopters of the intermediate portion come from the uncorrected myopia, and two diopters come from the prescription.

Patients with high myopia may simply remove their glasses for near tasks or may prefer inverted half-eyes with the distance correction in the top and no correction for near. A contact lens can be used as a microscope,[5] and this is discussed further in Chapter 17.

## Incorporating Prism for Eccentric Viewing

Some clinicians have tried incorporating prism into microscopes to assist patients with eccentric viewing. The concept was to allow patients to maintain their customary eye position and move the image to the seeing portion of the retina with prism.[6]

While there are reports of successful use of prism for this purpose, there is some controversy surrounding the explanation for why an improvement is found. Bailey[7] suggested that there would be no net gain since moving the image would cause the eye to shift, so, if a patient does better with prism, there must be another explanation. The technique has not been widely accepted, and interested readers are referred to the literature[6, 7, 8] for further information.

## ADAPTATION TO MICROSCOPES

Two major obstacles to successful adaptation to the use of a microscope are the near work distance and, for those with a central scotoma, inability to view eccentrically with efficiency. Patients often complain of headaches, neck aches, nausea, and an altered visual sense when first attempting to read with a high plus lens. These obstacles and symptoms can be remediated through the use of training programs[9] (Chapter 22) and other assistive devices including reading stands, reading guides, good lighting, and an emphasis on good reading posture. Patients should be encouraged to begin with larger print and progressively work toward their goal. It may be necessary to prescribe a weaker microscope first until they gain some facility in its use.

## DISPENSING AND FOLLOW-UP

Success in the office can easily become a failure at home if the patient does not receive adequate training with the microscope and if there is no planned follow-up. Patients should be reminded at dispensing to use good lighting, take frequent breaks, and build up their reading time slowly. They should demonstrate the correct use of the microscope before taking it home. Both the patient and family members should be reassured that it is not possible to damage one's eyes by using optical devices that require near working distances. A follow-up appointment for 1 to 2 weeks from the time of dispensing serves to remind patients that they are not being permanently dismissed and may also serve as encouragement to practice in order to demonstrate improved skills when they return.

As with all optical devices, care and cleaning are important aspects to address. Knowledge in this area should not be assumed. The correct adjustment of the microscope for lens position and comfort are, of course, integral to successful use.

## SUMMARY

The successful prescription of a microscope requires that the necessary power be dispensed in a usable form. The predicted power should serve as a starting point. It is not unusual to prescribe a slightly stronger lens than predicted in order to provide a margin of reserve reading ability. The final prescription should be determined with the actual task that the patient intends to use it for; for example, patients typically do not read continuous text as easily as they read individual letters of the same size on the acuity card. This is due to crowding of the letters, poor quality paper or print, and a continuous mixture of fonts as well as upper- and lower-case letters. Successful use of a microscope can be maximized with training and planned follow-up.

## REFERENCES

1. Alpern M: Types of movement, in Davson H (ed): *The Eye: Muscular Mechanisms,* Volume 3, 2 ed. New York, Academic Press, 1969, pp 65-174.
2. Faye EE: Problems in pathology, in Rosenthal BP, Cole RG (eds): A structured approach to low vision care. *Problems in Optometry* 3(3):408-415, 1991.
3. Bailey IL: Centering high-addition spectacle lenses. *Optom Monthly* 70:95-100, 1979.
4. Williams DR: An evaluation of the optical characteristics of prismatic half-eye spectacles for the low vision patient. *J Vis Rehab* 5(2):21-35, 1991.
5. Eldred KB: Use of a contact lens as a microscope. *J Vis Rehab* 3(2):23-28, 1989.
6. Romayananda M, Wong SW, Elzeneiny IH, Chan GH: Prismatic scanning method for improving visual acuity in patients with low vision. *Ophthalmol* 89:937-945, 1982.
7. Bailey I: Can prism control eccentric viewing? *Optom Monthly* 74(7):360-363, 1983.
8. Rosenberg R, Faye E, Fischer M, Budick D: Role of prism relocation in improving visual performance of patients with macular dysfunction. *J Optom Vis Sci* 66(11): 747-750, 1989.
9. Wheatley GP: Instructing the patient with low vision to use a microscope for reading and near tasks. *J Vis Rehab* 4(2):19-27, 1990.

## ADDITIONAL READING

Parkins TJ: I-Gard plastic hyperocular spectacle magnifiers. *Am J Opt* 33(11):624, 1956.
Westheimer G: The design and ophthalmic properties of binocular magnification devices. *Am J Opt* 31(11):578-584, 1954.
Wright V, Watson G: Reading level as a criterion for selecting materials for the adult reader with low vision. *J Vis Rehab* 5(1):23-35, 1991.

# HOW TO PRESCRIBE HAND AND STAND MAGNIFIERS

*Hand-held and stand magnifiers are considered together in this chapter because they fulfill similar needs for patients, but they have different optical properties that must be considered during the diagnostic trial. Hand-held and stand magnifiers are customarily labeled with a magnification, such as 4X, by the manufacturer. This value cannot be used because the magnification obtained by the patient depends on the circumstances under which the device is used. Similarly, the dioptric power given by the manufacturer is not necessarily the equivalent power. Hand and stand magnifiers are relatively inexpensive options, and most patients are familiar with how they should be used. Acceptance by the patient is usually easier than with more complex devices. Nevertheless, the use of prescription guidelines and a logical diagnostic sequence will maximize the patient-clinician interaction even with this simple device.*

*Stand magnifiers are preferred over hand-held magnifiers for patients who have physical infirmities that cause difficulty holding the lens steady and/or maintaining the correct lens-to-object distance. Because stand magnifiers have different optical properties than hand-held magnifiers, it is somewhat more difficult to determine the appropriate device for obtaining a given magnification. This problem is reduced considerably with the use of a computer program or spreadsheet, provided that the optical properties such as the enlargement and the image location are known for the magnifiers to be used. These were given for some magnifiers in Table 10–6. If the optical properties are not known, they can be determined easily for any stand magnifier as was explained in Chapter 10. Also, it is anticipated that most manufacturers will provide this information with their products in the near future. Meanwhile, the clinician should label all of the stand magnifiers in his or her inventory with the enlargement (E) and the image location (i).*

## A DIAGNOSTIC SEQUENCE FOR PRESCRIBING HAND-HELD AND STAND MAGNIFIERS

The recommended test sequence is as follows:

- Determine the best distance correction
- Measure the best corrected near acuity through the appropriate add
- Determine the goal acuity
- Calculate the magnification needed
- Demonstrate the appropriate device to the patient
- (Loan a device for home practice)
- Demonstrate the different options in which it can be prescribed

### Determination of the Goal Acuity and Required Magnification

As always, the goal acuity is determined by the patient's stated near goal. When general reading is the objective, a reasonable goal is to be able to read 1M continuous text with some measure of reserve. The magnification needed is determined by the patient's goal; however, the lens that will provide that magnification must be calculated differently for hand and stand magnifiers. The practitioner must be careful not to assume that if a patient needs a +20.00 diopter hand magnifier, he or she would also need a +20.00 stand magnifier. This would only be true if he or she held the hand magnifier the same distance from the print as the height of the stand magnifier, thus creating the same image size in the same location in either instance. For the stand magnifier, the total magnification is determined from the enlargement provided by the magnifier as well relative distance magnification based on the image location compared to the reference distance (Chapter 10). Since the image will be located a finite distance from the eye, presbyopic patients require an add to achieve the clearest possible focus. If the practitioner neglects a careful consideration of the patient's add strength and the image location when demonstrating a stand magnifier, a failure might result, forcing the patient to select another device when the stand magnifier would have been a better choice if it had been demonstrated properly. (*Have I made that point perfectly clear yet?*)

### Demonstration of the Appropriate Lens Power

Either type of magnifier is best demonstrated by using print somewhat larger than what the patient will eventually want to read. The hand magnifier is laid on the print and raised slowly until the print is as large and clear as possible. This should occur as the lens is raised to approximately its focal length, $f$, from the print or object of regard. Since this causes parallel light to leave the lens, presbyopic patients should view through the distance portion of their bifocals or with their distance correction in a trial frame. The use of a trial frame ensures that only the distance correction is used, and this may be helpful at first.

The clinician can be sure the lens is positioned properly by using a tape measure or ruler to measure the distance of the lens from the object. It was shown in Chapter 10 that the distance from the lens to the eye does not matter as long as the object remains near the focal point of the lens. Once the patient is able to use the lens effectively, smaller print can be demonstrated until the goal is achieved.

A stand magnifier requires that the patient accommodate or have the appropriate bifocal in order to see the image as clearly as possible. If the patient is not wearing the best correction and the appropriate add, it can be placed in a trial frame. The presbyopic patient must understand that it might be necessary to have a bifocal or reading lens designed specifically for using that particular magnifier. If the stand magnifiers available for demonstration have the image location and enlargement marked, the clinician will be able to select the one that offers the right magnification and will be able to determine the appropriate work distance and add for the patient. Example 14–1 demonstrates how the two types of magnifiers may be selected and demonstrated. Several other examples were given in Chapter 10.

■ **Example 14–1.** The clinician has a stand magnifier and a hand-held magnifier, each of which has an equivalent power of +10.00 D. She wishes to demonstrate the relative merits of each to a 65-year-old woman whose near reference acuity is 0.4/4M through best distance correction and a +2.50 add, which is what she is already wearing. Her goal is to be able to read a large print Bible that she has brought with her. The stand magnifier has been correctly marked as follows: $F_e$ = +10 D, E = 2.0X, and i = 20 cm. Can these magnifiers be used to achieve the goal, and if so, how?

The clinician measures the print size of several lower-case letters in the Bible and determines that they average 3 mm tall.

$$\text{M size} = \text{Letter height}/1.45 \text{ mm}$$
$$\text{M size} = 3 \text{ mm}/1.45 \text{ mm}$$
$$\text{M size} = 2.07 \text{ M } (\approx 2\text{M})$$
$$\text{Magnification required} = \text{Reference size}/\text{Goal size}$$
$$\text{Magnification required} = 4\text{M}/2\text{M}$$
$$\text{Magnification required} = 2\text{X}$$
$$\text{M} = \text{rF}$$
$$2 = (0.4)\text{F}$$
$$2/0.4 = \text{F}$$
$$+5 = \text{F}$$

If the hand-held magnifier is used, the patient should easily read 2M print when looking through her distance correction since its equivalent power is twice as strong as required. The fact that it is stronger than required is not necessarily bad since it may give her an important measure of reserve, but a lower power lens would be expected to have fewer peripheral aberrations and hence a larger usable field of view.

The stand magnifier must be used with an add, and the equivalent power of the system (add combined with stand magnifier) must be +5.00 diopters. The appropriate add is determined as follows:

$$F_e \text{ system} = E \times F_{add}$$
$$5 = 2 \times F_{add}$$
$$5/2 = F_{add}$$
$$+2.5 = F_{add}$$

It should be possible for the patient to read 2M print with the stand magnifier held 20 cm from a +2.50 add. The magnifier must be held 20 cm from the add because the image distance, i, is 20 cm from the magnifier; this puts the image at 40 cm, which is the focal point of a +2.50 add. Since she is already wearing her best correction and it has a +2.50 add, her current glasses will work in this situation. If the clinician wanted to have the same measure of reserve with the stand magnifier as with the hand-held magnifier, the add would have to be adjusted as follows:

$$F_e \text{ system} = E \times F_{add}$$
$$10 = 2 \times F_{add}$$
$$10/2 = F_{add}$$
$$+5 = F_{add}$$

The magnifier would have to be held literally against the add to position the image at the focal point of the add (20 cm), so the clinician decides to compromise with a +3.50 add. Will this work?

$$F_e \text{ system} = E \times F_{add}$$
$$F_e \text{ system} = 2 \times 3.50$$
$$F_e \text{ system} = +7.00$$
$$M = rF$$
$$M = 0.4(7)$$
$$M = 2.8X$$

This gives more magnification than is required, and it will work as long as the magnifier is held 8.57 cm from the add (20 + 8.57 = 28.57, the focal length of the add); however, this option requires that she obtain new glasses in order to have the correct add.

One final twist. The patient seems to prefer the hand-held magnifier and tries to use it with her +2.50 bifocal. Will this work?

If the magnifier is held 5 cm (one focal length) from her add, the system will have an equivalent power equal to the power of the magnifier itself, so, yes, +10 D is more than enough. The clinician can demonstrate the correct position by using a ruler to position the magnifier. If the magnifier is held closer than one focal length, the patient will get even more magnification; if it is held farther than one focal length away, she will get less magnification.

## Demonstration of Available Options

*Hand-held Versus Stand-mounted.* Hand-held and stand magnifiers are relatively easy to prescribe since there is no fabrication or lens design necessary by the practitioner. Also, there is little or no concern with whether or not the patient is binocular. There are, however, many available lenses of different size, shape, and design, and this can make the final decision difficult.

When considering hand-held devices in general, the main consideration is whether or not the patient prefers a stand magnifier as opposed to the truly hand-supported device. This depends on the patient's ability to hold the device in proper focus and is easily found out during the clinical trial. As a general rule, stand magnifiers are manipulated more easily than hand-held magnifiers by those who are either very young or relatively old. Any physical infirmity of the arms or hands suggests that the patient might perform better with a stand magnifier since it is supported by the material being viewed and is therefore maintained at its appropriate distance from the object. One pitfall to avoid when demonstrating the difference between hand and stand magnifiers is allowing the patient to compare two devices of the same dioptric power that actually provide different amounts of magnification. Ease of portability is a consideration in some cases since a stand magnifier is considerably more bulky and therefore more difficult to slip into one's pocket or purse. A variety of hand and stand magnifiers is shown in Figures 14–1 and 14–2 respectively.

The position of the lens in most stand magnifiers is fixed. Therefore, once the stand is placed on the material to be read, the lens is tilted with respect to the eye unless the material can be held at an angle. Reading stands or lap boards are useful for supporting the reading material and magnifier in a comfortable position. A tape measure is convenient for establishing and demonstrating the correct distance for the patient to hold the stand magnifier relative to his or her add.

A person will often lift a stand magnifier away from the page to achieve greater magnification, improve the focus, or get the lens closer to the eye for a bigger field of view. This defeats the purpose of the stand, which is to offer support. If the patient does it consistently, it may imply that more magnification is required, that the image is not positioned correctly for the add, or that a stand is not really necessary. If the stand is lifted only occasionally in order to see finer detail, this is not necessarily a problem. In fact, it is good for the user to know that this is an option.

*Field of View.* When a person moves a hand or stand magnifier farther away from the eye, the field of view diminishes. The linear field of view (FOV) for a

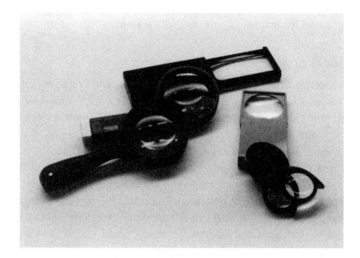

**Figure 14–1.** There is a large variety of hand-held magnifiers with different features such as aspheric surfaces, illumination, multiple lenses that can be combined to alter the total power, and a protective housing to shield the lens when it is not being used.

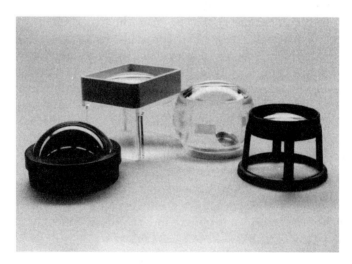

**Figure 14–2.** There is a large variety of stand magnifiers with different features, including a clear housing, illumination, and aspheric surfaces. The most important parameters to know are the equivalent power, the image location, and the enlargement factor (see text).

plus lens is equal to the aperture width (A) multiplied by the quotient of the focal length ($f$) and h, the distance of the lens from the eye.[1]

$$FOV = A(f/h)$$

Table 14–1 gives the field of view for a magnifier held different distances from the eye. It can be seen from examination of the formula for FOV and from Table 14–1 that the FOV is equal to the aperture of the lens when it is held one focal length from the eye, is equal to one-half of the aperture when held two focal lengths away, and so forth. Because the FOV decreases as the lens is moved farther from the eye, most persons typically prefer to hold it closer. The aperture is fixed for a given magnifier, and the only way to manipulate the FOV is to change the distance at which the lens is held from the eye. This works well for a hand-held magnifier with the object at the focal point of the lens, but changing the distance a stand magnifier is held from the eye also changes the magnification, as shown in Example 14–1. Even if magnifiers could be custom ordered with different aperture widths, the lens weight and peripheral lens aberrations would limit the effectiveness of specifying apertures much larger than those that are already available.

***Cost.*** Hand-held and stand magnifiers exist in a variety of forms and lens quality. As with most things, higher quality implies greater cost. Patients, however, may not appreciate improved visual function with the higher quality lens, so it is best to be able to demonstrate the difference prior to making the final decision. Batteries and bulbs used with illuminated systems have a finite life expectancy determined by the brightness of the illumination system and the type of battery. This adds to the expense of the system, which might not be insignificant if it is used frequently. Rechargeable batteries are a long-term cost-saving option but may not provide the same level of illumination as "disposable" batteries and may have a shorter useful life between charges.

***Optics and Illumination.*** Hand-held magnifiers are available with aspheric surfaces, tints, and antireflective coatings. These are probably good options, provided that they do not involve a lot of extra cost and seem to make a func-

**TABLE 14–1.** Field of view (FOV) for a +10 magnifier with an aperture of 6 centimeters when held different multiples of its focal length from the eye.

| F | f (cm) | A (cm) | h (cm) | FOV (cm) | h = xf |
|---|---|---|---|---|---|
| +10 | 10 | 6 | 5 | 12.0 | 1/2f |
| +10 | 10 | 6 | 10 | 6.0 | 1f |
| +10 | 10 | 6 | 20 | 3.0 | 2f |
| +10 | 10 | 6 | 30 | 2.0 | 3f |
| +10 | 10 | 6 | 40 | 1.5 | 4f |
| +10 | 10 | 6 | 50 | 1.2 | 5f |

F = lens power, f = focal length of the lens, A = aperture diameter, h = distance of the lens from the eye

tional difference for the patient. There are many hand and stand magnifiers available, but there is not a large variety for a particular equivalent power. Therefore, once equivalent power has been determined, the available options are somewhat limited.

When it seems clear that a hand or stand magnifier is the right device to prescribe but the patient performs poorly with it, the practitioner should evaluate an illuminated device. There are many devices available that incorporate an illumination system, including some with a choice between incandescent and halogen bulbs. The illumination is often the difference between success and failure. Eschenbach Optik (see Resources, Chapter 31) has developed an illumination system that can be clipped on a number of their magnifiers (Figure 14-3). This allows the clinician to demonstrate the value of illumination with a given magnifier, and the light source can be added or removed when desired. Another consideration relative to lighting is the thickness and color of the stand. Several designs recently have reduced stand size and shape in order to allow more light to reach the object of regard.

## ADAPTATION AND TRAINING

Hand-held magnifiers are familiar devices to most people, and they are usually used with relative ease. The major obstacles encountered are inability to hold the lens steady, difficulty maintaining the correct focal distance, and, for those who wear multifocals, not viewing through the correct part of the lens. As with all devices, the effort of using the device and the effort of trying to use the residual vision most effectively may cause fatigue. These obstacles and symp-

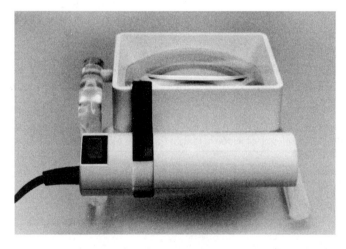

**Figure 14-3.** Eschenbach has developed a clip-on illumination system that attaches, reversibly, to a variety of their hand and stand magnifiers.

toms can be remediated through the use of training programs (Chapter 22) and assistive devices, including reading stands, reading guides, good lighting, and an emphasis on good reading posture. Patients should be encouraged to begin with larger print and progressively work toward the goal as facility improves.

If an illuminated system is being considered, it is worthwhile to teach the patient how to change the batteries and the bulb in order to avoid dependence on others. This may be difficult to perform with impaired vision, so the clinician may want to teach the patient how to do it tactually without using vision at all.

## DISPENSING AND FOLLOW-UP

Patients must know how to use a hand magnifier correctly before taking it home. Best results will be obtained if the patient is encouraged to use good lighting and to build up his or her reading time slowly. If an illuminated system is being dispensed, the patient should have an adequate supply of spare bulbs and batteries. A follow-up appointment should be scheduled to ensure that the device is being used correctly and effectively.

## SUMMARY

Hand-held and stand magnifiers are simple optical devices that have great utility in low vision rehabilitation. They are relatively inexpensive and are typically well received by patients. Because of this, it is easy for the clinician to become casual about prescribing these devices. This should be avoided. The best results are obtained by using an analytical approach to determining the most appropriate power and form to prescribe for the patient and by ensuring that the device can be used appropriately before being dispensed. Systematic prescribing and follow-up will ensure maximal success.

## REFERENCE

1. Bailey IL: Magnification for near vision. *Optom Monthly* 71:119–122, 1980.

## ADDITIONAL READING

Chung STL, Johnston AW: New stand magnifiers do not meet rated levels of performance. *Clin Exp Optom* 73(6):194–199, 1990.
Faye EE: Guide to selecting reading spectacles, hand magnifiers, stand magnifiers, telescopes, electronic aids, and absorptive lenses, in Faye EE (ed): *Clinical Low Vision,* 2 ed. Boston, Little, Brown and Company, 1984.

Johnston AW: The relationship between magnification and field of view for simple magnifiers. *Austr J Optom* 65:74–77, 1982.

Johnston AW: A further note on hand-held magnifiers. *Rehab Optom* 2(3):8–11, 1984.

Loshin DS, Bailey IL: Hand-held magnifiers. *Rehab Optom* 2(2): 29–32, 1984.

McMahon TT, Spigelman V: Reading with a stand magnifier: 1. Effect of text configuration and experience on normal subjects. *J Vis Rehab* 3:119–123, 1989.

Neve JJ: On the use of hand-held magnifiers during reading. *Optom Vis Sci* 66(7): 440–449, 1989.

Porter FI, Demer JL, Goldberg J, Jenkins HA, Schmidt K: Developing a methodology for predicting successful visual rehabilitation with spectacle magnifiers. *J Vis Rehab* 1(1):22–34, 1987.

Sloan LL, Brown DJ: Relative merits of headborne, hand and stand magnifiers. *Am J Ophthalmol* 58:594–604, 1964.

# HOW TO PRESCRIBE TELEMICROSCOPES

*If the patient is to receive a spectacle-borne low vision device for near, it will be a microscope or a telemicroscope. A telemicroscope is a telescope that has been modified to focus at a near distance either by adding a cap (permanent or removable) or by having a sufficiently large range of focus. A telemicroscope is prescribed to give near magnification at a more comfortable work distance than the equivalent microscope (see Example 10–21). The reader will recall from Chapter 10 that the work distance is the distance from the most anterior portion of the device to the required object distance.[1] This distance is measured from the cap or from the objective lens if the telescope is focusable for near. When the patient bases his or her choice on a comparison of the relative advantages and disadvantages of the two, the clinician must determine the optical parameters of both systems and demonstrate them to the patient as described below. Microscopes were considered in Chapter 13. Many of the considerations reviewed for telescopes and microscopes carry over to the telemicroscope and are not repeated here in the same detail.*

## A DIAGNOSTIC TEST SEQUENCE FOR PRESCRIBING TELEMICROSCOPES

The recommended test sequence is as follows:

- Determine the best distance correction
- Measure the best corrected near acuity through the appropriate add
- Determine the goal acuity

- Calculate the magnification needed
- Demonstrate the appropriate telemicroscope power to the patient
- Explain the options
- (Loan a device for home trial)
- Design the final prescription

## Determination of the Goal Acuity and Required Magnification

The goal acuity and required magnification are determined in exactly the same manner as described for telescopes and microscopes. What is different with telemicroscopes is how the system is designed to provide that magnification. The reader will recall that there is an infinite variety of theoretical telescope/cap combinations that will create a telemicroscope with the same equivalent power and the same magnification as a given microscope (Table 10–8); however, from a practical point of view, the choice is limited by the available telescopes. Example 15–1 demonstrates the clinical process. Some examples were given in Chapter 10.

■ **Example 15–1.** The clinician has three telescopes and a variety of caps for each. They are a 2.5X Galilean, a 3.0X Keplerian, and 4.0X Keplerian. She is working with a 60-year-old male who has a best corrected near acuity of 0.33/5M. His goal is to be able to read the daily newspaper, which is found to use 1M print. How could each telescope be used to accomplish his goal?

$$\text{Magnification required} = \text{Reference size/Goal size}$$
$$\text{Magnification required} = 5M/1M$$
$$\text{Magnification required} = 5X$$
$$M = rF$$
$$5 = (0.33)F$$
$$5/0.33 = F$$
$$+15.15 = F$$

This shows that he can accomplish his goal with 5X magnification and that it is provided by a lens or lens system with an equivalent power of +15.15. The equivalent power of a telescope/cap combination, as shown in Chapter 10, is equal to the product of the dioptric power of the cap multiplied by the magnification of the telescope. The work distance is the reciprocal of the cap.

$$F_e \text{ system} = F_{cap} \times M_{ts}$$
$$+15.15 = F_{cap} \times 2.5$$
$$+15.15/2.5 = F_{cap}$$
$$+6.06 = F_{cap} \text{ (Work distance} = 16.5 \text{ cm)}$$

$$F_e \text{ system} = F_{cap} \times M_{ts}$$
$$+15.15 = F_{cap} \times 3.0$$
$$+15.15/3.0 = F_{cap}$$
$$+5.05 = F_{cap} \text{ (Work distance} = 19.8 \text{ cm)}$$

$$F_e \text{ system} = F_{cap} \times M_{ts}$$
$$+15.15 = F_{cap} \times 4.0$$
$$+15.15/4.0 = F_{cap}$$
$$+3.79 = F_{cap} \text{ (Work distance = 26.4 cm)}$$

There is a significant difference in the work distance, and this may make it easy to decide which one to prescribe. Other factors are size, weight, appearance, optical quality, cost, and field of view. The Keplerian systems probably have the largest field of view because that is a feature of the Keplerian telescope compared to the Galilean telescope and because, for this example, they also require lower powered caps. Field of view is difficult to calculate but is relatively easy to determine clinically by simply measuring it using an Amsler chart, if it can be seen, or by moving a stimulus into view from each side while the patient fixates any near target (see Example 6–1).

## Demonstration of the Available Options

There is a large variety of available telemicroscopes from which the final prescription can be made. There are focusable telescopes that can give a clear image of near targets at many distances as well as caps for fixed-focus telescopes (Figure 15–1) that put that system in focus for a single near distance. In fact, any

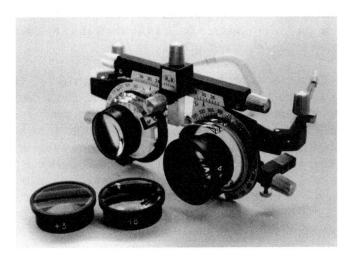

**Figure 15–1.** A telemicroscope may be made by placing a cap on a telescope. Two 2.2X fixed-focus telescopes from Designs for Vision, Inc., are shown in the trial frame, one with and one without a cap. A cap can be obtained with virtually any power desired, and more than one cap may be prescribed for different circumstances. Focusable telescopes may also serve as telemicroscopes if they focus to a near distance, and, of course, even a focusable telescope may be used with a cap.

telescope (focusable or not) can be modified for near by having a cap fabricated for it. A custom-designed system can be ordered that incorporates the power needed for any selected near distance into the objective lens. This eliminates the necessity of focusing or putting a cap off and on; however, it also eliminates the possibility of the device's being used as a telescope since the cap cannot be removed. Such dedicated systems are useful for a patient who requires frequent and prolonged use at a specific distance (such as a student for reading) or even for normally sighted surgeons and dentists requiring magnification for certain procedures. These systems are occasionally referred to as "surgical loupes" because of their frequent use by cardiovascular, thoracic, and neurosurgeons, among others.

Several factors influence the choice between a telescope that is focusable for near and one that requires a cap or caps. Caps may be difficult to keep track of. Also, since they are held in place by friction after being pressed in place, their housing will eventually loosen, and they will have to be replaced. A focusable telescope can be adjusted to a theoretically infinite number of near distances, whereas a fixed-focus telescope would require an infinite number of caps to accomplish the same flexibility. A focusable unit may be difficult for a patient to adjust properly. It may be easier for that person simply to press a cap in place. When an afocal telescope is focused for near, some of the power of the objective is being used as a cap. Since the power remaining creates a new objective lens that is lower in power than before, it produces a new telescope with higher magnification[2, 3] that probably has a somewhat smaller field of view. The change in power, compared to the afocal power, may be significant and is more so for lower powered Galilean systems than for higher powered Galilean systems or Keplerian systems.[3]

***Hand-held Versus Spectacle-mounted.*** A telemicroscope is most often prescribed as a spectacle-mounted device. A hand-held device can be useful for occasional spotting at intermediate distances such as window shopping or scanning the floor for a dropped object, but it is difficult to hold it steady enough for most near tasks that require discrimination of fine detail and/or a prolonged observation time. The spectacle-mounted device is more applicable in the latter case. There are telemicroscopes that can be clipped on to spectacles for short-term use and then removed as desired. These offer the advantages of both a hand-held telescope and a spectacle-mounted unit but are a compromise between the two since the clip-on unit increases the weight, interferes with using the device when hand-held, and does not offer as rigid a mounting when fastened to spectacles. When a telemicroscope is clipped onto glasses, the field of view is typically reduced since the exit pupil is farther from the eye than it would be if the device were used without the spectacles or if the telescope were mounted in a hole drilled through the lens.

***Monocular Versus Binocular.*** As before, a monocular device is prescribed for the patient when one eye is significantly better than the other. When there is good reason to consider a binocular system, the advantages must outweigh the disadvantages of increased weight and the higher cost of two devices, including the expense of determining and fabricating the precise placement and alignment that will allow binocular function. If the system is to be used binocularly, the optical axes of the telemicroscopes must converge at the point of fixation. This eliminates the possibility of having multiple near points of binocular focus, as in a monocular focusable system, or of using multiple caps since the angle of the telemicroscopes is fixed.

***Telemicroscopes Fabricated by the Manufacturer.*** Custom systems are available from Designs for Vision, Inc., that can be mounted in a specific manner at the practitioner's request. Telescopes with caps or with a built-in near focus are both available, and the patient's distance prescription can be incorporated in the ocular. Keeler Optical makes a variety of telemicroscopes that can be mounted to a bar fixed to a spectacle frame with the conventional prescription, mounted to a ring glued to the distance correction, or fastened through a hole drilled in the distance correction. One mounting style allows the telemicroscopes to be flipped up when not in use (Figure 15–2). With this system, the patient's prescription does not have to be incorporated in the ocular of the telescope. A similar design (Figure 15–3) is available from Orascoptic, Inc. (see Resources, Chapter 31).

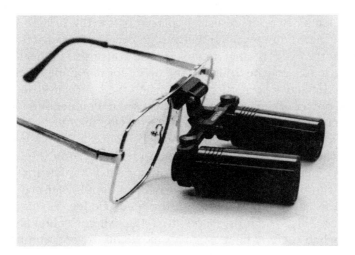

**Figure 15–2.** These telemicroscopes from Keeler are typically used by surgeons but could also be prescribed for reading or other near tasks. The hinge at the frame allows them to be raised if desired. Binocular systems similar to these are frequently referred to as surgical loupes.

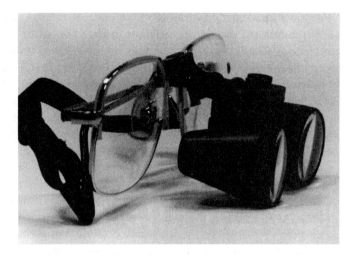

**Figure 15–3.** These telemicroscopes from Orascoptic Research are marketed primarily for dentists and surgeons but would also be useful for someone who is visually impaired.

***Telemicroscopes Fabricated by the Practitioner.*** The practitioner can mount telemicroscopes to the patient's spectacles just as described with telescopes. Many of the telescopes illustrated in Chapter 12 can serve as telemicroscopes because they are sufficiently focusable or because caps are available for them. They are mounted in the same manner as described in Chapter 12, with the exception that the placement and alignment are different as required by the near task. Telemicroscopes are usually placed below the straight-ahead line of sight and are angled downward and inward in order to be parallel with the line of sight when the eye is rotated downward and converged for near. Polycarbonate spectacle lenses may be drilled in the office for mounting telemicroscopes. The patient's refractive correction is lost when the hole is drilled, and some of the focusing power of the telemicroscope is used to compensate for the spherical component of the patient's refractive error. One in-office mounting option that preserves the patient's spectacle prescription is a double eyewire frame that allows a telemicroscope or telescope to be inserted in the front eyewire (Figure 15-4), but this is suitable primarily for small models that do not protrude very far through the lens. Telemicroscopes from Keeler may be mounted in a threaded ring glued to the front of the spectacle lens as described earlier for telescopes. This system preserves the refractive correction and is particularly useful when there is high astigmatism. Nikon Corporation has devised a system (available from The Lighthouse; see Resources, Chapter 31) that is mounted through a hole in the lens but has auxiliary lenses that can be attached to the back of the telescope or telemicroscope to correct the cylindrical portion of the refractive error.

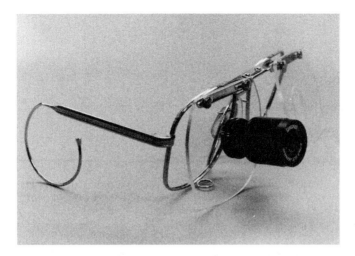

**Figure 15–4.** A double eyewire frame can be used to create a spectacle-mounted telemicroscope or telescope in the office. The patient's refractive error is preserved since the spectacle lens does not have to be drilled.

## DESIGN OF THE FINAL PRESCRIPTION

Telemicroscopes are usually prescribed monocularly for the better eye. They are usually mounted below the straight-ahead line of sight but may be mounted in the center of the lens, which might be necessary for a larger device, or even at the top if the patient has a particular need for viewing high or overhead objects at a near distance. An example of the latter is a maintenance worker who has to adjust wall-mounted thermostats.

The horizontal position must correspond with the line of sight for that eye when viewing at near. This might differ from the monocular pupillary distance if the patient views eccentrically. For continuous use or with full-diameter units, the telemicroscope is centered at the monocular pupillary distance. For intermittent use, the telemicroscope is usually placed below the line of sight and must be angled downward. The angle is predetermined for devices fabricated by Designs for Vision, Inc., but custom angles can be ordered. Other systems that can be mounted by the practitioner have special rings to adjust the angle of inclination.

If a binocular system is prescribed, the telemicroscopes must be angled inward so they converge at the point of near focus. Each unit is decentered to the respective monocular pupillary distance as measured when the patient is converging to the point at which the system focuses (Figure 15–5). This point is worth emphasizing again: *the pupillary separation must be measured while the patient is fixating at the desired near point of convergence.* Most people have a difference in the pupillary distance for each eye from the center of the

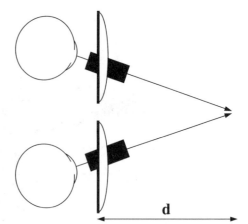

**Figure 15–5.** Telemicroscopes must be decentered to the monocular near pupillary distances and must be angled inward to be in line with the angle of convergence. The decentration and angle of convergence must be specific for the near point of fixation, which is specified as the distance from the spectacle plane (d).

bridge of the nose. This becomes an important consideration in the placement of the telemicroscopes since there is only a small area through which the patient can view. One technique for determining a close approximation to the near pupillary separation is that of Englemann.[4] It utilizes two red strips placed vertically in front of each eye in the spectacle plane. The strips are moved horizontally while the patient looks at a red card with a small green square in the center, held at the intended work distance. When the strip covers the red square, it appears dark. Each strip is adjusted monocularly and then compared and adjusted binocularly until the square remains dark with both eyes open. The monocular location of each strip is measured, and this gives the desired location of each telemicroscope in the frame (Figure 15–6). The pupillary separation can also be calculated (see Lens Decentration for Near, Chapter 13) or determined with a pupilometer, provided that it can compensate for the appropriate near work distance.

**Figure 15–6.** Englemann's technique for determining the monocular pupillary distances utilizes two transparent red plastic strips and a card with a green background and a red fixation square in the center. The card is held at the intended work distance from the spectacle plane, and the strips are decentered until they cover the red square, which then appears dark. The strips must be in the spectacle plane and can be attached to spectacles with rubber bands or can be glued to plano trial lenses for use with a trial frame. The monocular distances are measured from the center of each strip to the center of the bridge (+). The distances measured should be considered an approximation.

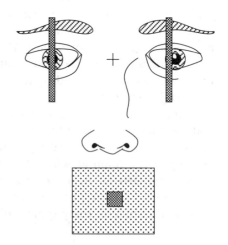

## ADAPTATION AND TRAINING

Telemicroscopes are probably prescribed less often than other devices for near because of their expense, weight, and appearance. They are also somewhat difficult to use and require a period of adaptation that, as discussed for other devices, is facilitated by training. Telemicroscopes have a short depth of focus and a small field of view, both of which are more significant as the equivalent power of the system is increased. These make adaptation difficult but do not preclude successful use. When the patient is sufficiently motivated and the advantage of increased work distance is the major consideration, a telemicroscope is the treatment of choice and may be used very successfully.

## DISPENSING AND FOLLOW-UP

Special attention must be paid to the frame adjustment of a spectacle-mounted telemicroscope. These devices are heavy, and maximum comfort is achieved with properly adjusted large nose pads. The vertex distance affects the field of view significantly, so the frame should be adjusted to place the unit as close to the eye as possible. The recipient should be reminded at dispensing to use good lighting, take frequent breaks, and build up his or her time of use slowly. Reading stands, reading guides, and other assistive devices may also be dispensed to enhance the patient's ability to use the device. Every patient should demonstrate the correct use of the telemicroscope before taking it home. A follow-up appointment for one to two weeks from the time of dispensing serves to remind patients that they are not being permanently dismissed and may serve as encouragement to practice in order to demonstrate improved skills when they return.

As with all optical devices, care and cleaning are important aspects to address. Knowledge in this area cannot be assumed. A telemicroscope should not be submerged in water. If condensation appears inside the unit, it should not be heated in the oven. The correct adjustment of the frame for lens position and comfort are integral to successful use.

When telemicroscopes are prescribed for surgeons or other health care providers, they should be reminded that they cannot be autoclaved. (Author's note: *Guess how I learned that!*)

## SUMMARY

The telemicroscope is the treatment of choice if the patient wants a spectacle-mounted device for near with the maximum work distance. Telemicroscopes have the disadvantages of increased weight, expense, and poor cosmesis but have the significant advantage of providing magnification at an extended work distance compared to the equivalent microscope.

## REFERENCES

1. *American National Standard for Ophthalmics—Low Vision Aids Requirements.* Merrifield, VA, Optical Laboratories Association, 1993, p 4.
2. Sloan LL: *Reading Aids for the Partially Sighted.* Baltimore, The Williams and Wilkins Company, 1977.
3. Smith G: Magnification of afocal telescopes when used focally. *Austr J Optom* 64(5): 202-205, 1981.
4. Englemann O: Subjective pupillary measurement. *Optom Weekly* September 28, 1961.

## ADDITIONAL READING

Bailey IL: Principles of near vision telescopes. *Optom Monthly* 72(9):32-34, 1981.
Bailey IL, Loshin DS: Keeler near vision telescopes. *J Vis Rehab* 3(2):19-21, 1985.
Jose RT, Morse SE: Telescopes: To cap or not to cap. *Rehab Optom J* 1(3):9-11, 1983.
Krefman RA: Working distance comparison of plus lenses and reading telescopes. *Am J Optom Physiol Optics* 57(11):835-838, 1980.
Loshin DS, Bailey IL: Standardization: Keeler near vision telescopes. *J Vis Rehab* 3(2):19-20, 1985.
Margach CB: Optical characteristics of focusable ophthalmic telescopes. *Opt J Rev Optom* 111(8):12-16, 1974.
Margach CB: Telescopic microscopes. *Opt J Rev Optom* 113(2):56-59, 1976.
Reich LN: Adjustable focus telescopes for near vision. *Optom Vis Sci* 68(3):183-188, 1991.
Williams DR: Magnification in telescopic loupes. *J Am Optom Assoc* 45(9):1068-1071, 1974.

# VERIFICATION OF OPTICAL DEVICES

> *Complex prescriptions and low vision devices often require special methods of verification. Just as with simple spectacles and contact lenses, it is not safe to trust that the laboratory will provide exactly what is ordered. It was also pointed out in earlier chapters that manufacturers often do not label their optical devices accurately and that there is some variability in optical properties among supposedly identical lenses. For these reasons, it is useful for the practitioner to be able to verify any optical device.*

## VERIFICATION OF TELESCOPE MAGNIFYING POWER

Telescope magnifying power can be verified in several ways. One method is to look through the telescope at a distant object and, keeping both eyes open, superimpose the magnified image over the unmagnified image in order to compare their relative sizes. This is not very accurate but is an easy way to estimate the power. A more accurate method is to measure the diameter of the entrance pupil and the diameter of the exit pupil and divide the latter into the former (Figure 16-1):

Magnification = Entrance pupil diameter/Exit pupil diameter

The diameter of the entrance pupil is the visible portion of the objective lens. The diameter of the exit pupil, however, is not the diameter of the visible part of the ocular. The exit pupil is seen by holding the telescope away from the eye and peering into the ocular. Within the diameter of the ocular, the exit pupil is seen as a small circle of light (Figure 16-2). It appears to be inside of a Galilean

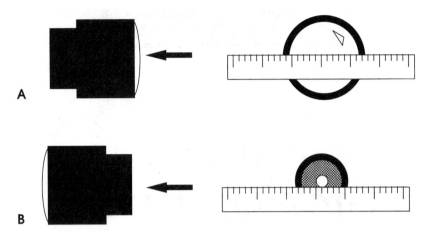

**Figure 16–1.** The magnifying power of a telescope is found by dividing the diameter of the entrance pupil by the diameter of the exit pupil. The diameter of the entrance pupil (**A**) is found by measuring the diameter of the visible opening at the objective lens. The diameter of the exit pupil (**B**) is found by measuring the small circle of light seen from the ocular side when holding the telescope away from the eye.

telescope and outside of a Keplerian telescope. In order to measure it accurately, the ruler should be in the same plane as the exit pupil. This is more difficult to visualize with a Galilean telescope since the exit pupil is within the housing of the device. The exit pupil is usually rather small, and this also makes an accurate measurement difficult; for example, a 5.0X telescope with a 20 mm objective diameter has an exit pupil diameter of only 4 mm, and a 1 mm error in measurement would give a significant error in the estimate of magnifying power.

For Galilean telescopes, Bailey[1] has shown a method of determining the power with the use of a lensometer. This technique is based on the vergence amplification property discussed earlier. A Galilean telescope that is either afocal or focused for distance should have a dioptric value of zero when read in the lensometer with the eyepiece against the lens stop (objective facing observer). When a +1.00 trial lens is placed against the objective, the emerging vergence is read in the lensometer. The expected value is based on the relationship:

$$A = M^2U/(1 - dMU)$$

where A is the vergence amplification, M is the magnification of the telescope, U is the vergence entering the telescope, and d is the length of the telescope in meters.[2] Since magnification is the unknown quantity, it can be found by solving the above equation for M.

$$0 = M^2U + AdUM + (-A)$$

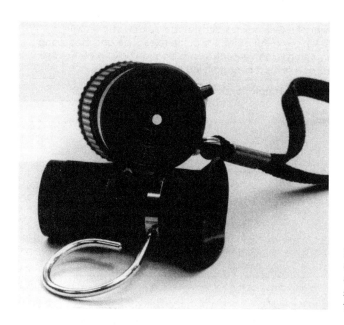

**Figure 16–2.** The exit pupil of the Keplerian telescope on top can be seen as a small circle of light within the diameter of the ocular.

The choice of a +1.00 D lens gives a value of +1.00 for U, and therefore

$$0 = M^2 + AdM + (-A)$$

This is a quadratic equation, and the general solution is

$$M = (-b \pm \sqrt{b^2 - 4ac})/2a$$

where, in this case, a = 1, b = Ad, and c = −A. Table 16-1 gives the magnification for a variety of measured amplification changes calculated on a spreadsheet. It is only necessary to know the length of the telescope, which can be measured with a ruler with acceptable accuracy by estimating the location of the objective and the ocular within the telescope housing. The reader should notice in Table 16-1 that, for a given vergence amplification, any error in measuring the length of the telescope has very little effect on the calculated magnifying power. Also, an error in reading the dioptric value of the vergence amplification has little effect on the outcome. Therefore, this is an inherently accurate procedure.

The lens separation, d, for a Keplerian telescope is less easily measured since the light path is altered by virtue of the image-erecting prism system. Because they are typically longer, Keplerian telescopes may not fit in a lensometer. An alternative method has been proposed[3, 4] for verifying the magnifying power of Keplerian telescopes based on the fact that the longitudinal magnification of an afocal telescope is proportional to the square of the angular magnifying power. In essence, the target is a plexiglass plate (n = 1.49) of known thickness

TABLE 16–1. The magnifying power of a Galilean telescope can be determined with a lensometer by placing a +1.00 D lens over the objective of the telescope and measuring the resultant back vertex power, which is the vergence amplification (VA). A comparison of VA with the length of the telescope gives the magnifying power.*

| | Length (cm) | | | | | |
|---|---|---|---|---|---|---|
| VA | 1 | 2 | 4 | 6 | 8 | 10 |
| 1.0 | 1.00 | 0.99 | 0.98 | 0.97 | 0.96 | 0.95 |
| 2.0 | 1.40 | 1.39 | 1.37 | 1.36 | 1.34 | 1.32 |
| 4.0 | 1.98 | 1.96 | 1.92 | 1.88 | 1.85 | 1.81 |
| 6.0 | 2.42 | 2.39 | 2.33 | 2.28 | 2.22 | 2.17 |
| 8.0 | 2.79 | 2.75 | 2.67 | 2.60 | 2.53 | 2.46 |
| 10.0 | 3.11 | 3.06 | 2.97 | 2.88 | 2.79 | 2.70 |
| 12.0 | 3.40 | 3.35 | 3.23 | 3.12 | 3.02 | 2.92 |
| 14.0 | 3.67 | 3.60 | 3.47 | 3.35 | 3.22 | 3.11 |
| 16.0 | 3.92 | 3.84 | 3.69 | 3.55 | 3.41 | 3.28 |
| 18.0 | 4.15 | 4.07 | 3.90 | 3.74 | 3.58 | 3.44 |
| 20.0 | 4.37 | 4.28 | 4.09 | 3.91 | 3.74 | 3.58 |

Example: A telescope that is 4 cm long and amplifies the vergence from a +1.00 lens to 18 D has a magnifying power of 3.90X.

*Based on the Bailey method[1] as described in the text.

(t) with a grid pattern on each surface. When the target is placed between the ocular and the location of the exit pupil with an illumination source behind it, two corresponding grid images will be located in front of the objective. Their separation is measured, and the magnifying power of the telescope is calculated as follows:

$$M^2 = \text{image separation}/(t/n)$$

This procedure, while not complex, is certainly not as convenient as the lensometer method described for Galilean telescopes and is therefore less likely to be used clinically.

## SPECTACLE Rx INCORPORATED IN A TELESCOPE OR TELEMICROSCOPE

If the patient's distance correction is incorporated in the ocular of a spectacle-mounted telescope, it can be verified with the lensometer by placing the frame in the lensometer in the usual manner and neutralizing the minified image. The image is minified because the telescope is reversed. A telemicroscope with a permanent "cap" built into the objective and the patient's prescription built into the ocular must be measured in two steps. First, a lens opposite in power to the cap power is placed against the objective of the telescope, and the patient's distance prescription is measured as described above. Next, the distance prescription is eliminated by holding the appropriate oppositely powered lens(es) against the ocular of the telescope, and the power of the cap is measured with the system reversed in the lensometer. This measures the front vertex power of the near focus lens, which is not the same as the equivalent power. These procedures can be practiced by using a small hand-held telescope that fits in the lensometer and holding lenses against the objective and/or ocular to simulate having the patient's prescription and/or a cap built into the system. The clinician should first verify that the telescope is afocal by focusing it on a very distant object and then fixing the focus adjustment with tape to ensure that it does not change.

Because of vergence amplification by a telescope, a significant measurement error may be introduced by a lensometer in which the reticle is not located precisely at the focal plane of the objective of the viewing system[5] even though the instrument seems to work fine for ophthalmic lenses. The function of a lensometer can be checked by using a telescope that is known to be afocal. The clinician can be sure that a telescope is afocal by focusing it on a very distant object. The eyepiece adjustment that gives a clear image through the afocal telescope can be marked on the lensometer for future reference.

A manual method can be used if the telescope does not fit in the lensometer. The procedure is to put a lens opposite in power to the presumed far or near correction (adjacent to the objective for a near correction or adjacent to the ocular for correction of ametropia) and then view a distant object. It should be in clear focus. The sensitivity of this method can be increased by using another telescope, known to be afocal, in tandem with the first. If the patient's telescope does not emit parallel light, the second telescope will amplify the vergence, and this will be obvious to the observer.

## HIGH PLUS OR MINUS LENSES

Most lensometers do not measure beyond 20 diopters in either direction, which makes it difficult to verify microscopes and high plus adds. Additionally, the lensometer measures vertex power, and we are often interested in equivalent power. The equivalent power ($F_e$) of any lens can be determined in the same manner as for stand magnifiers, by measuring the image size of a known object at a known distance and finding the equivalent focal length by similar triangles. This technique was presented in the section on stand magnifiers (Chapter 10) and will not be reviewed here. The equivalent power, $F_e$, can also be determined by measuring the curvature of the front and back surfaces and the center thickness ($F_e = F_1 + F_2 - (t/n)(F_1)(F_2)$); however, aspheric surfaces may not be measured accurately, and this will introduce a slight error in this result. If a quick approximation is desired for a convex lens, the image of a distant object can be focused on any surface and the distance from the surface to the lens measured. The measurement should be made from the position of the principal plane, which is not known. Therefore, this technique gives the approximate equivalent focal length. The reciprocal of this distance is therefore approximately equal to the equivalent power (Figure 16-3).

Neutralization is not a problem if the lensometer has sufficient range, but when it does not, there are some special techniques that can be used. A good lensometer will have an auxiliary cell for holding trial lenses (Figure 16-4). If the patient's glasses are +28.00 and the lensometer only reads to +20.00, it becomes necessary to use the auxiliary lens holder. If one had the equivalent of −8.00 in the auxiliary holder, it would be possible to neutralize the glasses by reading +20.00 and adding the power of the auxiliary lens; however, it is not quite as simple as placing any lens in the auxiliary holder. Since the auxiliary lens holder is not at the lens stop, any lens placed in it will have an effective power at the point of the lens stop that is different from its marked power. It is therefore necessary to place the auxiliary lens in the holder and read its effective power first by focusing the mire. Next, the glasses are inserted, and the resultant power is measured. This resultant power is adjusted for the effective power of the auxiliary lens to give the actual back vertex power of the glasses.

■ **Example 16-1.** A −10.00 D trial lens is placed in the auxiliary lens holder, and, when the mires are focused, it reads −7.25 D. The patient's glasses are now placed against the lens stop, and the resultant power is +17.50. What is the back vertex power *(bvp)* of the glasses?

$$+17.50 = bvp + (-7.25)$$
$$+17.50 - (-7.25) = bvp$$
$$+24.75 = bvp$$

If the lensometer does not have an auxiliary lens holder, it is possible to simply place a trial lens, of high enough opposite power, next to the spectacle

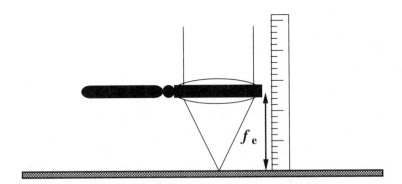

**Figure 16-3.** The equivalent power of a convex lens can be estimated by measuring its equivalent focal length. If a distant light source is focused on a flat surface, the distance from the lens to the surface is the equivalent focal length, $f_e$. This technique provides an approximation only since the measurement should actually be made to the principal plane, the position of which is unknown.

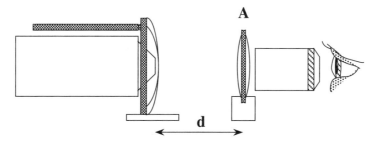

**Figure 16–4.** An auxiliary lens can be used to extend the range of a lensometer; however, since the auxiliary lens cell (A) is located some distance (d) from the lens stop, the lens will have an effective power that is different from its marked power. The effective power of the auxiliary lens should be measured with the lensometer before the ophthalmic device is neutralized.

lens and read the resultant back vertex power; however, this resultant power will not be exact due to the effective power difference caused by the trial lens being separated from the lens stop by the thickness of the lens being measured.

Adds must be neutralized in the correct manner to avoid rejecting glasses unnecessarily when they are returned from the laboratory. An add works in a different manner than the distance correction. The add takes divergent light and makes it parallel, while the distance correction takes parallel light and makes it converge or diverge (Figure 16-5). Because of this difference, one must determine the front vertex power of the add and the back vertex power of the distance correction. For low adds and/or low corrections, the add is measured in the same manner as the distance portion (that is, back vertex power). This rarely causes a problem since the power difference is negligible. The correct technique for neutralizing all adds, and high adds in particular, is to reverse the spectacles in the lensometer, read the distance portion, read the near portion, and take the difference as the correct power of the add (Figure 16-6).

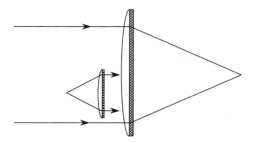

**Figure 16–5.** An add performs a different optical function from the distance correction. The add converts divergent light to parallel light, while the distance correction makes parallel light diverge or converge to be in focus on the retina. These two portions of the spectacle correction must be neutralized differently in the lensometer in order to determine the *front* vertex power of the add and the *back* vertex power of the distance correction.

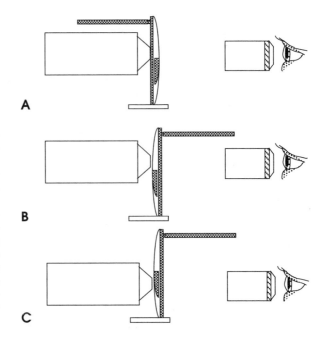

**Figure 16–6.** The correct procedure for neutralizing a spectacle correction with an add requires three steps. (**A**) The back vertex power of the distance portion is neutralized with the ocular surface of the lens against the lens stop. The glasses are then reversed, and the front vertex power is neutralized through the distance portion (**B**) and through the add (**C**). The difference between B and C is the correct power of the add.

This technique gives the front vertex power of the add. If the practitioner or assistant does not reverse the glasses to determine the add, there may be an apparent significant discrepancy between what was ordered and what was neutralized.

## VERIFICATION OF HAND AND STAND MAGNIFIERS

The reader will recall that the dioptric power of interest for magnifiers is equivalent power. The determination of equivalent power for any plus lens or lens system was covered in Chapter 10. Verification of the image location (i) and the enlargement factor (E) of a stand magnifier were also covered in Chapter 10. An approximation of $f_e$ (and hence $F_e$) for a hand-held magnifier may be made by imaging a distant light source on a flat surface as described previously in the section on high plus and minus lenses (see Figure 16–3).

## ANSI STANDARDS FOR LOW VISION DEVICES

The American National Standards Institute, Inc., has approved standards—designated as ANSI Z80.9-1993—for low vision aids.[6] These standards include definitions, specifications, design classifications, and methods for measurement of focal length, magnification of telescopes, telemicroscopes, transmittance, and prism power. They are available from the American National Standards Institute (see Resources, Chapter 31).

## SUMMARY

The parameters of low vision devices must be verified just as any other ophthalmic appliance must be. Manufacturers of "stock" items often label magnifying power and dioptric power according to different criteria than the clinician would use. Identical devices may have some degree of variation in their measured parameters due to relaxed quality control. Even custom-designed and fabricated lens systems are not always made as ordered. Just as with simple glasses, good clinical care includes verification of the optical parameters of any device before it is dispensed to the patient.

## REFERENCES

1. Bailey IL: A lensometer method for checking telescopes. *Optom Monthly* 70: 216-219, 1979.
2. Fried AN: Telescopes, vergences and accommodation. *Am J Optom Physiol Optics* 54:365-373, 1979.
3. Bailey IL: Measuring the magnifying power of Keplerian telescopes. *Applied Optics* 17:3520-3521, 1978.
4. Bailey IL: A new method for checking the power of common Keplerian telescopes. *Optom Monthly* 70:275-278, 1979.
5. Bailey IL: Checking the refractive correction in prescription telescopes. *Optom Monthly* 73(1):14-17, 1982.
6. *American National Standard for Ophthalmics—Low Vision Aids Requirements.* Merrifield, VA, Optical Laboratories Association, 1993.

## ADDITIONAL READING

Bailey IL: New method for determining the magnifying power of telescopes. *Am J Optom Physiol Opt* 55:203-207, 1978.
Bailey IL: Traditional methods for measuring the magnification of telescopes. *Optom Monthly* 70:127-131, 1979.
Bailey IL: Locating the image in stand magnifiers. *Optom Monthly* 72(6):22-24, 1981.
Bailey IL: Principles of near vision telescopes. *Optom Monthly* 72(9):32-34, 1981.
Bailey IL: Verifying near vision magnifiers, part 1. *Optom Monthly* 72(1):42-43, 1981.
Bailey IL: Verifying near vision magnifiers, part 2. *Optom Monthly* 72(2):34-38, 1981.

# CHAPTER XVII

# CONTACT LENS APPLICATIONS IN LOW VISION REHABILITATION

*For many conditions, contact lenses are the treatment of choice. Some examples include high refractive error as in pediatric aphakia, high astigmatism due to corneal toricity, reduced vision secondary to irregular corneas, reduced vision or monocular diplopia secondary to media abnormality, and a disfigured eye requiring cosmetic enhancement. Some disadvantages involved with prescribing contact lenses for people who are visually impaired are the difficulties involved with handling lenses and solutions that cannot be seen clearly and the tendency to overwear lenses when they offer a significantly better visual result compared to glasses.*

*Contact lenses can also be used as low vision devices or as part of an optical system as is described in the sections below on contact lens microscopes and telescopes.*

## CONTACT LENSES FOR MONOCULAR PATIENTS

When a contact lens is the treatment of choice for a person who is monocular, two major concerns are protection of the remaining eye with spectacles and the increased risk for loss of the remaining eye from contact lens-induced complications. Every person with monocular vision should wear protective spectacles. If a contact lens offers significantly better function or appearance, it should be prescribed in conjunction with protective spectacle lenses. One method used to ensure that the glasses are worn is to prescribe the majority of the correction in the contact lens and the remainder in the corresponding spectacle lens as an over-correction. If the person is presbyopic, the contact lens can have the full correction with the add placed in the spectacle lens. Someone with astigmatism might receive the spherical correction in the contact lens and the astigmatic correction in the spectacle. The patient must be carefully counseled about the potential result of losing the remaining eye and why protective lenses must be worn even with the contact lens.

A person who is visually impaired is less able to see potential contact lens-related problems such as redness of the eye, lens deposits or discoloration, and incorrect solutions with similar packaging. Also, if the lenses offer significantly better vision than glasses, they are more likely to overwear them. All of these potential problems are more acute with the monocular patient who cannot afford to place the remaining eye at increased risk for vision loss. Complications induced by contact lens wear can be minimized with more frequent follow-ups than would be required for someone who is normally sighted. The importance of this routine care must be emphasized, and contact lenses should not be considered for patients who do not appear to be good candidates from this point of view. Extended wear lenses should rarely, if ever, be considered for monocular patients. Even though the complication rate may be considered small, the possible consequences are not.

## THE CONTACT LENS MICROSCOPE

When a patient resists the appearance of a high plus add, it is possible to prescribe a "monovision" contact lens system in which the lens for near serves as a microscope rather than a conventional near add.[1] Cosmetically, this is a more pleasing option, although the near work distance may still make the user conspicuous. A disadvantage of this system that needs to be addressed is the loss of functional distance vision for a person who is already visually impaired; for example, the substantial monocular reduction in distance vision may affect mobility and safety. If the lens is to be worn only at the work station or during sedentary activities such as reading, this may not be a concern. The lens power is calculated in the same manner as for a spectacle microscope, and the total power must include the correction for the patient's refractive error. A power adjustment for the vertex distance of the microscope portion is not required since the lens is not for correcting a refractive error. It was shown earlier that a microscope functions the same regardless of where it is held as long as the print is maintained at the focal point of the lens.

## THE CONTACT LENS TELESCOPE

A Galilean telescope can be created with a high minus contact lens used in conjunction with a convex spectacle lens. The obvious advantages are that the system appears more normal compared to a spectacle-mounted telescope, and the exit pupil is as close to the entrance pupil of the eye as would be possible with any Galilean telescope except the IOL system. The obvious disadvantage is that the patient is constantly looking through a magnified system and must adjust to the altered visual space.

The ideal system would provide reasonable magnification and would have a vertex distance similar to ordinary spectacles. This may seem theoretically possible, but, unfortunately, there is an inherent optical problem. This is demonstrated in Table 17-1, in which it can be seen that for a normal vertex distance of 10 mm, the contact lens and spectacle lens powers must be very high in order to achieve reasonable magnification. This optical limitation necessitates the use of telescope systems that have low magnification, usually less than 2.0X. Lower contact lens powers require a longer vertex distance. This can be seen in Table 17-1 by comparing the vertex distances required for a given magnification and several different contact lens powers (for example, rows 1, 6, and 11). A vertex distance greater than ≈10 mm requires a special frame with extendable nose pads. Unfortunately, when these conditions are maintained, the powers of the contact lens and spectacle lens are so high that the system is virtually unusable. Example 17-1 demonstrates the procedure for designing a contact lens telescope and the inherent problems.

TABLE 17-1. Example parameters of selected contact lens telescope examples.

| Magnification | Vertex distance (m) | Contact lens (D) | Spectacle lens (D) |
| --- | --- | --- | --- |
| 1.2 | 0.010 | −20.00 | +16.67 |
| 1.4 | 0.010 | −40.00 | +28.57 |
| 1.6 | 0.010 | −60.00 | +37.50 |
| 1.8 | 0.010 | −80.00 | +44.44 |
| 2.0 | 0.010 | −100.00 | +50.00 |
| 1.2 | 0.015 | −13.33 | +11.11 |
| 1.4 | 0.015 | −26.67 | +19.05 |
| 1.6 | 0.015 | −40.00 | +25.00 |
| 1.8 | 0.015 | −53.33 | +29.63 |
| 2.0 | 0.015 | −66.67 | +33.33 |
| 1.2 | 0.020 | −10.00 | +8.33 |
| 1.4 | 0.020 | −20.00 | +14.29 |
| 1.6 | 0.020 | −30.00 | +18.75 |
| 1.8 | 0.020 | −40.00 | +22.22 |
| 2.0 | 0.020 | −50.00 | +25.00 |

Example: A 1.8X system with a 15 mm vertex distance requires a −53.33 D contact lens and a +29.63 D spectacle lens (ouch!).

■ **Example 17-1.** Design a contact lens telescope that allows a patient to read the equivalent of 20/60 if his reference acuity is 20/120 and his refractive correction with a contact lens is +10.00. Assume that the vertex distance (d) is 15 mm. The objective, $F_1$, is the spectacle lens, and the ocular, $F_2$, is the contact lens.

Magnification required = Reference size/Goal size
Magnification required = 120/60
Magnification required = 2.0X

$$M_{ts} = -F_2/F_1$$
$$M_{ts} = -(f_1/f_2)$$
$$2.0X = -(f_1/f_2)$$
$$-2.0f_2 = f_1$$

$$d = f_1 + f_2$$
$$15 \text{ mm} = f_1 + f_2$$
$$15 \text{ mm} = -2f_2 + f_2 \text{ (by substitution from above)}$$
$$15 \text{ mm} = -1f_2$$
$$15 \text{ mm} = -f_2$$
$$-15 \text{ mm} = f_2$$

$$F_2 = 1000/f_2$$
$$F_2 = 1000/-15$$
$$F_2 = -66.67 \text{ D}$$

$$M_{ts} = -F_2/F_1$$
$$2.0X = -(-66.67)/F_1$$
$$F_1 = +66.67/2.0$$
$$F_1 = +33.33 \text{ D}$$

For a 2.0X telescope with a vertex distance of 15 mm, he needs a +33.33 spectacle lens and a −66.67 contact lens, but since he also needs a +10.00 contact lens to correct his refractive error, the net power for the contact lens is:

$$-66.67 + (+10.00) = -56.67 \text{ D}$$

Other spectacle/contact lens combinations can be used to create a 2.0X telescope, but if lower powers are used, the vertex distance increases, and if higher powers are used, neither is wearable. The only other alternative is to reduce the magnification, which is why contact lens telescope systems are not particularly useful. While some practitioners report extraordinary results with these systems, they have not found general acceptance.

Finally, if the reader finds the sign convention confusing in the calculation of a contact lens telescope system, it is possible to simply ignore it and use all positive numbers, provided that one remembers that the contact lens is negative in power, the glasses are positive, and the vertex distance, d, is the difference of the two focal lengths, both expressed as positive numbers (Figure 10-1). This allows the following formulas to be used:

$$\text{Magnification required} = \text{Reference size/Goal size}$$
$$M_{ts} = F_2/F_1 \text{ (all positive)}$$
$$M_{ts} = f_1/f_2 \text{ (all positive)}$$
$$d = f_1 - f_2 \text{ (all positive)}$$
$$F_2 = 1000/d \text{ (remember that } F_2 \text{ is negative)}$$

## NYSTAGMUS

Contact lenses have been considered as a potential treatment for nystagmus. One theory is that edge rub against the palpebral conjunctiva would provide feedback inhibition and lessen the amplitude of the eye movement. It is also possible that an improved retinal image might contribute to lessening the amplitude of the nystagmus. A contact lens telescope system has also been used for image stabilization in an attempt to reduce nystagmus. Contact lenses have not found general acceptance as a treatment for nystagmus, and there have been no adequate clinical studies to support a therapeutic effect. Image stabilization and other contact lens applications for nystagmus are covered in greater detail in Chapter 27.

## OTHER APPLICATIONS

It is assumed that the reader is familiar with the traditional uses of contact lenses to improve cosmesis and correct refractive errors. An opaque contact lens with an artificial pupil may also be used for illumination control for persons with aniridia, albinism, or other conditions causing photophobia. They should be considered for infants who are exposed to excessive light levels and who do not tolerate glasses. Artificial pupils have also been used for treating monocular diplopia and polyopia,[2] and a totally opaque lens may be used for intractable diplopia or polyopia.

In a nontraditional application, the author has used a minus powered hard contact lens as the ocular of a Galilean telescope by cementing it to a peripheral portion of a patient's spectacle lens. The patient can then use a hand-held plus lens as the objective lens for occasional spotting or separately as a simple magnifier for reading (Figure 17-1).

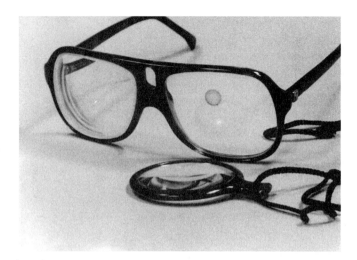

**Figure 17–1.** A negative power contact lens glued to a spectacle lens serves as the ocular of a Galilean telescope. A hand-held convex lens serves as the objective for occasional spotting and can be used otherwise as a simple magnifier.

## SUMMARY

Contact lenses have many applications in vision rehabilitation. In addition to certain conditions where they are the treatment of choice, they may be used to create microscope and telescope systems. They have important roles in improving cosmesis for those who have disfigured eyes, in management of diplopia or polyopia, and in illumination control for those with photophobia or who are at increased risk for excessive light exposure. The value of contact lenses in the control of nystagmus requires more definitive clinical studies.

## REFERENCES

1. Eldred KB: Use of a contact lens as a microscope. *J Vis Rehab* 3(2):23–28, 1989.
2. Crews J, Gordon AG, Nowakowski RW: Management of monocular polyopia using an artificial iris contact lens. *J Am Optom Assoc* 59:140–142, 1988.

## ADDITIONAL READING

Abadi RV, Papas EB: Visual performance with artificial iris contact lenses. *J Brit Contact Lens Assoc* 10:10–15, 1987.
Baglien JW, Middleton RV: Telescopic device with corneal contact lenses. *Optom Weekly* 43:39, 1952.

Bettman JW, McNair GS: Contact-lens telescopic system. *Am J Ophthalmol* 22:27, 1939.

Byer A: Magnification limitations of a contact lens telescope. *Am J Optom Physiol Optics* 63:724–732, 1986.

Jose RT, Browning R: Designing a bioptic contact lens telescopic system. *Am J Optom* 60(1):74–79, 1983.

Jose RT: Contact lens telescopic system—Part 2. *Optom Weekly* 67(23):624–625, 1976.

Lewis HT: Parameters of contact lens-spectacle telescopic systems and considerations in prescribing. *Am J Optom Physiol Optics* 63:387–391, 1986.

Ludlam WM: Clinical experience with the contact lens telescope. *Am J Optom Arch Am Acad Optom* 37(7):363–372, 1960.

Piccolo M, Jose RT: Contact lenses for the multiply impaired. *Rehab Optom J* 1(2):7–8, 1983.

Rosenbloom AA: The controlled-pupil contact lens in low vision. *J Am Optom Assoc* 40(8):836–840, 1969.

Weiss NJ: CL telescopic system—with a soft lens!—Part 1. *Optom Weekly* 67(22): 597–600, 1976.

Williams CE: Contact lenses as used in subnormal vision. *J Am Optom Assoc* 32(8): 636–637, 1961.

Woo G: Use of contact lenses in low vision. *Optom Weekly* 66(29):768–771, 1975.

# CHAPTER XVIII

# VISUAL FIELD ENHANCEMENT

A loss of visual field can be as debilitating as a reduction in visual acuity or even more so. Even with good central acuity, a person with very constricted visual fields is functionally impaired with respect to mobility. The ability to read is also hampered if the loss makes it difficult to track across the page or visualize more than a few letters in a word.

Just as it is not possible to restore vision with optical devices, it is not possible to restore a person's lost visual field. It is therefore not appropriate to refer to this area of treatment as field expansion. A person's visual field cannot be expanded. However, the ability to utilize the remaining field more effectively can be enhanced, and this mode of treatment is therefore referred to as field enhancement rather than field expansion. If patients do not understand this subtle difference, they may expect much more than can be provided and hence may reject an otherwise useful treatment option.

A partial field loss and an overall field constriction are distinguished with respect to which type of therapy is considered first. Although any field enhancement technique may be helpful in either case, different techniques should be considered first for each type. Reversed telescopes and concave lenses may be most useful for an overall restriction, whereas Fresnel prisms and hemianopic mirrors are more often useful for partial field loss; however, these are generalizations, not absolute rules.

A measure of the visual field that does not include both central and peripheral isopters is not adequate for assessing the potential need for field enhancement. The tangent screen and some automated perimeters do not provide adequate measures of the peripheral extent of the visual field. Confrontation fields provide information about the peripheral field but should be considered only a gross form of assessment. Conversely, a threshold visual field, if it can be accomplished, may be misleading with respect to the functional implications of a subtle field depression. The measured visual field may be suggestive of functional limitations but is not the definitive test. Most *people seem to function well with a field as narrow as 20° in widest diameter. Once the field is restricted to 10° in widest diameter, difficulties with mobility and other activities typically emerge. Between these two values, there is considerable variation in function. When the clinician is considering whether or not to try field enhancement, it is important to obtain some indication about whether or not the patient's function is impaired. This cannot be determined simply by a measurement of the visual field, although that is certainly an important part of the overall evaluation. Functional ability can be established by a careful interview with respect to daily activities, particularly those related to mobility. Patients should be asked about problems such as difficulty crossing the street, bumping into objects, finding their way around in unfamiliar areas, tracking while reading, seeing the food on their plate, or seeing items on the desk or dinner table. Problems in these areas are also related to visual acuity, and an attempt should be made to distinguish whether the patient believes his or her problems are based on inability to distinguish objects clearly or rather inability to see them at all. Family members or care givers should be able to offer additional observations that will be helpful. The clinician can also take advantage of the opportunity to watch the patient move about the office setting. A formal assessment of mobility can be obtained by a certified orientation and mobility instructor.*

## SCANNING

Perhaps the simplest method of enhancing one's visual field is to use effective techniques of scanning. When the field of view is restricted, it is necessary to learn systematic approaches to scanning the environment in order to encompass the area of concern adequately. While simple techniques can be taught to the patient by a clinician, this is an area in which the assistance of a certified orientation and mobility instructor can be most effective. He or she is trained to teach these techniques systematically, in a real world setting, by accompanying the patient while traveling on planned lessons in the community.

## REVERSED TELESCOPES

When a person looks through a telescope in the reverse direction, there is an apparent increase in the field of view approximately equal to the power of the telescope; for example, a 2X telescope provides approximately twice the field when the telescope is reversed as opposed to viewing without it. A significant disadvantage of this technique is that the object of regard is minified by the same amount; therefore, the patient effectively has a reduction in acuity equal to the power of the telescope (Example 18-1). This limits the usefulness of the technique, and, in general, only lower power telescopes can be used effectively. Reversed telescopes can be mounted in spectacles or held in the hand for occasional spotting. When mounted in spectacles, they have the additional disadvantages of weight and poor cosmesis, although these can be reduced by using smaller telescopes. A patient might use a reversed hand-held telescope for spotting by pausing at the entrance to a room or building and scanning the area for obstacles before entering. While reversed telescopes are primarily useful for improving mobility, other uses have been mentioned by patients such as being able to view an entire chessboard at once rather than having to scan multiple times to complete the view.

A spectacle-mounted reversed telescope developed by Designs for Vision, Inc., incorporates a cylindrical effect in such a manner that the vertical dimension retains its normal size while the horizontal dimension is minified.[1] The design theory was that a person could adapt better if there were one meridian with size constancy. This device, the Amorphic® lens (Figure 18-1), is expensive, bulky, and cosmetically displeasing, and has not found wide usage. It is available in the following powers: $-1.2$, $-1.4$, $-1.6$, $-1.8$, and $-2.0X$. The manufacturer's use of the negative sign is to indicate minification, not an inverted image.

■ **Example 18-1.** A patient has best corrected acuity of 20/100, and her visual field is restricted to 5° in widest diameter. What will the apparent field increase be with a reversed 2.5X telescope, and what will the apparent reduction in visual acuity be when spotting through that telescope?

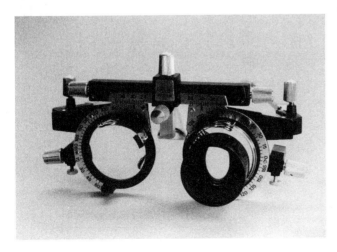

**Figure 18-1.** The Amorphic lens from Designs for Vision, Inc., was designed for field enhancement. The field is primarily compressed in the horizontal meridian, while normal size constancy is preserved in the vertical meridian. This cylindrical effect is suggested by the elliptical aperture visible within the lens. These lenses are meant to be permanently mounted in spectacles and are available in a trial ring as shown here.

The reversed telescope allows 2.5X more visual field to be included at one time for an apparent increase to 12.5° (2.5 × 5° = 12.5°). When spotting through the telescope, the visual acuity is effectively reduced to 20/250 (100 × 2.5 = 250) since everything seen through the telescope is reduced 2.5X.

The apparent reduction in visual acuity may seem more dramatic to the clinician than to the patient. The acuity of 20/250 for the patient in Example 18-1 may still be adequate for spotting obstacles and for general mobility. After all, the purpose of the reversed telescope is to enhance mobility, not read an acuity chart. Obstacles such as cars, tables, lamps, and other people are still large enough to be detected.

## FRESNEL PRISMS

Fresnel prisms are used to move the image of an object in the patient's nonseeing area closer to the functional retinal area. This is accomplished by placing a prism in front of the eye, with the base in the direction of the field loss (Figure 18-2). This allows the person to see the object with a smaller eye and/or head turn than would otherwise be necessary. In other words, no effect is appreciated until the gaze is actually shifted into the prism, but the shift in gaze required to detect the object is less than would be required without the prism. A prism on the order of 15$^\Delta$ to 25$^\Delta$ in power is usually needed to produce a noticeable effect. Therefore, it is necessary to use the Fresnel membrane type prisms to reduce weight and thickness. These prisms are applied to the back surface of the spectacle lens, and, since they are easily removed, it is possible to

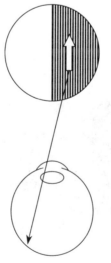
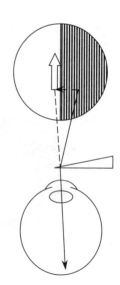

**Figure 18-2.** A prism can be used for field enhancement. It is placed before the eye with the base in the direction of the field loss. The image of an object in the nonseeing area is displaced towards the apex and hence is closer to the seeing portion of the retina. The viewer is able to see the object by looking into the prism, which requires a smaller eye movement than would have been required without the prism.

experiment with different powers until a satisfactory amount is found. Powers up to 30$^\Delta$ may be used successfully. The prism is typically applied to only part of the lens and is placed in such a manner that the apical edge is just outside of the patient's line of sight in straight-ahead gaze. The prism usually covers the remainder of the lens on the side of the field loss, although it is possible to use smaller portions if desired. Figure 18–3 shows the placement of a Fresnel prism before the right eye of a patient with a right hemianopsia. It is usually easier, in the author's experience, for the patient to adapt to one prism at a time, although any induced diplopia must be ignored when looking through the prism. A second prism can be added for the opposite eye, but placement becomes somewhat more difficult in order to allow the patient to enter both prisms simultaneously with lateral gaze. The principle of placing the prism with the base in the direction of the field loss is applicable to other field losses, in different directions than for the right hemianopsia as illustrated in Figure 18–3. An arrangement that has worked for some patients with very constricted fields secondary to retinitis pigmentosa is two narrow strips on either side of the pupil for each eye. Similarly, the prism could be applied above and/or below the line of sight for an altitudinal loss.

Fresnel prisms have some disadvantages. There is an induced scotoma and "jack-in-the-box" image jump when the patient's gaze enters and leaves the prism as well as chromatic aberration and image degradation. Each of these is more noticeable with higher power prisms. Fresnel prisms may also be less useful if the patient has a high plus or minus spectacle correction because of the additive effect of peripheral aberrations. The appearance is more acceptable cosmetically if the spectacle lens is tinted a light tan, which makes the prism(s) much less noticeable. Fresnel prisms may be difficult to clean and may have to

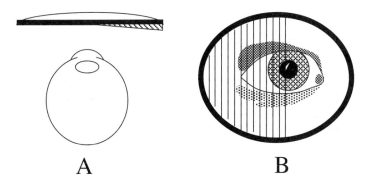

A                           B

**Figure 18–3.** (**A**) A Fresnel prism, used for field enhancement, is placed on the posterior surface of the lens. (**B**) For a right hemianopsia, the prism is placed over the temporal portion of the right lens with the apex just lateral to the viewer's line of sight in straight-ahead gaze.

be reapplied periodically. The patient can be taught to reapply the prisms and to clean them gently with a cotton-tipped applicator or soft cloth.

The Fresnel prism is probably the most successful form of therapy for field enhancement. One review of 22 patients fitted with Fresnel prisms over a four-year period found an acceptance rate of 86.3% (19 patients), with periods of continuous use varying from two to 26 months.[2] It is important to note that each of these patients had received extensive training in the use of the prism.

■ **Example 18-2.** A clinician decides to try a single 15$^\Delta$ Fresnel membrane for a patient with a bilateral left hemianopsia. How would the prism be oriented on the patient's glasses?

Because the field loss is to the left, the prism would be oriented base-out on the temporal half of the left lens.

### How to Apply a Fresnel Prism

Figure 18-4 illustrates and describes how to cut and shape a Fresnel prism for the most cosmetically pleasing end result. The orientation of the base should be determined such that it will be in the correct direction when applied to the *back* of the spectacle lens. The Fresnel membrane is applied to the back of the lens because it adheres better to a concave surface. The desired location of the apex is marked on the spectacle lens while the patient is wearing it in the normal manner. The Fresnel membrane is cut vertically with a razor blade and a straight edge because cutting with scissors invariably makes a crooked line. Filing the peripheral excess may seem inefficient, but it results in a smooth edge, which looks best, gives a better fit at the edge, and helps the prism stay in place longer. The excess membrane comes off in a long, thin strip. The end result is a membrane that is cut to match exactly the shape of the spectacle lens and is beveled parallel with the lens bevel. Both the membrane and the lens are then cleaned thoroughly and placed under water in a sink or bowl. All bubbles are pressed out from the center toward the edge as the membrane is pressed in place against the lens. When this has been accomplished, the lens with the adherent membrane is placed in a secure spot and allowed to dry. Until it has dried, the membrane is not firmly adherent and can be slipped out of place with light pressure. Once dry, the spectacle lens can then be replaced in the frame. Drying can be hastened with a blower and/or by applying the Fresnel with alcohol instead of water.

### MIRRORS

A small plano mirror can be fastened to a patient's frame to reflect the image of an object in the nonseeing area closer to the functional retinal area. The principle applied here is much the same as that for the Fresnel prism but with the sig-

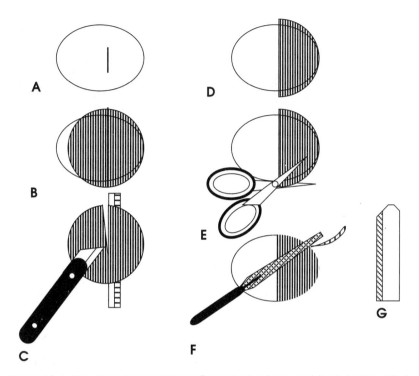

**Figure 18–4.** Directions for applying a Fresnel prism to an ophthalmic lens. (**A**) A mark is made on the spectacle lens where the apex of the prism will be located. (**B**) A corresponding mark is made on the prism, making sure that the base is in the correct direction. (**C**) The membrane is cut along the apex line with a sharp razor blade and straight edge. (**D**) The membrane is pressed in place, dry, on the posterior surface of the lens, and (**E**) most of the excess is removed with scissors. The remainder of the excess membrane is removed by holding the prism in place and filing carefully around the periphery (**F**) to match the bevel of the lens (**G**). The membrane is then applied wet and allowed to dry (see text). (The author is indebted to Mr. Al Pierce, who taught him this technique.)

nificant disadvantage that the mirror must be placed so that it actually blocks some of the remaining useful visual field (Figure 18-5). This may preclude successful use by monocular patients. The image is also reversed, but this can be adapted to readily, much as drivers do with their rearview mirrors. The mirror is more noticeable than the Fresnel prism and may be rejected by patients concerned with cosmesis. Small clip-on mirrors are available from the Jardon Institute (see Resources, Chapter 31) for diagnostic evaluation, or they may be dispensed as the final prescription form, which has the advantage of providing a device that is easily removable for intermittent or selective use (Figure 18-6). The mirrors used by cyclists can also be adapted for trial use. A mirror is usually a better choice than a prism when the desired amount of image displacement is

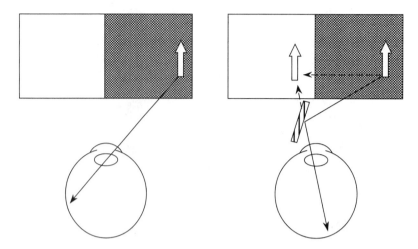

**Figure 18–5.** A mirror used for visual field enhancement displaces the image of an object in the nonseeing area closer to the seeing area. The main disadvantage, compared to a Fresnel lens, is that the mirror blocks part of the remaining visual field.

large. This general rule is primarily a consequence of the increasing chromatic aberration associated with increasing prism power.

The final prescription is usually provided in a metal frame to which the mirror housing can be soldered (Figure 18-7). The metal frame can be removed later if desired. With a metal mount it is easy to alter the direction of the mirror

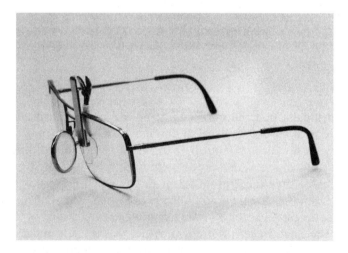

**Figure 18–6.** These clip-on mirrors from Jardon Eye Prosthetics, Inc., can be used to demonstrate the effect of a hemianopic mirror that may be permanently mounted if the trial is successful.

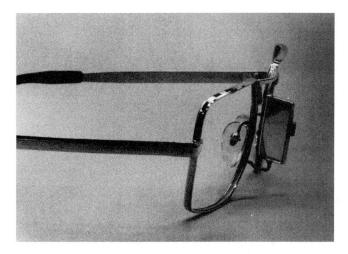

**Figure 18–7.** This permanently mounted hemianopic mirror was prescribed for a person with a right hemianopsia.

to the precise viewing angle. The mirror is usually applied to the front of the frame but can also be applied to the back, although this carries some risk of injury to the globe in the event of an accident. A mirror in a plastic housing can be applied to a plastic frame with acetone using an acetate strip,[3] but adjustment of the angle is more difficult, and removal of the mirror leaves a cosmetic defect that is more difficult to repair satisfactorily than a soldered joint on a metal frame.

Semireflective mirrors have been used to reduce the effect of blocking the remaining visual field. The user sees two images simultaneously, the one reflected from the nonseeing area being dimmer. A full-field semireflective mirror has been used with some success by one author.[3, 4]

## CONCAVE LENSES

A concave lens creates a minified image and can provide the user with a larger field of view, much like the reversed telescope, with overall minification. Because the lens is hand-held, it is used as a spotting device to orient the patient to obstacles, landmarks, or objects of interest on a short-term basis (Figures 18–8 and 18–9).

Kozlowski et al.[5, 6] proposed the use of a large-diameter concave lens, hand-held at a specific distance in front of the eye, and presented a procedure for determining the appropriate lens and distance at which it should be held. When a negative lens is held in front of the eye for viewing a distant object, the image is minified and located a finite distance in front of the lens. The eye must

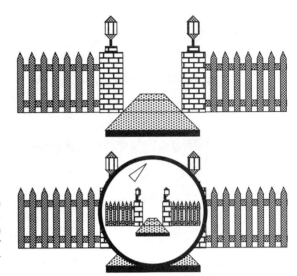

**Figure 18–8.** A concave lens can be used for field enhancement. The minified image seen through the lens gives an effectively larger field of view but a concomitant reduction in apparent acuity.

accommodate to see the image clearly, and the combination of a concave lens (F) and the plus lens of the accommodating eye (A) forms a reversed Galilean telescope. The relationships that follow are illustrated in Figure 18–10. The apparent increase in the visual field is equal to the magnification of the system, which is F/A. In order to utilize the entire lens, it should be held at a point

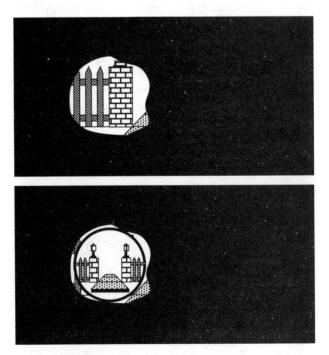

**Figure 18–9.** A concave lens may be useful for mobility by allowing the user to spot obstacles before proceeding.

where it is at least as wide as the visual field (V). For any diameter lens (d) the distance it should be held from the eye (h) to achieve this relationship is given by h = (d/2)/tan(V/2). Once h is known, F is given by F = (M − 1)/h, and A is given by A = F/M. The patient must be able to accommodate sufficiently to have a clear image or an add will be required. He or she must also be able to hold the lens comfortably at the distance h. One method proposed to assist the patient in holding the lens at the correct distance is to suspend the lens on a cord to be worn around the neck such that the lens is at distance h when the cord is taut. Just as with a reversed telescope, the image is minified, and the patient's acuity must be adequate to perceive useful detail within the minified image. Examples of selected concave lenses and the system parameters are given in Table 18-1.

■ **Example 18–3.** A young man's visual field (V) is restricted to 10° in widest diameter. What power concave lens, 60 mm in diameter, will give him an apparent 50° visual field, and how much will he have to accommodate when using it?

$$M = 50°/10°$$
$$M = 5X$$
$$h = d/2/Tan(V/2)$$
$$h = (60/2)/Tan(10°/2)$$
$$h = 30/Tan(5°)$$
$$h = 30/0.08749$$
$$h = 342.89 \text{ mm, or } 0.3429 \text{ m}$$
$$F = (M − 1)/h$$
$$F = (5 − 1)/0.3429$$
$$F = 11.67 \text{ D } (−11.67 \text{ actually})$$
$$A = F/M$$
$$A = 11.67/5$$
$$A = 2.33$$

Therefore, he will get 5X field enhancement from a −11.67 D lens held 34.29 cm from the eye, and he will have to accommodate 2.33 D. This result

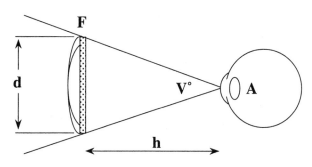

**Figure 18–10.** A concave lens, used for visual field enhancement, is essentially a reversed Galilean telescope. The lens, F, is held at a distance h that allows the diameter of the lens, d, to fill the visual field, V°, at that distance. The second lens, A, is provided by accommodation or an add. The calculation of these various parameters for a given degree of field enhancement is described in the text.

**TABLE 18–1. Concave lenses for field enhancement: the effect of changing lens diameter on power, eye-lens distance, and accommodation.***

|                            | #1      | #2      | #3     | #4      | #5      | #6     |
| -------------------------- | ------- | ------- | ------ | ------- | ------- | ------ |
| Field of view              | 10°     | 10°     | 10°    | 10°     | 10°     | 10°    |
| Minification desired       | 5X      | 5X      | 5X     | 5X      | 5X      | 5X     |
| Diameter of lens (mm)      | 30      | 40      | 50     | 60      | 70      | 80     |
| Lens power needed          | −23.33  | −17.50  | −14.00 | −11.67  | −10.00  | −8.75  |
| Eye-to-lens distance (cm)  | 17.15   | 22.86   | 28.58  | 34.29   | 40.01   | 45.72  |
| Accommodation required†    | 4.67    | 3.50    | 2.80   | 2.33    | 2.00    | 1.75   |

Example: A person with a 10° field will achieve 5X field enhancement with a 60 mm diameter concave lens of −11.67 D held 34.29 cm from the eye but must accommodate 2.33 D. The reader should note that using a large diameter lens to achieve the same level of enhancement requires less power and less accommodation, but it must be held farther from the eye.
*Based on the technique of Kozlowski[5, 6] as described in the text. †Accommodation can be replaced by the appropriate add.

can also be found from column #4 in Table 18-1. If this form of therapy is used frequently enough, the calculations can be simplified by entering the formulas in a computer spreadsheet.

Hand-held negative lenses can be obtained by simply ordering lens blanks from the laboratory. The edge of an uncut lens blank is often sharp, so it is a good idea to have it beveled smooth. An ophthalmic laboratory can cut the blank to a circular pattern of any diameter and bevel the edges. It is simple to drill a small hole through the periphery for attaching a cord or ribbon. Concave lenses with an attached cord, similar to a monocle, are also available from the Lighthouse in New York (see Resources, Chapter 31).

## IMAGE RELOCATION WITHOUT FIELD RESTRICTION

Some patients benefit from image relocation even though they do not have a visual field loss. Patients who are bedridden or who have restricted movement of the head may require relocation of the image for an object to be viewed. An example, in the case of bedridden patients, is the use of prisms such as the NAP prism[7] in order to view a television at the foot of the bed even though the face is turned toward the ceiling. The NAP prism deflects the beam approximately 90° but keeps the image erect. Other examples of conditions potentially necessitating image relocation are torticollis, synostosis, and spinal curvature secondary to osteoporosis. Prisms and mirrors can each be used successfully in these instances.

## READING WITH A FIELD LOSS

A right hemianopsia, or other substantial field loss to the right, can make reading difficult because the patient must track into the blind area. Simple compensating devices such as a reading guide or ruler may facilitate tracking (Figure 18–11). Reading guides are referred to as typoscopes.[8] While some are available for purchase, they also can be made from black construction paper with a razor blade. The typoscope actually offers several advantages to the reader: the black surround reduces glare, the cut-out area defines the target, and the straight edge facilitates tracking.

An alternative approach to the use of a reading guide is to have the patient reorient the print in order to track into a seeing area or even to keep the print entirely within the reading area; for example, a patient with a right hemianopsia might hold the book so that the print is oriented vertically and hence contained entirely within the seeing area (Figure 18–12). It is also possible to hold the print upside down and backwards in order to track into the seeing area, although the eyes must still return toward the nonseeing area to pick up the next line (Figure 18–12). While it may seem difficult to read print at oblique orientations, one can adapt to it with practice.

An individual who has suffered head trauma or a stroke may have difficulty reading because of alexia as well as a field loss. Any attempt at rehabilitation with prosthetic devices should take this into account before declaring a device unsuccessful.

## TRAINING

Regardless of the type of therapy recommended for a patient with a field restriction, the possibility of success is positively correlated with the degree of training provided. The training regimen can be adapted from that pro-

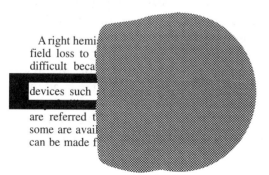

**Figure 18–11.** A reading or tracking guide may be useful when trying to read in the direction of a field loss.

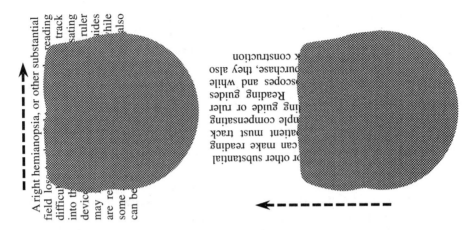

**Figure 18–12.** When reading is complicated by a field loss to the right, it is possible to orient the print in a different direction, even upside down and backwards, to allow the reader to track (dotted arrow) in a seeing direction.

posed for those who learn to use a spectacle-mounted telescope for driving (Chapter 23).

The effect of a reversed telescope, mirror, or concave lens is usually immediately apparent to the user. A Fresnel prism, however, may require a planned demonstration in order for the patient to appreciate its effect. This can be accomplished by using a hand-held prism with an object, such as the examiner's face, just outside the patient's field of view. When the prism is inserted, the object should "jump" into view. This demonstration can be performed with the patient in straight-ahead gaze but is more effective if he or she is gazing in the direction of the field loss.

The induced scotoma caused by looking into a prism may represent a hazard if the patient is not made aware of it and taught how to compensate for it. A technique for compensating is to look into the prism, scan toward the field loss by turning the head, look out of the prism, and scan back to straight ahead. This procedure produces two scotomas—one when looking into the prism and one passing back out of the prism. The missed areas are covered by the head turns. The first scotoma is covered when the head is rotated back to straight-ahead gaze with the line of sight out of the prism. The second induced scotoma was already covered when the head was rotated to the right while looking through the prism.

## SUMMARY

Field enhancement is useful for those who experience a functional problem caused by their field limitation, regardless of the measured extent of the visual field. In order to design a field enhancement therapy, it is necessary to measure the complete extent of the central and peripheral field. Fresnel prisms are the most successful optical form of therapy for field enhancement. Whether an optical aid is prescribed or not, the patient may benefit from evaluation and training by a certified orientation and mobility instructor.

## REFERENCES

1. Hoeft WW, Feinbloom W, Brilliant R, Gordon R, Hollander C, Newman J, Noval E, Rosenthal, B, Voss E: Amorphic lenses: A mobility aid for patients with retinitis pigmentosa. *Am J Optom Physiol Opt* 62(2):142–148, 1985.
2. Hoppe E, Perlin RR: The effectivity of Fresnel prisms for visual field enhancement. *J Am Optom Assoc* 64(1):46–53, 1993.
3. Goodlaw E: Rehabilitation of the patient with homonymous hemianopsia. *J Vis Rehab* 7:13–16, 1993.
4. Goodlaw E: Rehabilitating a patient with bitemporal hemianopia. *Am J Optom Physiol Opt* 59(7):617–619, 1982.
5. Kozlowski JMD, Mainster MA, Avila MP: Negative-lens field expander for patients with concentric field constriction. *Arch Ophthalmol* 102:1182–1184, 1984.
6. Kozlowski JMD, Jalkh AE: An improved negative-lens field expander for patients with concentric field constriction. *Arch Ophthalmol* 103:326, 1985.
7. Smith G, Johnston AW, Maddocks JD: The NAP prism. *Optom Vis Sci* 67:133–137, 1990.
8. Mehr EB: The typoscope of Charles Prentice. *Am J Optom Arch Am Acad Optom* 46(11):885–887, 1969.

## ADDITIONAL READING

Bailey IL: Field expanders. *Optom Monthly* 69:813–816, 1978.
Bailey IL: Prismatic treatment of field defects. *Optom Monthly* 69:1073–1078, 1978.
Bell E Jr.: A mirror for patients with hemianopsia. *JAMA* 140:1024, 1949.
Burns TA, Hanley WJ, Pietri JF, et al.: Spectacles for hemianopia: A clinical evaluation. *Am J Ophthalmol,* 35:1489–1492, 1952.
Campbell MCW, Ellison PJ, Strong JG, Lovasik JV: Unexpectedly large enhancement of a severely constricted field with reverse Galilean telescopes. *Optom Vis Sci* 66(5):276–280, 1989.
Ciuffreda KJ: A new field expander. A preliminary report. *Optom Weekly* 68(5):29–30, 1977.

Cohen JM, Waiss B: An overview of enhancement techniques for peripheral field loss. *J Am Optom Assoc* 64(1):60-70, 1993.

Drasdo N: Visual field expanders. *Am J Optom Physiol Optics* 53(9):464-467, 1976.

Ferraro J, Jose RT: Training programs for individuals with restricted fields, in Jose RT (ed): *Understanding Low Vision.* New York, American Foundation for the Blind, 1983, pp 363-376.

Frith MJ: The use of field expanders for patients with pigmentary degeneration of the retina. *Austr J Optom* 63:60, 1979.

Hoeft WW: The management of visual field defects through low vision aids. *J Am Optom Assoc* 51:863-864, 1980.

Jose RT, Smith AJ: Increasing peripheral field awareness with Fresnel prisms. *Opt J Rev Optom* 113(12):33-37, 1976.

Jose RT, Spitzberg LA, Kuether CL: A behind the lens reversed (BTLR) telescope. *J Vis Rehab* 3(2):37-46, 1989.

Kennedy W, Rosten J, Young L, Ciuffreda K, Levin M: A field expander for patients with retinitis pigmentosa: A clinical study. *Am J Optom Physiol Optics* 54(11):744-755, 1977.

Krefman RA: Reversed telescopes on visual efficiency scores in field restricted patients. *Am J Optom Physiol Optics* 58:159-162, 1981.

Mehr EB, Quillman RD: Field "expansion" by use of binocular full-field reversed 1.3X telescopic spectacles: A case report. *Am J Optom Physiol Optics* 56:446-450, 1979.

Nooney TW Jr.: Partial visual rehabilitation of hemianopic patients. *Am J Optom* 63: 382-386, 1986.

Rickers KS: Visual field wideners: A personal report. *J Vis Impair Blind* 72(1):28-29, 1978.

Swann PG: Extending the restricted visual field. *Austr J Optom* 57(10):299-305, 1974.

Weiner A: A preliminary report regarding a device to be used in lateral homonymous hemianopsia. *Arch Ophthalmol* 55:362, 1926.

Weiss NJ: An application of cemented prisms with severe field loss. *Am J Optom,* 49:261-264, 1972.

# ILLUMINATION AND GLARE CONTROL

*It is easy to fall into the habit of thinking that a brighter level of illumination will assist seeing clearly. For normally sighted individuals this is often true, but there are types of vision impairment in which the person may prefer lower illumination, including progressive cone dystrophy, rod monochromatism, albinism, aniridia, and cataracts on the visual axis, especially the posterior subcapsular type. Varying levels of illumination can also be difficult for patients to adapt to. Those with retinitis pigmentosa often report delayed adaptation, and hence difficulty, when moving from indoors to outdoors and vice versa.*

*Apart from the functional concerns is the mounting body of evidence that bright levels of light can cause ocular damage[1, 2, 3, 4] and that some individuals with predisposing ocular conditions are especially susceptible, either because they have lost some of their natural protection, as in aphakia, or because the nature of their condition somehow renders them more prone to damage. The wavelengths of greatest concern are ultraviolet (UV), short wavelength visible, and to a lesser extent infrared (IR). Filters for these wavelengths are available in ophthalmic lenses. The ideal broad spectrum filter would eliminate both ends of the spectrum while maintaining the remaining visible spectrum, beyond the short wavelength visible blue, for normal color vision. A tint or neutral density filter, which was not wavelength-specific, would then reduce the remaining visible spectrum to the desired transmission level. This idealized transmission curve is approximated by some ophthalmic lenses, but there can be major deviations. The importance of knowing the transmission curve of any lens, before it is prescribed, was made very apparent when it was shown that some sunglasses actually reduced the transmission of the visible spectrum while allowing significant amounts of UV and IR through the lens.[5]*

## OPHTHALMIC FILTERS

As suggested in the introduction, there are two major concerns with respect to ophthalmic filters: the uniform attenuation of light across the spectrum and the wavelength-specific attenuation of light. Functional and organic concerns related to light are addressed as a natural part of the evaluation and management of someone who is visually impaired who, by nature of his or her condition, is more likely to be at risk for photophobia or photic damage or who may show a functional improvement with ophthalmic filters. There is a wide variety of ophthalmic filters available to be prescribed, but, with few exceptions, there is little scientific rationale to support prescribing specific filters for specific conditions.

The NoIR lenses from NoIR Medical Technologies (see Resources, Chapter 31) are so labeled as an acronym for "no infrared." These lenses eliminate much of the infrared as well as substantial amounts of UV and reduce the visible spectrum. Many different models are available with different transmission curves; these transmission curves are available from the company. The lens material is plastic. Unfortunately, it is too soft to be surfaced, so prescription lenses are not available. These lenses are prescribed in ready-made plano spectacle form, available in different sizes and shapes. Since these are not available in prescription form, a large size is available that fits over a conventional frame so the patient can wear both pairs, simultaneously, for best correction and light attenuation. A smaller size is available for solo wear for those who wear contact lenses or are emmetropic. Also available are an infant-size frame and children's clip-on filters. Lens blanks can be ordered and edged for any frame. The same company also offers UVShields, which selectively absorb broad portions of the UV spectrum and reduce the visible spectrum but have little or no effect on longer wavelengths.

Corning Medical Optics manufactures a series of lenses that are glass photochromics. These lenses, the Corning® Glare Control™ Lenses, significantly reduce UV but allow substantial IR to pass. Since the lenses are glass, they can be surfaced for the patient's prescription. The fact that they are photochromic offers an advantage to those who adapt poorly to differing levels of illumination. The lenses are currently available in five transmissions: CPF 550, CPF 550 dark, CPF 450, CPF 527, and CPF 511. In each case, the number indicates the approximate wavelength cutoff point in nanometers. CPF™ stands for Corning Photochromic Filter. As one would predict, the lenses are distinctly colored because of their transmission characteristics, with the 550 being quite red and the 450 rather yellow. This causes some patients to reject the lenses based on their appearance as well as the color effect when viewing through them. The CPF 550 "dark" is simply the 550 coating on a darker photochromic base. Polarizing filters are effective in reducing some types of glare but by themselves are not specifically restrictive of specific wavelengths. A polaroid lens may protect against UV or IR if the polarizing filter is laminated with a base that acts as the UV or IR filter.

The most important feature of any lens, in order to prescribe it selectively for protection, is the availability of the transmission curve. Descriptive literature can often be misleading; for example, statements such as "90% reduction in UV" are essentially meaningless since it is the wavelength-specific filtering that is of importance.

Ophthalmic filters must be prescribed with some caution. The filtering characteristic that makes them desirable also can impair the user's function.[6] A deep red or green lens can make it impossible to distinguish red from green in traffic signals[7] and can impair a person's ability to function in a job that requires good color discrimination. Lenses with very low transmission percentages can impair a person's ability to function in the lower levels of illumination encountered during dusk, dawn, or inclement weather. When this is a concern, several lenses with different transmission characteristics can be prescribed for different environmental conditions. The actual lenses selected depend on the person's needs and are best determined by a trial period with one or more possible types. Clip-on examples are available for the CPF series. The NoIR lenses and UVShields are sufficiently inexpensive that a small inventory can easily be maintained for loan to patients. The user should be warned of the possible effect on color perception and the inherent danger associated with reduced ability to distinguish traffic signals as a pedestrian or driver.

Filters may be prescribed for use with other optical devices; for example, a plano cap with a filter could be made for a telescope. NoIR Medical Technologies has introduced a series of hand-held magnifiers, called NoIR Contrast Magnifiers, with various tints. Just as with glasses, the value of such tinted magnifiers and the rationale for prescribing one versus another are presently undetermined.

## Glare Control and Contrast Enhancement

Filters with certain transmission characteristics *may* improve visual performance related to glare disability and/or contrast sensitivity. Short wavelength filters have been recommended for many years under the assumption that reducing short wavelength light in eyes subject to intraocular Rayleigh scattering would improve visual function. Rayleigh scattering is that in which particulate matter, considerably smaller than the wavelength of light, scatters shorter wavelengths of light more than longer wavelengths. The requisite particulate matter in an eye might include aggregates of protein present in a cataract or very small aggregates of fluid as in corneal or retinal edema.

There are reports in the literature to support a functional improvement with short wavelength filters and others that refute it. Vision tests on a series of elderly human subjects with either cataracts, pseudophakia, no pathology, or macular degeneration showed that a filter with a 480 nm cutoff improved contrast sensitivity and visual clarity.[8] Another study found a statistically significant improvement in contrast sensitivity with commercially available yellow lenses and with yellow lenses fabricated by an optician.[9] Contrast sensitivity was measured with the Vision Contrast Test System (VCTS 6500) with and without the yellow lenses. The transmission curves were not specified for either lens. Using neutral density filters and the Corning CPF 550, 527, and 511 lenses, Leat et al.[10] measured grating visual acuity with targets of various contrast for 46 adults who had a variety of visual impairments. Their general conclusion was that long wavelength pass filters improved low contrast acuity in a variety of ocular conditions compared to neutral density filters. The improvement was primarily in those with preretinal conditions that would reasonably be expected to produce intraocular scattering. The optimal result was found most often with the CPF 511 lens. This latter study was performed under artificial lighting, and all of these studies together involved relatively small patient populations. Evidence against the reported benefit of long wavelength pass filters was presented in a study of light scatter in the eyes of normal young, elderly, and cataractous subjects.[11] The results indicated that wavelength-dependent scatter was of little significance in any of the three study groups. The investigators concluded that the transmission characteristics of a filter across the *visible* spectrum were not important when considering disability glare.

So who is right? That remains to be seen. It is reasonable to think that both results are correct for some subjects and that it has not yet been established what ocular conditions and what visible wavelengths may interact to reduce function. There is evidence that UV-induced fluorescence of the lens may affect visual function.[12] Therefore filters that reduce or eliminate this nonvisible portion of the spectrum may be beneficial for some people. Meanwhile, it is a simple matter to test the effect of a filter using a contrast sensitivity chart indoors or outdoors. A documentable improvement in performance on that test might form a basis for rational prescribing, but the implications for functional improvement in activities of daily living remain speculative. More research is needed.

## ARTIFICIAL LIGHTING

Occasionally someone is helped by a suggestion as simple as increasing the wattage of the bulb in the favorite reading lamp at home. Consideration should also be given to the spectrum emitted from a given light source. Fluorescent lights emit a high UV and short wavelength content that is more prone to scatter and may produce glare in patients with cataracts or hazy ocular media. The advantage of fluorescent bulbs is that they are much cooler than incandescent bulbs, which is important if the person requires a close light source. Incandescent bulbs, in general, have a more continuous emission spectrum than fluorescent bulbs but are much hotter. The two types of lighting can be used together to produce more even illumination and can be made more comfortable if the incandescent source is farther away. Single light bulbs such as the Chromalux® bulb, which has a nyodymiun element, have been designed to provide a more natural spectrum, similar to daylight, and can be demonstrated as another alternative.

Virtually all optical devices reduce illumination either directly or indirectly. A microscope, for example, reduces illumination indirectly through the near work distance since the patient's head and nose interfere with the light source. The patient's hand and the housing of a hand or stand magnifier may also interfere with the illumination source. Solutions for these problems include illuminated magnifiers and a lamp with an adjustable arm that can direct the light source around the obstacle. New designs for some magnifiers have utilized clear housings and thinner housings, which block less light. It is easy to forget that the patient will be using the device at home under circumstances that might differ considerably from the office. Questions about lighting and lamps available in the home or work place may reveal potential problems that can be solved with the use of an adjustable lamp of sufficient brightness.

## ILLUMINATED MAGNIFIERS

Hand and stand magnifiers are available that have a built-in illumination source that either is battery powered (Figure 19–1) or can be plugged into the wall receptacle (Figure 14–3). When a very high powered device is required, this additional illumination may be necessary because the close working distance causes other light sources to be blocked by the patient's head. An illuminated device should also be considered when a patient does not perform as well as expected with the calculated degree of magnification. When illuminated magnifiers are

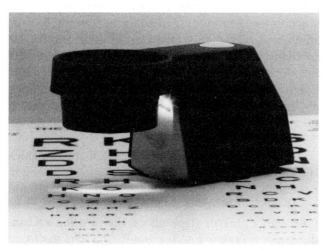

**Figure 19–1.** An illuminated magnifier should be considered when performance is less than expected based on equivalent power. This illuminated stand magnifier from COIL (Model #5228) uses batteries as the power source.

considered, the expense and nuisance of replacing batteries and bulbs should also be considered. While this should not preclude prescribing an illuminated magnifier, it certainly warrants a discussion of the logistics with the patient in order to avoid false expectations. Some bulbs have a very short life expectancy, as do most batteries. While rechargeable batteries may reduce cost over time, they may not produce as bright a light source as other types of batteries, and the charge may dissipate rapidly. Battery replacement is eliminated if the unit can be powered from a wall receptacle, but this limits the places where it can be used conveniently.

## NONOPTICAL AIDS

Several nonoptical aids that may be helpful in controlling illumination include visors and hats or caps with broad brims. There are clip-on visors and side shields for spectacle frames that can reduce ambient light. A typoscope or black reading guide reduces the glare from a page of print as well as providing a guide for eye tracking (Figure 18-11). Commercial typoscopes are available, but any size can be custom made quickly from black construction paper with a razor blade. A yellow acetate sheet has been advocated for years as an overlay for printed materials and for the closed circuit television screen to improve contrast and hence visibility, presumably under the same rationale as discussed previously in the section on glare disability and contrast enhancement. There is presently insufficient scientific evidence to support this concept, but it is a simple matter to try it for a given patient if one so desires.

### Pinhole Glasses

Lenses with one or more pinholes may be used for uniform attenuation of light reaching the pupil. They have the additional advantage of creating a sharper image for those with an irregular optical surface or media who cannot be corrected in the traditional manner with glasses or contact lenses. The diameter of the pinhole must be smaller than the pupil yet not so small that it effectively blocks all or most of the light. If more than one pinhole at a time allows light to enter the pupil, the potential for multiple images exists.[13] Clearly this depends not only on the spacing between the pinholes but the vertex distance at which the glasses are worn and the amount of defocus caused by uncorrected refractive error.

In the simplest sense, a lens with multiple pinholes restricts the transmission to a percentage equal to the sum of the areas of the individual holes compared to the overall area of the lens. This is an approximation only and should be considered the maximum possible transmission since the ability of light to reach the eye after passing through a pinhole depends on the position and angle of the hole (actually a short tunnel) relative to the pupil. The lens has to be curved appropriately, or the holes drilled at increasing angles towards the edge of the lens, in order for the peripheral pinholes to allow the same amount of light to pass as a central hole aligned with the visual axis. In order to provide as clear an image as possible, the holes have to be the appropriate size, and they must be spaced sufficiently far apart to avoid creating diplopia yet not so wide that the user must search for each hole.

Pinhole eyewear, unfortunately, has been the subject of considerable controversy based on public attempts to claim unwarranted advantages.[13] While this may have created a negative mind-set for some, pinhole eyewear still has utility for some persons who are visually impaired both for improving the sharpness of the retinal image and for the attenuation of light.

## SUMMARY

A common complaint with low vision devices that are loaned or dispensed is that they worked much better in the doctor's office than in the patient's home. One possible explanation is that the lighting was much better in the doctor's office. The lighting required for successful use of optical devices is an important part of the patient's education about the devices prescribed and the circumstances under which they can be used most effectively. If it is clear that the lighting at home or on the job is not adequate, the appropriate modifications should be discussed.

Glare, photophobia, light damage, and comfort are areas of concern for which ophthalmic filters may be prescribed. Filters are typically prescribed on the basis of patient preference as there presently is little scientific rationale, beyond UV protection, that directs the clinician in prescribing specific filters on the basis of their transmission curve. As more is learned about the potential for ocular damage from light and about how different parts of the spectrum affect function for people with specific impairments, filters will be prescribed with a more scientific rationale and with greater benefit to the patient.

## REFERENCES

1. Lanum J: The damaging effects of light on the retina. Empirical findings, theoretical and practical implications. *Surv Ophthalmol* 22:221–249, 1978.
2. Brod RD, Olsen KR, Ball SF, Packer AJ: The site of operating microscope light-induced injury on the human retina. *Am J Ophthalmol* 107:390–397, 1989.
3. Waxler M, Hitchins VM: *Optical Radiation and Visual Health.* Boca Raton, FL, CRC Press, 1986.
4. Young R: Solar radiation and age-related macular degeneration. *Surv Ophthalmol* 32:252–269, 1988.

5. Anderson WJ, Gebel RK: Ultraviolet windows in commercial sunglasses. *Applied Optics* 16:515-517, 1967.
6. Kuyk TK, Thomas SR: Effect of short wavelength absorbing filters on Farnsworth-Munsell 100 hue test and hue identification task performance. *Optom Vis Sci* 67: 522-531, 1990.
7. Whillans MG, Allen MJ: Color defective drivers and safety. *Optom Vis Sci* 69(6): 463-466.
8. Zigman S: Vision enhancement using a short wavelength light-absorbing filter. *Optom Vis Sci* 67:100-104, 1990.
9. Rieger G: Improvement of contrast sensitivity with yellow filter glasses. *Can J Ophthalmol* 27(3):137-138, 1992.
10. Leat SJ, North RV, Bryson H: Do long wavelength pass filters improve low vision performance? *Ophthal Physiol Opt* 10:219-224, 1990.
11. Whitaker D, Steen R, Elliott DB: Light scatter in the normal young, elderly and cataractous eye demonstrates little wavelength dependency. *Optom Vis Sci* 70(11): 963-968, 1993.
12. Elliott DB, Yang KCH, Dumbleton K, Cullen AP: UV-induced lenticular fluorescence: Intraocular straylight affecting visual function. *Vision Res* 33:1827-1833, 1993.
13. Wittenberg S: Pinhole eyewear systems: A special report. *J Am Optom Assoc* 64(2): 112-116, 1993.

## ADDITIONAL READING

Aarnisalo E: Effects of yellow filter glasses on colour discrimination of normal observers and on the illumination level. *Acta Ophthalmol (Copenh)* 65:274-278, 1987.
Abrahamsson M, Sjöstrand J: Impairment of contrast sensitivity function as a measurement of disability glare. *Invest Ophthalmol Vis Sci* 27:1131-1136, 1986.
Clark BAJ: Near infrared absorption in sunglasses. *Austr J Optom* 65(5):192-193, 1982.
Hoeft WW, Hughes MK: A comparative study of low vision patients: Their ocular disease and preference for one specific series of light transmission filters. *Am J Opt Physiol Optics* 58:841-845, 1981.
Lindquist TD, Grutzmacher RD, Gofman JDL: Light-induced maculopathy. *Arch Ophthalmol* 104:1641-1647, 1986.
Lipman RM, Tripathi BJ, Tripathi RC: Cataracts produced by microwave and ionizing radiation. *Surv Ophthalmol* 33:200-210, 1988.
Luria SM: Vision with chromatic filters. *Am J Optom* 49(10):818-829, 1972.
Lynch DM, Brilliant R: An evaluation of the CPF 550 lens. *Optom Monthly* 75:36-42, 1984.
Meyers SM, Bonner RF: Yellow filter to decrease the risk of light damage to the retina during vitrectomy. *Am J Ophthalmol* 94:677, 1982.
Morrissette DL, Mehr EB, Keswick CW: Users' and nonusers' evaluations of the CPF 550 lenses. *Am J Opt Physiol Optics* 61:704-710, 1984.
Regan D, Giaschi DE, Fresco BB: Measurement of glare susceptibility using low-contrast letter charts. *Optom Vis Sci* 70(11):969-975, 1993.

# CHAPTER XX

# THE CLOSED CIRCUIT TELEVISION

The closed circuit television (CCTV) provides electronic magnification. It has proven to be a very effective device for those who are visually impaired and has replaced the projection magnifiers used in the past. It consists of a monitor and a camera. The material to be viewed is placed beneath the camera, and the image is formed on the screen of the monitor (Figure 20–1). Monitors are available that are black and white, green, or amber, or with a full color capability. Specific advantages of the CCTV include the ability to enlarge the image over a wide range of sizes, very high maximum enlargement, variable contrast and brightness, and the ability to reverse contrast (white letters on a black background) by reversing polarity. It is also possible to use a CCTV for writing or working on small objects. If the camera can be tilted and has an appropriate lens, the system can be used to view distant objects such as the blackboard in a classroom. The major disadvantages are size, weight, and expense. Compact models exist that are considered portable but are still quite heavy. A small CCTV (Figure 20–2) that is truly portable exists, but, naturally, it sacrifices total enlargement capability because the screen is small. Since most models are not truly portable, they must be used in a fixed location. Therefore, it might be necessary to have more than one if a person needs it at multiple locations; for example, a student may need one at home and one in the classroom. Given the expense of the device, it is important to have an opportunity for extended evaluation prior to making a decision to purchase one.

Just as with other devices, it is important to provide training in the proper use of the CCTV when it is prescribed, especially if the model is different from the one patients used prior to purchasing their own. The user should understand all of the features and how to use them appropriately to maximize function. Perhaps the most difficult aspect of using a CCTV is moving the object in a coordinated manner for efficient viewing since the relative motion on the screen is different than would be expected with direct viewing of the object. Some units come with an X-Y table that requires considerable practice in order to track effectively while reading. A foot-operated electric X-Y table is available.

The CCTV should be placed at an appropriate height that will allow the patient to maintain a comfortable reading posture. This might require a special table and chair. Anyone who cannot accommodate must have the appropriate add for the viewing distance. Some users report that the image seems more discernible with an amber filter. Tinted lenses or a plastic filter over the screen can be used when this is considered worthwhile. If the preferred unit is available with an amber screen, this might create the same effect. Again, an appropriate trial before purchasing the unit should include a consideration of screen color and concomitant use of filters. Even though a better response may be obtained initially with an amber screen, some users are bothered by this color with prolonged usage. An appropriate chance to try different options prior to purchase should determine if this will be a problem.

While it is possible to use other optical devices with the CCTV, this is not generally recommended since it defeats the purpose of the unit; however, there are exceptions. A user might prefer to use a hand magnifier to view a section of smaller print on the screen rather than change the setting on the camera back and forth when different sizes of print are encountered.

The CCTV makes an excellent in-office training device even for patients who will not get one for personal use. The convenience of adjusting image size, contrast, and brightness is particularly useful for training patients to use their residual vision more effectively.

It is easy to think that the most appropriate users for a CCTV are those with the least vision; however, others who might benefit significantly are those who have large reading demands and those who perform significantly better with the CCTV regardless of their acuity.

## MAGNIFICATION

The magnification provided by a CCTV for a specific patient cannot be determined simply by measuring the size of the image on the screen and comparing it to the size of the object. As usual, magnification is relative and must be compared to the reference acuity and the distance at which that acuity was measured (the reference distance). There are two components to the total magnification that the patient obtains when viewing the CCTV: the amount by which the CCTV enlarges the image of the object and the relative distance magnification (RDM) achieved by the final viewing distance compared to the reference distance. The magnification provided by the CCTV alone ($M_{CCTV}$) can be

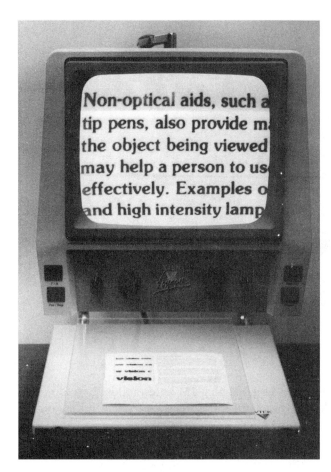

**Figure 20–1.** A closed circuit television consists of a monitor and a camera. The object is enlarged electronically on the monitor, and, on most models, the viewer can control contrast, brightness, magnification, polarity, and focus. Reversing polarity allows the viewer to have white print on a black background. Some models have an adjustable mask that allows a line or lines to be isolated.

determined by measuring the image size with a ruler and dividing that by the size of the object. A good target to use is a ruler itself, while using another ruler to measure the image size. If "one inch" on the object ruler is enlarged to four inches when measured on the screen, then the $M_{CCTV}$ is 4X (M = Image size/ Object size = 4/1 = 4X). This is the enlargement, or magnification, by the CCTV only, *not* the final magnification for the viewer.

■ **Example 20–1.** A woman with age-related maculopathy has a best corrected near acuity of 3M print at 10 cm with a +10.00 add. The 3M print is now placed under the camera, and the image on the screen is enlarged until she is just able to read it while sitting 40 cm from the screen. The image on the screen is measured, and it is found to be 21.75 mm tall. What is the total magnification she will receive?

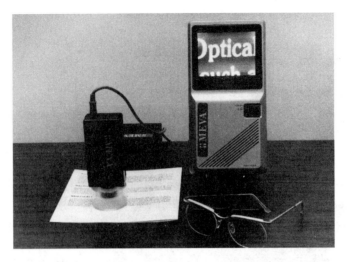

**Figure 20–2.** The MEVA was the first truly portable CCTV, although this particular model has recently been discontinued. The main advantage is portability, but this may be offset by the small screen, which limits the size of the magnified field.

■ **Solution.** A 3M letter is 3 times larger than a 1M letter and is therefore 4.35 mm tall (3 × 1.45 = 4.35). The total magnification is the product of the component parts, as given by the formula below.

$$M_{total} = M_{CCTV} \times RDM$$
$$= 21.75/4.35 \times 10 \text{ cm}/40 \text{ cm}$$
$$= 5 \times 0.4$$
$$= 2X$$

This answer might seem too low given how much taller the letters are on the screen; however, she is also 4 times farther away than the reference distance, which in effect counteracts some of the enlargement by the CCTV. Since she is now 40 cm from the image, she would have to use a +2.50 add to see the screen as clearly as possible, not the +10.00 add used for her reference acuity.

■ **Example 20–2.** A male with nuclear sclerosis has a best corrected near acuity of 0.20/4M with a +5.00 add. He wants to read a book that has 1M print. How large will it have to be on a CCTV screen in order for him to see it if he sits 50 cm away?

■ **Solution.** He will be able to read the 1M print if it is enlarged enough on the screen at a 50 cm viewing distance to be equivalent to the 4M letters he reads at 20 cm (that is, if their height subtends the same angle at the eye).

$$\text{Magnification required} = \text{Reference size/Goal size}$$
$$= 4M/1M$$
$$= 4X$$

$$M_{total} = M_{CCTV} \times RDM$$
$$4X = M_{CCTV} \times 20 \text{ cm}/50 \text{ cm}$$
$$10X = M_{CCTV}$$

$$M_{CCTV} = \text{Image size/Object size}$$
$$10X = \text{Image size/Object size}$$
$$10X = \text{Image size}/1.45$$
$$14.5 \text{ mm} = \text{Image size}$$

Of course, he will need his best correction and a +2.00 add in order to see as clearly as possible at the 50 cm viewing distance.

■ **Alternate Solution.** This same problem can be solved with similar triangles as follows. The image on the screen must subtend the same angle as the 4M letters at 20 cm in order to be visible. A 4M letter is 5.8 mm tall ($4 \times 1.45 = 5.8$), and by similar triangles we have:

$$\text{Object size/Object distance} = \text{Image size/Image distance}$$
$$5.8/20 = \text{Image size}/50$$
$$0.29 \times 50 = \text{Image size}$$
$$14.5 \text{ mm} = \text{Image size}$$

It may seem unnecessary to calculate the image size when all the person has to do is enlarge the image until it becomes readable; however, enlarging the image to the exact size required prevents overmagnification with resultant loss of field. As always, the clinician should have a clear understanding of how the system works based on the clinical data.

## PRESCRIPTION CONSIDERATIONS FOR CCTVS

It is not necessary to keep an inventory of CCTVs in order to have this option available for patients. One CCTV should be acquired for demonstration and training. Other models can be discussed and shown initially through the use of brochures. If the person wishes to pursue this option, he or she can be put in contact with representatives of the various companies for home demonstration and purchase.

### Cost

Most people's initial reaction to the CCTV is enthusiasm until the price is revealed. It may help to put the expense in perspective as in the following examples. The clinician can make a comparison of the cost of a CCTV relative to other medical appliances such as braces for teeth. It may be helpful to create a picture of the cost when amortized over the years of its expected useful life. The average daily cost is relatively insignificant if the CCTV were to be used for five to 10 years; for example, a unit that costs $2,500 and lasts for five years costs approximately ("only") $1.37 per day. If the CCTV is for a college student, the expense is a comparatively small part of the overall cost of a college education, especially if that is the one device that allows him or her to compete successfully in class. When the CCTV is to be used in the person's place of employment, again it is a relatively small investment compared to his or her potential income if the CCTV is the one item that lets him or her function in that occupational setting.

Many older patients reject the possibility of purchasing a CCTV because of the cost yet continue to maintain a car, worth as much as or more than a CCTV, that they can't drive because of their reduced vision. The clinician might suggest that such patients consider selling their car if he or she believes that the CCTV would be of significant use to them. The car, even though unused, may be symbolic of continued hope for complete independence, so selling it might be a very difficult decision. This subject should be approached tactfully and in a manner that allows the patient to draw his or her own conclusion. For example, the clinician might ask, "Do you still own an automobile? How much do you use it? Does anyone use it? What do you think it would be worth if you were to try to sell it? How much do you think it will be worth in several years?"

None of the preceding discussion is meant to imply that the clinician should emphasize a sales-oriented approach to prescribing a CCTV, but some guidance may assist the patient in making a difficult financial decision. This is not unlike the cost-benefit discussion that takes place before ordering an MRI or any other expensive diagnostic test or treatment.

## Glasses

The user who is presbyopic will require an add for the intended viewing distance. All of the considerations that enter into prescribing glasses for someone who uses a computer apply to the user of a CCTV. The arrangement of the work station with respect to screen height and viewing distance will determine the type of glasses (single vision, multifocal, and so forth) that are prescribed. Lighting, screen glare, posture, and comfort are also factors that determine how successfully the device is used.

## Training

As with other low vision devices, most people who obtain a CCTV will benefit from a training program designed to maximize their effectivity in using the device. The training program should include learning to use all of the controls, proper posture and viewing distance, concomitant use of a near add if necessary, and extensive practice in coordinating reading with moving the object beneath the camera. Training in the use of residual vision, such as eccentric viewing training, should also be considered apart from the actual operation of the CCTV.

## SUMMARY

The CCTV and similar alternative devices are excellent aids for many people. The main drawbacks are cost, size, and weight, while the main advantages are variable magnification and control of brightness, contrast, and polarity. Most potential users will benefit from some degree of training in the use of this device, and comprehensive training will ensure maximum effectivity.

## ADDITIONAL READING

Cunningham PJ, Johnston AW: New closed-circuit television magnifier for the low vision patient. *Austr J Optom* 63:60, 1980.

Ehrenberg R: Projection magnifier. *Am J Opt* 33(6):324, 1956.

Ellerbrock VJ: Instrument review: The opaque projection magnifier for subnormal vision. *Am J Opt* 30:273, 1953.

Ellerbrock VJ: Instrument review: The opaque projection magnifier for subnormal vision. *Opt J Rev Optom* 90:58, 1953.

Genensky S: Some comments on the closed circuit television system for the visually handicapped. *Am J Optom Physiol Optics* 46(7):519–524, 1969.

Genensky SM, Petersen HE, Moshin HL, Clewett RW, Yoshimura RI: *Advances in closed-circuit TV systems for the partially sighted.* Rand Corporation Report R-1040-HEW/RC April, 1972.

Genensky SM, Petersen HE, Clewett RW, Moshin HL: *Information transfer problems of the partially sighted: Recent results and project summary.* Rand Corporation Report R-1770-HEW June, 1975.

Goodrich GL, Mehr EB, Darling NC: Parameters in the use of CCTVs and optical aids. *Am J Optom & Arch Am Acad Optom* 57(12):881–892, 1980.

Kasik M: Evaluation of the A.O. projection magnifier. *Opt Weekly* 49:1756, 1958.

Mehr EB, Frost AB, Apple LE: Experience with closed circuit television in the blind rehabilitation program of the Veterans Administration. *Am J Optom & Arch Am Acad Optom* 50(6):458–469, 1973.

Turner PJ: The place of the CCTV in the rehabilitation of the low vision patient. *The New Outlook for the Blind* 70:206–214, 1976.

Turner PJ: The application of the CCTV to the working environment. *Austr J Optom* 61:66–71, 1978.

Watson G, Berg VR: Near training techniques, in Jose RT (ed): *Understanding Low Vision.* New York, American Foundation for the Blind, 1983, pp 317–362.

# PROSTHETIC EYES

A number of people who are visually impaired have lost one eye and have a prosthesis. Because of this, the low vision practitioner should be comfortable with the in-office management of a patient who has a prosthetic eye. The fabrication and modification of prosthetic eyes is a highly skilled craft practiced by ocularists and is not part of the professional training for eye care specialists. The clinician should, however, be able to evaluate the fit and cosmetic features of a prosthetic eye, assess the health of the orbit, remove and insert the prosthesis smoothly, polish it when required, instruct the patient in proper care and handling, and make appropriate referrals for replacement or adjustment when indicated. These skills are discussed in this chapter along with an overview of prosthetic eyes, surgical procedures for eye removal, and adaptation to monocular vision.

## INCIDENCE OF EYE LOSS

The National Society to Prevent Blindness reported from unpublished data of hospital discharge summaries that in 1976 there were 771,000 eye operations, with 11,000 of them for removal of an eyeball.[1] The most frequent occurrence in the latter series was in the age group 15 to 44, and there were two times more males than females. The enucleation rate for a geographically defined population was reported by Erie et al.[2] They reviewed records for Olmstead County, Minnesota, covering a 33-year period (1956 to 1988). The mean annual incidence, age-adjusted to the 1980 white population in the United States, was 4.32 per 100,000. The most common reasons for enucleation were trauma (39%), neovascular glaucoma (29%), and tumor (17%). The visual acuity of the fellow eye at the time of the enucleation was 20/50 to 20/100 in 10.9% and 20/200 or worse in 11.9%. At the time of last follow-up, the visual acuity of the fellow eye was 20/50 to 20/100 for 8.9% and 20/200 or worse for 17.8%. These represent minimum percentages since the acuity of the fellow eye was unknown for eight individuals at the time of enucleation and for 15 individuals at the time of last follow-up. The large percentage of those with reduced acuity in the fellow eye emphasizes the fact that a number of people who are visually impaired will have, or require, a prosthetic eye.

When an eye is lost, it is replaced with an implant and a prosthetic eye. The prosthesis is usually made of polymethylmethacrylate (PMMA) plastic, although glass prostheses are still made and are required by those who cannot tolerate plastic. Herman Snellen tried to produce artificial eyes to fill in the space left by enucleation. Under his encouragement, hollow prostheses were first blown from glass successfully in 1892 by the Müller brothers in Wiesbaden, Germany.[3] A person who makes prosthetic eyes is called an ocularist. The American Society of Ocularists provides board certification in this specialty.

## SURGICAL PROCEDURES FOR EYE REMOVAL

There are three basic types of surgery for removal of an eye or the contents of the globe. An *enucleation* is the removal of the entire globe. This procedure became common during the latter half of the 19th century and necessitated that thicker prostheses be developed that could fill in the remaining space, unlike the thinner shell prostheses that were used over atrophic eyes.[3] An *evisceration* is the removal of the contents of the globe, with the sclera and perhaps part of the cornea remaining. An *exenteration* is more radical and involves the removal of the globe, orbital contents, and parts of the bony orbit.

When an eye is enucleated or eviscerated, the mass of the lost tissue is replaced with an implant (Figure 21-1). The implant is placed within the remaining tissue. The globe (if it remains) or tenon's capsule and the conjunctiva are closed over the implant, so the implant is no longer visible unless the tissue thins or, in the case of an evisceration, there is enough clear cornea remaining to see into the globe. An evisceration gives the best cosmetic result since much of the eye remains and, more importantly, the extraocular muscles are functional and can provide more natural movement of the prosthetic.

At the time of enucleation or evisceration, a conformer is placed in the socket after the implant has been enclosed. The conformer is very much like a thick contact lens (Figure 21-1) and has fenestrations to allow fluid movement between the anterior and posterior aspects. A conformer serves several important functions.

1. It provides the sense of fullness that the prosthetic eye will give and therefore conditions the patient for this sensation.
2. It helps maintain the implant in place while the tissue heals.

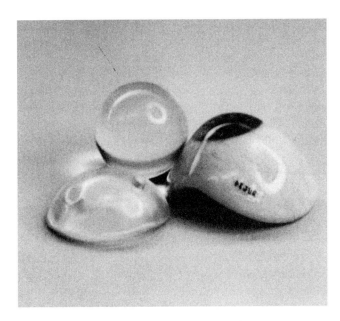

**Figure 21-1.** Shown, from left to right, are a conformer, a Berens clear acrylic spherical implant, and a Monoplex prosthetic eye from American Optical.

3. It keeps the lids away from the sutures to prevent irritation.
4. It helps fill the void of lost orbital contents preventing contraction of the surrounding tissues until the prosthesis is fitted one to three months later.

## Implants

Implants are typically round and have been made of a variety of materials including glass, gold, silicone, plastic, and, most recently, a new material called hydroxyapatite. Hydroxyapatite is a form of calcium carbonate manufactured from sea coral and is extremely porous.

The implant cannot usually be seen unless the overlying tissue has thinned. When an artificial eye is provided, its movement with excursion of the opposite eye depends on friction between the prosthesis and the tissue overlying the implant. As might be imagined, this gives some movement but not a lot. Several early attempts to achieve better movement and hence a more cosmetically pleasing result were innovative but unsuccessful. One approach was to have a combined implant/prosthesis. This was a single sphere painted on one half to simulate the fellow eye. The opposite half had a wire mesh to which the remaining orbital tissue and muscles were attached. Unfortunately, since complete closure around the wound was not possible, infection eventually caused extrusion of the prosthesis. Another approach was to use an implant, part of which protruded through the remaining tissue and contained an opening into which a prosthetic eye with a stalk could be inserted. Again, incomplete wound closure around the protruding portion eventually led to infection and extrusion. Extrusion may also occur with implants that are completely sealed within the orbital tissue. While it is not common, it is also not rare. The indirect joining of an implant with a prosthesis has also been attempted through the use of a magnet imbedded within the implant.[4]

Implants made of hydroxyapatite (Hydroxyapatite Ocular Implant) may finally solve the dilemma of connecting the implant with the overlying prosthesis.[5, 6] The material is similar to natural bone and is porous, allowing fibrovascular tissue to grow into the implant. Ingrowth has been confirmed in humans within four weeks of implantation.[7] A small hole can be drilled into the implant and an artificial eye with a stalk inserted. Similarly, a ball and socket approach utilizes a stalk with a ball end inserted into the implant and an artificial eye with a "socket." Either approach gives an artificial eye attached to the implant (reversibly) such that the prosthesis moves in conjunction with the fellow eye, provided that the extraocular muscles did not have to be surgically removed when the eye was lost. The fact that the implant becomes integrated with the orbital tissue also reduces migration of the implant within the orbit, a rather common problem with other types of implants. When an implant does shift within the orbit, it affects the cosmetic result by altering the fit of the prosthesis and may require surgical correction. If an implant is not placed at the time of enucleation (a primary implant), the cosmetic result is much poorer since there is less movement of the prosthesis compared to the remaining eye.[8] An implant can be inserted surgically at a later time, even years after the original enucleation, and this is referred to as a secondary implant.

## FITTING PROSTHETIC EYES

The development of facial and ocular prostheses has a long and interesting history and makes fascinating reading.[9, 10, 11] The loss of an eye is a tragic event not only for the loss of sight but for the altered cosmesis; however, the advances made in restoration of facial disfigurement have been remarkable. There are three ways in which modern prosthetic eyes are fitted. The most convenient method, although less desirable from a cosmetic point of view, is to have a diagnostic kit of ready-made eyes and to make the best choice from this kit. American Optical (AO) makes prosthetic eyes in their Monoplex eye department, and it is possible to have a kit consisting of different shapes, sizes, and basic colors (Figure 21-2). Different eyes are tried, and the final selection is ordered from AO by their numerical code corresponding to the best shape, size, and color match.

A custom fit is the most desirable approach. First the socket is molded to produce a form. The prosthetic eye is then built to match the form and adjusted until the best possible fit is achieved. An artist, or the ocularist, paints the iris and sclera to match the fellow eye as closely as possible. Since the patient is

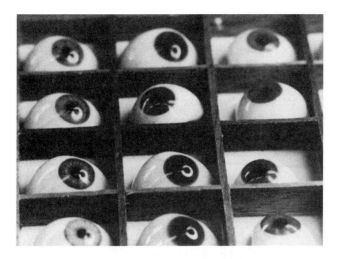

**Figure 21-2.** This fitting kit of prosthetic eyes from American Optical contains 16 combinations of the standard sizes and shapes for right and left eyes. A similar kit can be used to fit someone with a prosthesis directly, or, if a good match cannot be made, several different eyes can be used to find the best size, shape, and color. Then the prosthetic that combines those features can be ordered.

present for the artist and the process is a custom fit from scratch, the best possible cosmetic result is achieved.

A third approach, which could be called the semicustom method, utilizes a ready-made eye as the starting point. It is built up or reduced in size and shape as necessary to achieve the final fit. The iris may or may not be custom painted depending on the closeness of the match with stock colors. In most cases, a custom or semicustom eye can be fabricated in a single day.

## IN-OFFICE PROTOCOL FOR EXAMINING A PROSTHETIC EYE

The cosmetic evaluation begins with observing the prosthesis compared to the fellow eye and evaluating the overall size, pupil size, iris color, scleral color, scleral vascularization, lid position, and movement. The goal is to have a prosthetic eye that matches the fellow eye so closely that it is unnoticeable. The most difficult part of achieving this goal is to have good movement of the prosthesis when the fellow eye moves. This can be evaluated by observing "versions." Movement of the prosthesis depends on friction with the underlying tissue, and if the two are not closely adjacent, no movement is possible. Similarly, a prosthesis that is too large or too small will not move in a natural manner and will not position the lids symmetrically compared to those of the fellow eye.

Examination of the orbit is part of the routine evaluation and requires removal of the prosthesis. This can be accomplished by asking the patient to remove the eye. The clinician should observe the method by which it is done to be sure that the patient is capable of this act. It also can be informative for the clinician to remove the eye. Rubber gloves should be worn to protect the clini-

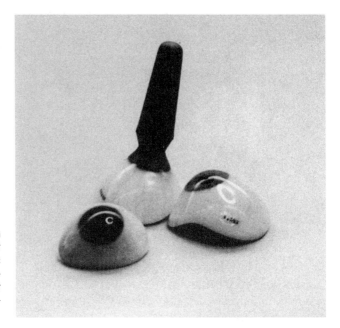

**Figure 21–3.** A large suction cup is required to support the weight of a prosthetic eye. The suction cups typically used for contact lenses do not have sufficient holding power.

cian since there is contact with body fluids. The prosthesis can be removed by hand or with the aid of a suction cup (Figure 21-3). The standard suction cup used for contact lens insertion and removal is too small to hold a prosthesis. Removing the prosthetic eye provides an opportunity to move it about the orbit slightly to check for soreness, which may be indicative of sharp edges or areas of irritation. This is best accomplished with the aid of the suction cup. In order to remove the prosthesis, the lower lid is pulled down slightly and pressed backwards beneath the edge of the prosthesis. If a suction cup is not being used, the hand should immediately be cupped under the eye because the prosthesis will soon be in that general location. Once the eye is removed, it should be cleaned and then checked for scratches with the slit lamp and for sharp edges by observation and by feel. The surface of a PMMA prosthesis will eventually become rough, even if it is not visible clinically, and this has been shown with the scanning electron microscope.[4] Periodic polishing is recommended to prevent discomfort and infection. Chronic or recurrent infections are often associated with a rough surface, which presumably breaks down the protective barrier of the adjacent tissue and serves as a point to harbor bacteria. The orbit is examined for infection, areas of irritation, implant placement, and the appearance of any abnormalities. It is infrequent, but an implant can be extruded if the tissue surrounding it thins or breaks down from infection or necrosis. This is easily checked with the slit lamp. The implant should also be evaluated for migration within the orbit. Also included in the slit lamp inspection are the palpebral aspects of the conjunctiva for signs of giant papillary conjunctivitis.

If the prosthesis is scratched, it can be polished in the same manner, and with the same tools, as a hard contact lens. In general, the plastic layers are thick enough that polishing cannot damage them, but with multiple polishings it is possible to expose the threads used to represent surface blood vessels or to produce a small cavity at the point of fusion for two layers of plastic. Any crack or crevice represents a point to sequester bacteria and should be polished out or repaired. For once, the clinician need not worry about adding positive or negative power by pressing too hard while polishing on the contact lens wheel.

If the prosthesis is a stock model such as a Monoplex eye from AO, there will be a series of numbers on the side that should be recorded. In the event that the eye is lost, a new one can be ordered, exactly the same in every respect, by that numerical code.

The prosthesis can be reinserted by the patient, which allows the clinician to evaluate how the procedure is performed. It is easier to remove a prosthesis than it is to insert it, so it is not safe to assume that a patient can do both until he or she demonstrates it. A prosthesis is inserted easily by elevating the upper lid and placing the temporal aspect of the prosthesis, held vertically, under the lid and then rotating it temporally beneath the lid. The lower lid is now pulled down, and the lower edge of the prosthesis is tucked behind it. The suction cup is more useful to the clinician for insertion than it is for removal.

Care and handling of the prosthesis should be reviewed with each person regardless of how long he or she may have worn one. In general, he or she should be encouraged to handle the prosthesis as little as possible. It is meant to remain in the socket continuously, and it is removed for cleaning only when necessary. Excessive cleaning and handling will cause scratches and subsequent discomfort. Constant drying and rewetting will cause the plastic to crack and necessitate earlier replacement. If the patient insists on removing the eye each night while sleeping, it can be placed in a glass of water or wetting solution to maintain hydration. Thirsty patients should put the glass someplace far away. Ordinary contact lens solutions work fine for cleaning and wetting prosthetic eyes, although there are some cleaners and lubricants designed specifically for them. Annual evaluations are appropriate for asymptomatic patients.

## PROTECTION OF THE REMAINING EYE

**All patients with a prosthetic eye should have safety glasses prescribed for full-time wear!** This is also true for anyone who has two eyes, one of which is substantially better than the other. The primary value in having two eyes is to have a spare. Monocular patients have lost their spare, and loss of the remaining eye would render them sightless. According to the NSPB[1] there are 288,000 product-related eye injuries annually, and it is estimated that 90% of these could be prevented through the use of protective eyewear. The most common products implicated are metal pieces, motor vehicles, and then chemicals.

If the patient desires a contact lens for the fellow eye because of a high refractive error or other compelling reason, he or she should be told that safety glasses are still mandatory even with the contact lens. One way to ensure that the glasses are worn is to provide only a partial correction in the contact lens and the rest in the spectacle lens. This approach works especially well for patients with significant astigmatism by prescribing a spherical contact lens and placing the astigmatic correction in spectacles.

## COSMETIC OPHTHALMIC OPTICS

Glasses can be prescribed for cosmetic enhancement as well as for protection. A prosthesis, in spite of the ocularist's best efforts, may still appear different from the fellow eye. Some cosmetic improvement may be obtained by prescribing a spectacle lens specifically for the prosthesis. If the prosthetic eye is too large or small compared to the fellow eye, it can be made to appear smaller or larger by prescribing more or less power in the corresponding spectacle lens. The effect can be demonstrated and evaluated with trial lenses, although they are typically too small in diameter to allow an optimum evaluation.

Prism can be used to make the prosthetic eye appear, or appear to look, higher or lower. The base is oriented opposite to that which would be used for a strabismus or phoria; for example, a prosthesis that appeared to look up might be corrected or improved with base-up prism. Minor differential tinting can be used to match the patient's iris color more closely. Darker tints and gradient tints are useful to mask any poor cosmetic result that cannot be improved by modifying the prosthesis.

Cosmetic optics are effective for small adjustments in appearance, but some caution is advised as the clinician can easily create conspicuous glasses in place of a conspicuous prosthetic eye.

## ADAPTATION TO MONOCULAR VISION

There are many examples of monocular people who have led not only successful lives but extraordinary lives such as Sandy Duncan (entertainer), Sammy Davis, Jr. (entertainer), and Wiley Post (pilot) to name a few. These and others should serve as examples that loss of an eye need not be a handicapping condition, although it is certainly a more significant event when the remaining eye is visually impaired.

One of the more important aspects of the management of patients who have lost an eye is assisting them with adaptation to monocular vision. Many people feel completely handicapped when the sight of one eye is lost. In fact, most of the visual function is preserved provided that the other eye has normal sight. The loss of visual field is only approximately 15°. This can be demonstrated effectively to other family members by having them move a hand forward on one side, with both eyes open, until it can just be seen and then closing the eye on that side and continuing to advance the hand until it is seen again. The lost portion of the visual field is surprisingly small.

Depth perception is not lost when one eye is lost, but stereopsis is. There are many monocular clues to depth perception such as perceived size, brightness, overlap, and parallax. These can be explained, along with hints about daily activities, to minimize the period of adaptation; for example, where one chooses to sit in a restaurant can minimize the risk of an accident caused by gesturing into the path of an oncoming overladen waiter. When reaching for a glass of wine, one can slide his or her hand along the table top until it touches the base of the stem. Shaking hands need not be a problem if the monocular patient simply extends his or her hand part of the way and waits for the other person to actually make the contact. These and other hints about adaptation are discussed in a small text that is suitable reading for both clinicians and patients.[12]

Monocular persons can drive legally in all 50 states, although at this time they cannot obtain a commercial interstate license. There are thousands of legally licensed monocular pilots, including commercial pilots. It might seem surprising that pilots can fly with one eye since landing a plane appears to require very precise utilization of binocular vision, but this is not the case.[13] An interesting study[14] was performed in which binocular private pilots, with low flying time, were evaluated on their ability to land aircraft accurately ("spot" landing) when the dominant eye was occluded and under binocular conditions. The actual landings were judged equally accurate, although the landing approaches were flown differently, being higher and steeper under monocular conditions.

A consideration for those who are monocular and presbyopic, especially if there is also a field restriction, is that a bifocal may impair mobility by reducing the visual field even further. Some people who are monocular prefer a single vision lens for distance and a separate bifocal or single vision lens for near tasks.

A counseling session—covering what the loss of one eye, or the sight of one eye, really means and how one adapts to monocular vision—is an important therapeutic activity for the person who has lost an eye. It should not be assumed that this was addressed by the ophthalmic surgeon or the ocularist, nor should it be assumed that the patient will figure it out on his or her own.

## SUMMARY

Adaptation to the loss of an eye varies and is dependent on the amount of remaining vision in the fellow eye. Adaptation to a prosthesis can be facilitated by assisting the patient to obtain the best possible cosmetic result. A competent ocularist will provide the best possible prosthesis, but the clinician may be able to improve the result with glasses designed specifically to protect the remaining eye and to enhance the appearance of the prosthesis. The continuing management of the patient includes counseling about adaptation, periodic review of the care and handling of the prosthesis, evaluation of its fit, and evaluation of the health of the remaining orbital tissue.

## REFERENCES

1. *Vision Problems in the United States.* New York, National Society to Prevent Blindness, 1980.
2. Erie JC, Nevitt MP, Hodge D, Ballard DJ: Incidence of enucleation in a defined population. *Am J Ophthalmol* 113(2):138–144, 1992.
3. den Tonkelaar I, Henkes HE, van Leersum GK: Herman Snellen (1834–1908) and Müller's 'reform-auge'. A short history of the artificial eye. *Doc Ophthalmol* 77(4): 349–354, 1991.
4. Mishima K, Matsunaga N, Amemiya T: Methylmethacrylate implants: A scanning electron microscopic study. *Annals Plastic Surg* 26(6):561–563, 1991.
5. Perry AC: Advances in enucleation. *Ophthalmol Clin North Am* 4(1):173–182, 1991.
6. Dutton JJ: Coralline hydroxyapatite as an ocular implant. *Ophthalmol* 98(3): 370–377, 1991.
7. Shields CL, Shields JA, Eagle RC, De Potter P: Histopathologic evidence of fibrovascular ingrowth four weeks after placement of the hydroxyapatite orbital implant. *Am J Ophthalmol* 111(3):363–366, 1991.
8. Smit TJ, Koornneef L, Groet E, Zonneveld FW, Otto AJ: Prosthesis motility with and without intraorbital implants in the anophthalmic socket. *Brit J Ophthalmol* 75(11):667–670, 1991.
9. Reisberg DJ, Habakuk SW: A history of facial and ocular prosthetics. *Adv Ophthal, Plas & Reconstructive Surgery* 8:11–24, 1990.
10. Danz W Sr.: Ancient and contemporary history of artificial eyes. *Adv Ophthal, Plas & Reconstructive Surgery* 8:1–10, 1990.
11. Trester W: The history of artificial eyes and the evolution of the ocularistic profession. *J Am Soc Ocularists*, 12 ed, pp 5–13, 1981.
12. Brady FB: *A Singular View.* Oradell, NJ, Medical Economics Company, 1979.
13. Mayer HB, Lane JC: Monocular pilots—a followup study. *Aerosp Med* May: 1070–1074, 1973.
14. Grosslight JH, Fletcher HJ, Masterton RB, Hagen R: Monocular vision and landing performance in general aviation pilots: Cyclops revisited. *Hum Factors* 20(1): 27–33, 1978.

# TRAINING IN THE USE OF LOW VISION DEVICES AND RESIDUAL VISION

Most people who are visually impaired can benefit from systematic training in the use of residual vision and in the proper use of the prescribed, or intended, low vision devices. Training in both areas can be provided by the low vision practitioner or the practitioner's staff. It may be necessary to provide training before deciding on the final treatment plan for patients with severely limited vision. The most frequent disorder that is amenable to improvement through training is macular degeneration with its resultant central scotoma. It might seem reasonable that someone with this disorder would learn to view eccentrically as an automatic process, but this is often not the case. Those who are older have had a lifetime of reinforcement for central fixation and are reluctant to change this pattern of viewing. Methods of reinforcing eccentric viewing have been developed and used for many years.

Others who might benefit from training in the use of residual vision are those with field losses (Chapter 18), those using telescopes for driving (Chapter 23), and children with severe vision impairments who have been treated as essentially blind and have not developed visual concepts. Training a child or adolescent who has not had an opportunity to learn to use his or her residual vision requires a more involved and extensive program since basic visual concepts may be lacking. This type of training is not within the scope of this text.

No matter what happens in the office, it is what happens at home that is most important. If the patient cannot practice effectively outside of the *office, progress may be stalled. One form of assistance for patients and family members to use at home is a printed instruction sheet. Several examples of such forms, which can be modified as desired, are included in this chapter. This same information can be recorded on a cassette for those who prefer an auditory format.*

*Finally, whenever a low vision device is prescribed, the patient should be trained in its proper use in order to achieve the maximum therapeutic benefit. Even patients who seem to use a device effectively might do better with additional training.*

## TRAINING ECCENTRIC VIEWING

The initial step in training eccentric viewing is to help the patient find the eccentric viewing angle that affords him or her the best visual performance. There are many ways to do this, but all are variations on the same theme, which is to present targets in different areas of the patient's visual field until the area of best vision is determined. This can be demonstrated for an intermediate distance with the tangent screen or for near with targets of one's own design placed against a reading stand. The tangent screen can be used by having the patient fixate centrally (that is, placing the central scotoma in the center of the tangent screen) and presenting targets, such as numbers or letters, corresponding to the patient's visual acuity level in different areas until the region of best vision is approximated (Figure 22–1). It can then be refined by moving the target around this area until the exact location for best vision is located. The direction and angle of eccentric viewing is read directly from the tangent screen; this angle can then be used for all distances. The patient must learn that even though the eccentric angle of viewing is the same for all distances, the linear distance from the point of fixation to the object of regard will be different for each target distance. This can be demonstrated by walking toward the patient with the target at the appropriate eccentric angle and pointing out the decreasing lateral distance from the line of sight to the target as it gets closer.

An alternative approach to establishing the eccentric viewing angle is to have a clock-like target and ask the patient to fixate the center and state which "time" appears the clearest. This can be performed with the tangent screen or a similar target. With homemade targets it is helpful to have markings that allow an angle to be specified exactly. It is also possible to have a target placed centrally. The clinician asks the patient to move his or her eyes around systematically until the target is as clear as possible (Figure 22–2) and remember what "time" he or she was looking at as a future reference. In this latter case, it is

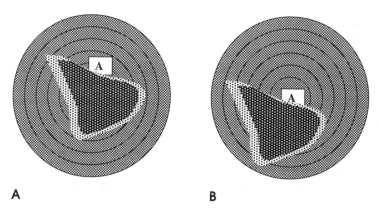

A                                    B

**Figure 22–1.** The tangent screen can be used to teach eccentric viewing. (**A**) The person is instructed to fixate the center of the screen, and the examiner moves a target peripherally until the area of best vision is located. (**B**) The target can also be placed centrally, and the person is asked to move his or her eye around until it is seen as clearly as possible.

harder to specify the angle of eccentric viewing since it is not obvious exactly where the person is viewing in order to see eccentrically.

Once the eccentric viewing angle is established, it is necessary to reinforce it with programmed exercises such as reading. An infinite number of exercises can be devised to accomplish this task and should be presented from

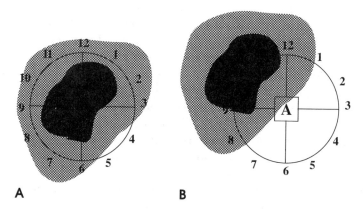

A                                    B

**Figure 22–2.** A clock-like target gives the viewer a familiar frame of reference for establishing the best angle for eccentric viewing. (**A**) The person is asked to place his or her scotoma in the center of the target and report what "time" appears clearest, or (**B**) the person views eccentrically and reports what "time" he or she is looking at when a target in the center is seen as clearly as possible.

easier to harder with respect to both eye movements and the discrimination level necessary to distinguish the target. Some are available commercially.[1] Techniques used for orthoptics that lend themselves well to training eccentric viewing include tracking exercises and fixation reinforcement with afterimage generation. The recent development of computer-generated orthoptic training programs should provide additional material for some training sessions.

Whenever training is provided, success is best measured with a valid pre- and posttest. Since reading is a frequent goal, it is possible to use standardized reading tests for speed and comprehension. It may be necessary to have the test reprinted in larger print if the person is unable to read standard size text with his or her optical device. One test that was developed specifically for those who are visually impaired is the Pepper Visual Skills Analysis Test.[2] The use of periodic performance measurements allows the practitioner to have a rational basis for continuing or suspending training. These measures also give the patient feedback on the progress made. If the exercises are properly chosen and sequenced, every patient should have some initial success. This positive reinforcement may provide sufficient motivation to continue the process until maximum benefit is realized.

## TRAINING IN THE PROPER USE OF LOW VISION DEVICES

Techniques for specific devices are presented below. Some aspects of training have already been covered in earlier chapters concerned with prescribing optical devices. For all devices it is appropriate to give the patient or other family member a page of instructions that will reinforce correct use at home and may prevent unnecessary calls to the practitioner. An "information sheet" or brochure about each device that is prescribed can be an effective means of helping the patient use the device to maximum advantage. The instructions should include information about the proper care and cleaning for any optical device. Other information that might be helpful is the required work distance, whether or not the device is to be used in conjunction with glasses or a bifocal add, what it is not useful for (for example, some telescopes do not work for near), which eye to use, the minimum size print to use, and the correct or recommended use of lighting. These instructions may be particularly helpful for teachers of visually impaired students. The information sheet may also be used as a guide by a member of the office staff when telephoning the patient for a progress report a few days after the device is dispensed.

It is most useful if the instructions are given to the patient in printed form to take home for review and for other family members or care givers to read. Many personal computers can print in large font sizes, and this is ideal for patient handouts. Examples of such information sheets are given below. The information sheet can be read to the patient by another family member, or, if printed in a large enough font, it may be read by the patient. If it is read by other family members, it will help them to understand how the device is to be used and may allow them to reinforce key points to the intended user. All of the points should also be discussed with the individual when the device is dispensed in the office and during the in-office training session(s). Again, if other family members are present during these sessions, their observations may serve to help reinforce the points at home.

## Microscopes

The major consideration with a microscope is that the user understand how close the object of regard must be held in order to be in focus. Not everyone understands what is meant by, "The focal point is at 5 cm," so it may be necessary to provide a drawing of a line 5 cm long, made with a broad felt-tip pen. It is also possible to attach a pipe cleaner to the temple that protrudes 5 cm to the front until the person learns to hold print this close automatically. It is often easier to find the clearest image by moving the print in too close and then backing out rather than moving the print in until it seems as clear as possible. The patient can be told to move the print in until it literally touches the nose and then to back it out slowly until it is as clear as possible. If this procedure is not used, the natural tendency to hold things farther away may preclude ever getting close enough to be in focus.

---

### SAMPLE INFORMATION SHEET

#### Microscopes

The optical device your doctor has prescribed for you is called a microscope. It is to be used for near activities only. Things that are far away will not be in focus and cannot be seen clearly with your microscope.

You may find that it is harder to use the microscope at home than it was when you were in the doctor's office. That is because the doctor uses the best possible lighting along with high quality printed reading cards and makes sure that you hold the print at exactly the right distance from the lens. Most common books, newspapers, and magazines do not have the same quality of print and paper and are therefore harder to read. Also, many people have low wattage light bulbs, such as 60 or 75 watts, in their lamps at home, even though much stronger ones are available. The following are some hints to help you use your microscope effectively.

1. When you want to look at something with your microscope, you must hold it approximately _____ inches from the front of the lens. Try moving the object slightly closer and farther until it appears as clear as possible, and then maintain that position while reading.

2. Use good lighting. You should try different types of lamps to determine what works best for you. Some people prefer lamps with fluorescent bulbs since regular bulbs may be too hot when they are nearby. Adjustable lamps allow you to position the light in the best location. For some people, a combination of lamps works better than just one. For example, a lamp with a fluorescent bulb combined with one having a standard bulb may provide a better light source than either one alone. Natural daylight is an excellent light source, so you might try to establish a reading area near a window.

3. When reading with a microscope, try to move the print and not your head. This is different from how you are used to reading, but it will make it easier to keep your place and use the microscope effectively.

4. Reading guides are very helpful when using a microscope. A simple reading guide can be made using the edge of a piece of black construction paper. Position the edge beneath the print in order to follow the line across the page. You may also cut a rectangle out of the paper so there will be a line above as well as below. Some people find it helpful to use their finger as a marker in order to find their place when moving to a new line of print.

5. A reading stand may be useful to assist you with holding the print in a comfortable position. You should also adjust your table and chair in order to find the most comfortable position for reading since using a microscope may cause you to tire after a few minutes.

6. Reading with a microscope may be tiring at first. Be sure to take frequent rest periods and build up your reading time gradually; for example, begin by practicing for only five minutes several times each day. It is best to begin with larger print such as headlines in the newspaper and then read progressively smaller print as you learn to use the microscope. With practice, it should become easier to read for longer periods of time and to read faster.

Many books are printed in large print and are available at the library as well as bookstores.

7.  A microscope may be used for reading recipes, price labels, labels on medicine bottles, bills, and letters. But reading is not the only thing it can be useful for. Some other possible uses are looking at photographs of family members and friends, looking at your wrist watch to tell the time, checking your fingernails, adjusting the heating and cooling thermostats, identifying foods in the kitchen or store, seeing playing cards in your hand, identifying cosmetics, tuning the radio, looking at pictures in magazines, and so on. If you try looking at everything you can hold close to the lens, you will discover many other uses for your microscope.

8.  Your microscope has a high quality optical lens, and it must be cared for carefully. When you are not using it, be sure to keep it in its case. The lens can be cleaned with a liquid lens cleaner and a soft piece of cloth such as a clean diaper or T-shirt. Do not use tissues such as Kleenex® since they may scratch the lens surface.

9.  Remember that using your eyes to read with your microscope, or any other optical device, will not harm your eyes or your vision in any way. If you have any questions, please feel free to call the clinic.

## Hand-Held Telescopes

The user of a hand-held telescope must know how to focus it, how to locate a target that was seen with the unaided eye, and how to scan systematically while looking through the telescope. The correct focusing should be practiced for targets at a variety of distances. It may also be helpful to demonstrate how the tube gets longer when a telescope is focused for near. It may be difficult, especially with a high magnification telescope, to locate an object in the field of the telescope that was first seen with the unaided eye. One technique is to have patients look at the object without the telescope, then move their head down along a straight line to look at their own feet, and then raise their head slowly in the direction of the object with the telescope before the eye. This back-and-forth motion along a straight line should bring them in alignment with the object of regard. Another technique is to move systematically from an object that is easier to spot until the object of regard is in view; for example, a distant sign next to a building might be located by finding the building and then following its exterior wall until the sign is found just to the side of it. Certain objects can be found in predictable locations even if they are not first spotted by the unaided eye; for example, traffic signals are usually in similar locations throughout a city. The person should be reminded of this in order to develop a systematic scanning procedure for finding them.

With higher strength telescopes, it is difficult to hold them steady enough to have the clearest image possible. A technique for holding a telescope steady is to place the opposite hand across the stomach or waist with a clenched fist and place the elbow of the hand holding the telescope on that clenched fist for support.

---

### SAMPLE INFORMATION SHEET

## Hand-Held Telescopes Used for Distance Only

The optical device your doctor has prescribed for you is called a hand-held telescope. It is to be used for looking at things that are far away. Things that are closer than 10 to 20 feet will not be in focus and cannot be seen clearly with your telescope.

You may find that it is harder to use the telescope at home than it was when you were in the doctor's office. That is because the doctor used high quality printed reading cards and made sure that you held the telescope steady and focused it correctly. The following are some hints to help you use your telescope effectively.

1. When you want to look at something with your telescope, you should first spot it without the telescope and then raise the telescope into position without moving your head or eyes. Rotate the focusing knob slowly in each direction to obtain the clearest possible image.
2. If you have difficulty locating objects through the telescope, try following real or imaginary paths. For example, to spot a traffic signal on a street corner you might be able to spot the curb and then follow it to the corner and up the light pole. Notice surrounding landmarks such as a nearby tree or building. When those are seen through the telescope, you have a better idea of which direction to move and how far. If there are no convenient landmarks, trace an imaginary path with your hand before spotting through the telescope, and then follow that same motion with the telescope. With practice you will become much better at spotting objects. Begin by spotting large stationary objects and then progressively smaller objects.
3. When scanning with a telescope, try to move slowly because the image may appear to move much faster than you seem to be turning.

4. It may be helpful to support the arm holding your telescope in order to keep the image steady and to keep your arm from getting tired. One technique is to place the elbow of the arm holding the telescope on your opposite fist, which is held firmly against your body at about waist level.

5. Using a telescope may be tiring at first. Be sure to take frequent rest periods and build up your time gradually; for example, begin by practicing for only five minutes several times each day.

6. A telescope may be used for spotting traffic signals, building and house numbers, and bus numbers and signs and for identifying friends' faces from a distance. Students may use a telescope for seeing the blackboard or watching slides and filmstrips. Some people use them to watch television, but it is difficult to hold a telescope steady for an extended period of time. Try sitting closer to the television. This usually works better. Some other places you might use your telescope are the zoo, botanical gardens, parks, and the beach. Try watching birds, animals, people, and cars. If you try using your telescope to look at as many distant objects as possible, you will find many more uses.

7. Your telescope is a high quality optical instrument, and it must be cared for carefully. When you are not using it, be sure to keep it in its case. The lenses can be cleaned with a liquid lens cleaner and a soft piece of cloth such as a clean diaper or T-shirt. Do not use tissues such as Kleenex® since they may scratch the lens surface. Never submerge the telescope underwater to clean it.

8. Remember that using your eyes with your telescope, or any other optical device, will not harm your eyes or your vision in any way. If you have any questions or problems, be sure to call the clinic.

## Hand-Held Magnifiers and Stand Magnifiers

The hand-held magnifier is typically prescribed to be used with an object located at or close to its focal point. The easiest way for a patient to find this spot is to lay the magnifier on the page or object and then raise it slowly until the image is as large as possible. When a stand magnifier is used by a presbyopic patient, the key point is to hold the lens the correct distance from the add in order to have the clearest possible image and the prescribed amount of magnification. Both magnifier types may be used more effectively with adjustable lighting, reading guides, and a reading stand. The instructions should also remind patients if they are to use their glasses in conjunction with the magnifier and if they are to look through the distance portion or the add. When a magnifier cannot be used as well as expected, it may be because the patient is not an effective eccentric viewer. Training in techniques to improve this skill might be required first.

---

### SAMPLE INFORMATION SHEET

#### Hand-Held Magnifiers

The optical device your doctor has prescribed for you is called a hand-held magnifier. It is to be used for looking at things that can be held or positioned close to the lens. Things that are far away will not be in focus and cannot be seen clearly with your hand-held magnifier.

You may find that it is harder to use the hand-held magnifier at home than it was when you were in the doctor's office. That is because the doctor uses the best possible lighting along with high quality printed reading cards and makes sure that you hold the print at exactly the right distance from the lens. Most common books, newspapers, and magazines do not have the same quality of print and paper and are therefore harder to read. Also, many people have low wattage light bulbs, such as 60 or 75 watts, in their lamps at home, even though much stronger ones are available. The following are some hints to help you use your hand-held magnifier effectively.

1. When you want to look at something with your magnifier, you must hold it approximately _____ inches from the front of the lens. Try moving the magnifier slightly closer and farther until the object appears as clear as possible, and then maintain that distance from the object.

2. You should wear your glasses when using your hand-held magnifier. You should look through the top portion of your glasses to get the clearest image. The magnifier can be held close to your eye or farther away. If you hold it closer, you will have a larger field of view, but it may be less comfortable than holding it farther away. Try different distances and find out what works the best for you. (Author's note: *This paragraph can be deleted or expanded depending on the individualized prescription for each patient.*)

3. Use good lighting. You should try different types of lamps to determine what works best for you. Some people prefer lamps with fluorescent bulbs since regular bulbs may be too hot when they are nearby. Adjustable lamps allow you to position the light in the best location. For some people, a combination of lamps works better than just one. For example, a lamp with a fluorescent bulb

combined with one having a standard bulb may provide a better light source than either one alone. Natural daylight is an excellent light source, so you might try to establish a reading area near a window.

4. Reading guides may be helpful when using a hand-held magnifier. A simple reading guide can be made using the edge of a piece of black construction paper. Position the edge beneath the print in order to follow the line across the page. You may also cut a rectangle out of the paper so there is a line above as well as below. Some people find it helpful to use their finger as a marker in order to find their place when moving to a new line of print.

5. A reading stand may be useful to assist you with holding the print in a comfortable position. You should also adjust your table and chair in order to find the most comfortable position.

6. Reading with a hand-held magnifier may be tiring at first. Be sure to take frequent rest periods and build up your reading time gradually; for example, begin by practicing for only five minutes several times each day. It is best to begin with larger print such as headlines in the newspaper and then read progressively smaller print as you learn to use the magnifier. With practice, it should become easier to read for longer periods of time and to read faster. Many books are printed in large print and are available at the library as well as bookstores.

7. A hand-held magnifier may be used for reading recipes, price labels, labels on medicine bottles, bills, and letters. But reading is not the only thing it can be useful for. Some other possible uses are looking at photographs of family members and friends, looking at your wrist watch to tell the time, checking your fingernails, adjusting the heating and cooling thermostats, identifying foods in the kitchen or store, seeing playing cards in your hand, identifying cosmetics, tuning the radio, looking at pictures in magazines, and so on. If you try looking at everything you can hold close to the lens, you will discover many other uses for your magnifier.

8. Your hand-held magnifier has a high quality optical lens, and it must be cared for carefully. When you are not using it, be sure to keep it in its case. (Author's note: *Some hand-held magnifiers do not come with a case but will fit in a spectacle case.*) The lens can be cleaned with a liquid lens cleaner and a soft piece of cloth such as a clean diaper or T-shirt. Do not use tissues such as Kleenex® since they may scratch the lens surface.

9. Remember that using your eyes to read with your magnifier, or any other optical device, will not harm your eyes or your vision in any way. If you have any questions or problems, be sure to call the clinic.

## SAMPLE INFORMATION SHEET

### Stand Magnifiers

The optical device your doctor has prescribed for you is called a stand magnifier. It is designed to be placed directly on the page of print that you wish to read.

You may find that it is harder to use the stand magnifier at home than it was when you were in the doctor's office. That is because the doctor uses the best possible lighting along with high quality printed reading cards and makes sure that you hold the print at exactly the right distance from the lens. Most common books, newspapers, and magazines do not have the same quality of print and paper and are therefore harder to read. Also, many people have low wattage light bulbs, such as 60 or 75 watts, in their lamps at home, even though much stronger ones are available. The following are some hints to help you use your stand magnifier effectively.

1. When you want to look at something with your stand magnifier, you should place the base of the magnifier directly on the page and keep it there. The page should be approximately _____ inches from your glasses, and you should view through the bifocal (bottom part of your glasses).
2. Make sure that you have the clearest possible image by slowly moving the magnifier and print closer and farther until you see it the best. When you do this, make sure that the base of the magnifier stays firmly against the page and that you are looking through the right part of your glasses. If you find that it becomes necessary to pick the magnifier up from the page in order to see better, you should call the office. It may be necessary to prescribe a different magnifier for smaller print, or it might indicate that your vision has changed and needs to be checked by your doctor.
3. When you use the stand magnifier for reading, slide it slowly along the line of print without picking it up from the page. This

will help you keep the image in focus and will also help you to keep your place.

4. Use good lighting. You should try different types of lamps to determine what works best for you. Some people prefer lamps with fluorescent bulbs since regular bulbs may be too hot when they are nearby. Adjustable lamps allow you to position the light in the best location. For some people, a combination of lamps works better than just one. For example, a lamp with a fluorescent bulb combined with one having a standard bulb may provide a better light source than either one alone. Natural daylight is an excellent light source, so you might try to establish a reading area near a window.

5. Reading guides may be helpful when using a hand-held magnifier. A simple reading guide can be made using the edge of a piece of black construction paper. Position the edge beneath the print in order to follow the line across the page. You may also cut a rectangle out of the paper so there will be a line above as well as below. Some people find it helpful to use their finger as a marker in order to find their place when moving to a new line of print.

6. A reading stand may be useful to assist you with holding the print in a comfortable position. You should also adjust your table and chair in order to find the most comfortable position.

7. Reading with a stand magnifier may be tiring at first. Be sure to take frequent rest periods and build up your reading time gradually; for example, begin by practicing for only five minutes several times each day. It is best to begin with larger print such as headlines in the newspaper and then read progressively smaller print as you learn to use the magnifier. With practice, it should become easier to read for longer periods of time and to read faster. Many books are printed in large print and are available at the library as well as bookstores.

8. A stand magnifier is most useful for looking at flat objects because the base is designed to be held against the object; however, it may be used for looking at other objects. Try using your magnifier for reading recipes, price labels, labels on medicine bottles, bills, and letters. Reading is not the only thing your stand magnifier can be useful for. Some other possible uses are looking at photographs of family members and friends, looking at your wrist watch to tell the time, checking your fingernails, adjusting the heating and cooling thermostats, identifying foods

in the kitchen or store, seeing playing cards in your hand, identifying cosmetics, tuning the radio, looking at pictures in magazines, and so on. If you try looking at everything you can hold close to the base of the stand, you will discover many other uses for your magnifier.

9. Your stand magnifier has a high quality optical lens, and it must be cared for carefully. When you are not using it, be sure to keep it in its case or in a small box. The lens can be cleaned with a liquid lens cleaner and a soft piece of cloth such as a clean diaper or T-shirt. Do not use tissues such as Kleenex since they may scratch the lens surface.

10. Remember that using your eyes to read with your magnifier, or any other optical device, will not harm your eyes or your vision in any way. If you have any questions, please feel free to call the clinic.

## ORIENTATION AND MOBILITY

Orientation refers to knowing one's physical location in the environment relative to significant landmarks and objects. Mobility refers to the ability to travel efficiently and safely from one location to another. Both orientation and mobility are more difficult without good sight and are taught to blind and visually impaired persons by orientation and mobility (O&M) specialists. These specialists have college training at the master's or bachelor's level. There is a national certification program for this specialty.

Anyone who is blind or severely visually impaired should benefit from O&M training. A person with good central acuity but very restricted fields is also a good candidate for training. Training for night travel can be important for someone who has reasonable function during the day but limited vision in low levels of illumination. A comprehensive training program in O&M is labor intensive and may require several months for an adventitiously blinded adult or even years for a congenitally blind child.

Some common techniques and instruments used to enhance mobility are discussed in the following sections.

### The Sighted Guide

A visually impaired person may travel with the use of a sighted guide who leads the way. Proper technique requires that the follower grasp the guide's arm just above the elbow and walk slightly behind and to the side. The guide's grasped arm should hang freely by the side. The guide can help the follower avoid obstacles or traverse a narrow passage by moving the arm slightly behind, indicating that the follower should move to that position. Stairways should be announced, including the direction of movement, and then entered smoothly and rhythmically. When passing through doorways, the guide must communicate which side the door is on and the direction in which it opens, in order that the follower may hold the door when passing through and avoid being struck as it closes. These techniques are taught by an O&M specialist. Each low vision practitioner, as well as some of the staff, should be versed in the basic skills for being a sighted guide. This ability helps in getting patients about the office effectively and contributes to a sense of confidence in the practitioner's expertise in dealing with the problems encountered by those who are visually impaired.

Before assuming that patients who are visually impaired will need assistance in traveling, it is appropriate to ask if they need assistance; for example, "May I assist you in moving to the examination room?" Allow them the opportunity to accept or decline. If they travel independently, careful observation of their movement to the examination room will indicate how successful they are and gives an initial indication if referral for O&M training might be appropriate.

## The Guide Dog

There are several schools in the United States that train a variety of species of dogs to serve as guides to those who are blind or severely visually impaired. These dogs are very carefully screened for suitability and then subjected to a rigorous training program before they are matched to the user. It is important to realize that these dogs are intended to be a working partner with the recipient and not a pet. The dogs are taught basic skills involved in travel such as avoidance of obstacles and safe crossing of streets; however, they do not function independently and must receive some direction from the user. This requires that the recipient spend time in the training program with the dog prior to taking it home. The dogs can be taught certain routes in order to guide the user over a fixed pattern of travel, but they cannot be taught to go to some new location by verbal command. Consequently, the user must have some travel skills in order to use the dog effectively for travel to a wide variety of locations. Effective use of the guide dog requires that it be used routinely in order to maintain its physical fitness. Recipients who do not maintain their dog in prime physical condition with exercise, proper feeding, and grooming may have it taken away. This understanding is part of the original agreement prior to receiving a guide dog.

## The Long Cane

The long cane is a tool that assists the user to travel independently. It is used to avoid obstacles and detect changes in the terrain. The user learns to sweep the cane back and forth in front of the line of travel in a systematic manner. The long cane offers a number of advantages compared to a guide dog: it does not have to be groomed or fed; it doesn't shed; it is light, portable, and inexpensive; and it doesn't do "you know what," which has to be cleaned up. However, just as with a guide dog, one must learn to use a cane effectively, and this requires a comprehensive training program. Correct use of the cane requires the learning of sophisticated skills.

The long cane also serves as a means of identification that the holder is visually impaired when painted in the internationally recognized pattern of white with approximately six inches of red at the tip. Some visually impaired persons seek a cane simply for identification. This is probably not a good idea since an improperly used cane poses certain risks to the user.

## Electronic Travel Devices

Several travel assisting devices have come about through the application of new technology. The Mowatt Sensor is a hand-held device that emits an ultrasonic wavefront and vibrates in the user's hand in response to near obstacles. A typical application would be to find a hall, doorway, or large obstacle when traveling within a building. Another application of ultrasound technology resulted in the Sonic Guide. This device is a pair of spectacles that emit an ultrasonic wavefront and give auditory feedback to the wearer when obstacles are encountered.

A "laser cane" was created to increase the usefulness of the long cane; for example, the long cane cannot identify obstacles above the plane in which it is used, such as a low hanging tree branch. The laser cane emits three beams at different angles from the cane that are reflected back to the cane if an object is encountered. The user receives auditory feedback of differing pitches for each of the beams. Although the concept seems useful, it has certain limitations. In a crowded area such as a busy intersection, the user is literally overwhelmed with feedback.

The Nightscope, originally developed by ITT, was designed to assist persons with nightblindness. Essentially, it is a hand-held monocular that amplifies ambient light manyfold and hence allows the person with a rod dysfunction to perform better in areas of dim illumination. It was initially thought that this device would be of great benefit to persons with retinitis pigmentosa; however, experience has shown that a strong flashlight performs just as well and is considerably less expensive.

## SUMMARY

Training plays an important part in the rehabilitation process. The most common types include training in techniques of eccentric viewing, training in the correct use of a specific device, and orientation and mobility training. Even when a patient seems to function well with a device, there is an excellent chance that performance can be enhanced further by systematic training. The difference between success and failure for any individual may be the time spent reinforcing the basic skills necessary to use an optical device or residual vision more effectively.

## REFERENCES

1. Freeman PB, Jose RT: *The Art and Practice of Low Vision.* Boston, Butterworth-Heinemann, 1991.
2. Baldasare J, Watson GR, Whittaker SG, Miller-Shaffer H: The development and evaluation of a reading test for low vision individuals with macular loss. *J Vis Impair Blind* 80(6):785-789, 1986.

## ADDITIONAL READING

Barraga N: Effects of experimental teaching on the visual behavior of children with low vision. *Am J Optom & Arch Am Acad Optom* 42(9):557-561, 1965.

Barraga N: Learning efficiency in low vision. *J Am Optom Assoc* 40(8):807-810, 1969.

Goodrich GL, Mehr EB, Quillman RD, Shaw HK, Wiley JK: Training and practice effects on performance with low vision aids: A preliminary study. *Am J Optom Physiol Optics* 54(5):312-318, 1977.

Goodrich GL, Quillman R: Training eccentric viewing. *J Vis Impair Blind* 71:377-381, 1977.

Hoeft W: Bioptic telescopes: Training and adaptation. *Optom Monthly* Sept:71-74, 1980.

Holcomb JG, Goodrich GL: Eccentric viewing training. *J Am Optom Assoc* 47(11): 1438-1443, 1976.

Jose RT, Browning R: Training with the expanded field bioptic telescope. *Rehab Optom J* 1:5-6, 1983.

Jose RT, Watson G: Increasing reading efficiency with an optical aid/training curriculum. *Rev Optom* 15(2):41-48, 1978.

Jose RT, Butler JH: Training a patient to drive with telescopic lenses. *Am J Optom Physiol Optics* 52(5):343-346, 1975.

Jose RT, Carter K, Carter C: A training program for clients considering the use of bioptic telescope for driving. *J Vis Impair Blind* 77(9):425-428, 1983.

Kelleher DK: Training low vision patients. *J Am Optom Assoc* 47(11):1425-1427, 1976.

Newman JD, Pogoda A: An overview of visual rehabilitation and training of the low vision patient. *J Am Optom Assoc* 49(4):423-426, 1978.

Rosenberg R: Training in low vision practice. *J Am Optom Assoc* 39(1):57-60, 1978.

Watson G, Jose RT: A training sequence for low vision patients. *J Am Optom Assoc* 47(11):1407-1415, 1976.

Wheatley GP: Instructing the patient with low vision to use a microscope for reading and near tasks. *J Vis Rehab* 4(2):19-28, 1990.

# DRIVING WITH IMPAIRED VISION

It should come as no surprise that many patients express driving as their main goal. What may be surprising, however, is how many people with low vision continue to drive even though their acuity is well below that required to obtain a legal license in their state. The usual justifications are that they "only drive a short distance to the store, only drive in familiar places, do not have anyone to drive them, or do not want to impose on their friends or family members." Our society is mobile and status-oriented, and it places great value on the ability to own and use an automobile. No one wants to give up this facet of his or her life, even though there has been a decrease in vision. For youngsters with impaired vision, there is an equally strong desire to acquire the right to drive. The social burden, fueled by peer pressure, of not achieving this milestone in development weighs heavily on teenagers' thoughts. The clinician working with such people, young and old, has to walk a fine line to ease them into accepting the possibility that they might never be able to drive or that they might have to give up driving.

Courts in Texas and Pennsylvania have ruled that visually impaired drivers have the right to individual driving performance evaluations and that driving privileges cannot be denied solely on the basis of a visual disability or the use of a prosthetic device. This is consistent with the Rehabilitation Act of 1973, Section 504 (Nondiscrimination Under Federal Grants), which states:

No otherwise qualified handicapped individual in the United States, as defined in section 7(6), shall, solely by reason of his handicap, be excluded from the participation in, be denied the benefits of, or be subjected to discrimination under any program or activity receiving Federal financial assistance.

Since portions of state highway programs are federally funded, this section is applicable to driving.

## VISION REQUIREMENTS FOR DRIVING

There is disparity among the various states with respect to vision requirements for legal driving. This highlights the fact that there is not universal agreement with respect to what acuity and field are necessary to be a safe driver. People drive under such widely, and often rapidly, varying conditions that it is difficult to determine how a specific vision loss will affect their performance. Such variable conditions include illumination, weather, speed, traffic, windshield cleanliness, road condition, vehicle maintenance, attention to task, complexity of the route, and familiarity with the area. It seems clear that a normally sighted person can drive adequately at night in the rain, so why can't a moderately visually impaired person drive safely on a sunny day or at a lower rate of speed? Such variables have yet to be studied adequately in order to determine a true measure of the vision requirements for driving. Some states require periodic testing of vision, while others do not, which allows some people to drive well past the time when their vision loss puts them, and others, at definite risk.

While most states have a visual field requirement for operating a motorized vehicle, applicants are rarely tested as part of routine vision screenings when renewing or applying for a license. Similarly, relatively little has been published about driving with a field restriction (see Additional Reading: Danielson, Johnson, and Keltner), but some adaptations, such as special mirrors mounted on the vehicle,[1] have been tried. A vignette concerning driving with a lateral field restriction appears in Chapter 30.

## DRIVING WITH TELESCOPES

More than one-half of the states have allowed visually impaired drivers to obtain a legal license if they use a telescope mounted in spectacles to improve their functional spotting acuity. Such a policy has been firmly rejected by other states, including some that have allowed it on an experimental basis. The optical device most often considered for driving is a spectacle-mounted "bioptic" telescope to be used for spotting. Those who have argued against driving with telescopes have expressed five major concerns:

1. People who need such a device have vision that is so bad that they should not be driving anyway.
2. It is not possible to drive while looking through a telescope because of the alteration in apparent movement of objects.
3. If a person is 20/200 without the telescope, then he or she would be legally blind at all times while driving since the *acuity* would be impaired without the telescope and the *field* would be impaired to less than 20 degrees when spotting through the telescope.

4. The telescope housing creates a large ring scotoma that represents a significant hazard while using it.
5. The person will use the telescope to obtain a legal license but then will drive without it.

Proponents of driving with bioptic telescopes have presented the following counterarguments:

1. The acuity required for safe driving is not established, and it probably is not 20/20.
2. The person does not drive around looking through the telescope but rather uses it as a spotting device, much like a rearview mirror.
3. An acuity of 20/200 would not qualify for most of the special driving programs anyway.
4. The scotoma caused by the telescope housing blends in with the scotoma caused by the hood of the vehicle inferiorly, is several feet above the road superiorly, and, at a reasonable distance, is beyond the edge of the road laterally. Hence the induced scotoma is not as serious an obstruction as the opponents would have one believe.
5. The telescope will be a legal requirement for driving, just as glasses might, and the photograph on the driver's license could include the telescope.

New York legalized driving with bioptic telescopes in 1977. The major restrictions applied to the use of telescopes were that the visual acuity must be at least 20/40 through the telescope and at least 20/100 through the carrier lens with a horizontal field of vision no less than 140 degrees without benefit of any compensating device. Additionally, the person must have been fitted with telescopes, must have had them in their possession at least 60 days prior to renewal or first licensure, and must have received training (equal to a suggested protocol) designed to adjust the user gradually to the use of the telescopic device, first under simulated, and finally under actual, driving conditions.

A similar law in Virginia, effective July 1, 1986, required visual acuity of 20/200 or better in one or both eyes through the carrier and 20/70 or better through the spectacle-mounted bioptic lens. The field of view without assistive devices had to be 70 degrees or better. Driving was restricted to daylight hours only.

## EXPERIMENTAL PROGRAMS FOR DRIVERS WHO ARE VISUALLY IMPAIRED

Some experimental driving programs for those who are visually impaired were established in order to evaluate the feasibility of driving with telescopic lenses. Enrollment was extremely selective for mature and responsible subjects. Such selectivity was considered essential since a bad outcome might have caused the opportunity to be lost for all people with visual impairment. One early concern was that the limited number of drivers in these programs meant that even one fatality or serious accident would seem statistically significant in terms of the usual comparisons such as "accidents or fatalities per man-hour of driving." The first report of driving with telescopes appeared in 1970.[2] It presented 128 cases over a six-year period with an accident rate lower than that for the general population. In spite of excellent safety records from various programs, many states have refused to allow licensing of visually impaired drivers.

## Training Protocols

Various training protocols have been developed, but presently there is no scientific body of evidence to support their effectivity, although it seems intuitively logical to expect that more effective use of a bioptic telescope for driving could be developed through sequential training from less complex tasks to more complex tasks. Chapman[3,4] suggested the following protocol:

1. Target practice
   a. spot stationary targets from a stationary position
   b. spot and track moving targets from a stationary position
2. In-car training as observer, not driver
   a. spot stationary targets while moving
   b. spot and track moving targets while moving
3. In-car training as driver
   a. controlled access highway driving
   b. residential street, 25 to 35 mph speed limit
   c. major traffic artery, 45 to 55 mph speed limit
   d. residential street, 40 mph speed limit
   e. downtown rush hour traffic
   f. street, 35 mph speed limit
   g. random mixtures of all of the above
   h. four-lane highway
   i. two-lane highway
   j. city freeway

The sequence of street and traffic experiences above is selected to provide increasing complexity of the driving task with respect to traffic, roadside clutter (signs, parked cars, pedestrians, and so on), and speed. It might seem unusual to begin driving on a controlled access highway, but the author points out that this situation has less clutter to interpret, fewer potential hazards such as pedestrians or entering traffic, and less need for driving adjustment since traffic travels at a rather uniform speed. The New York statute allowing drivers to be licensed for driving with bioptic telescopes required a similar training protocol prior to final approval.

Park et al.[5] reported on a comprehensive, multidisciplinary assessment and training program designed to provide the visually impaired driver a means to demonstrate and substantiate safe driving skills. The multidisciplinary team included a low vision practitioner, orientation and mobility specialist, occupational therapist, and a certified driving instructor. Those who were referred to the program must have met the visual driving requirements for the state of Michigan prior to a prescreening. The prescreening included a review of medical and health history, current medications, and previous driving history as well as tests for visual perception (the Motor Free Visual Perception Test), scanning, lateral neglect, midline orientation deficits, color perception, glare recovery, depth perception, night vision, and reaction time. Cognitive evaluations were performed if deficits were suspected. A telescopic evaluation that averaged 20 hours was performed on a standardized course. The duration of the evaluation depended primarily on prior experience and analyzed such skills as ability to locate stationary and moving objects while the user was stationary and/or moving. The telescopic evaluation was followed by training as a "co-pilot" in a vehicle approximately four weeks after the telescope was dispensed. The user was then evaluated while actually driving. The road evaluation included an assessment of a large number of skills such as identification of hazards, compensation for blind spots, utilization of defensive driving skills, and proper operation of the vehicle. Skills evaluated specifically with respect to the use of the telescope included object identification and recognition, compensation for blind spots, scanning, spotting, localization, and fixation. Based on these evaluations, a plan was established for training sessions to maximize safe driving skills.

In spite of the apparent logic of providing training to compensate for a disability or impairment, the adaptation of any required training protocol for those who are visually impaired that is not required for those who are normally sighted may be challenged as discriminatory.

## ACCIDENT RATES FOR VISUALLY IMPAIRED DRIVERS

Accident rates for drivers with bioptic telescopes have been reported in five states. They are consistently higher than rates for normally sighted control groups (Table 23–1), with the exception of Illinois during 1988.[6,7] A flaw in these studies is the failure to adequately define the accident with respect to cause, fault, fatalities, amount of property damage, and so forth in order to make reasonable comparisons. If one is to make meaningful comparisons, it is also necessary to identify a control population that is matched for age, sex, and

TABLE 23-1. Accident rates for users of bioptic telescopes (BTS) compared to other drivers in that state.

|  | New York* | California* | Maine* | Texas*,† | Illinois† |
|---|---|---|---|---|---|
| BTS sample size | 168 | 229 | 14 | 64 | 101 |
| Control sample size | all drivers | 21,064 | all drivers | 64 | all drivers |
| Accident rate for BTS users | 2–3 | 1.5 | 1.4 | 1.34 | 0.98 |

Example: The general accident rate for users of bioptic telescopes in California was 1.5 times that of the control group of 21,064 drivers.
*Lippman, Corn, and Lewis[6] †Age and sex matched ‡Taylor[7]

driving exposure. This is particularly important and is often neglected in statistical reports as demonstrated in Table 23-1. When visually impaired drivers are compared to drivers with other disabilities, the accident rates appear more favorable (Table 23-2).

## SUMMARY

The desire to continue driving or to obtain a driver's license is a goal commonly expressed by persons who are visually impaired. Opportunity exists, in some states, to drive legally with impaired vision. For those who live in states where it is not allowed, changing residency is the only viable alternative. Visually impaired drivers have performed well using spectacle-mounted telescopes. While their accident rates appear to be somewhat higher than those for drivers without impaired vision, they may actually have a lower rate than drivers with other disabilities. Any comparison of accident rates or driving performance should categorize the etiology and severity of the accidents and should use appropriately matched controls. Failure to do so is a fault with a number of previous studies.

The information presented in this chapter has emphasized vision, but, of course, that is not the only variable that affects driving performance. Many

TABLE 23-2. Accident ratios for disabled drivers in Texas for one year after review by the medical advisory board.[6]

| Etiology of Disability | Ratio per 100 Drivers |
|---|---|
| Neurological | 8.50 |
| Cardiovascular | 5.63 |
| Visual impairment | 4.86 |

other environmental, physical, and mental factors contribute to driving. These should also be considered in studies of driving safety that determine whether or not those who are visually impaired are allowed to drive. The use of bioptic telescopes and training programs is a natural and logical consideration since visual acuity has always been considered an important test for obtaining a driver's license; however, neither the effectiveness of using a telescope as opposed to driving without it nor the effectiveness of specific training programs has been proven.

Further research is needed to provide scientifically based guidelines for mandating the visual performance levels necessary for safe driving with an unrestricted license as well as the conditions (lighting, speed, and so forth) under which those guidelines might safely be relaxed for those with various levels of impaired vision.

## REFERENCES

1. Weiss NJ: Adapting an automobile for driving with hemianopsia. *Rehab Optom* 2(3):7, 1984.
2. Korb D: Preparing the visually-handicapped person for motor vehicle operation. *Am J Optom Physiol Optics* 47(8):619-628, 1970.
3. Chapman BG: Techniques and variables related to driving—Part 1. *Rehab Optom* 2(2):18-20, 1984.
4. Chapman BG: Techniques and variables related to driving—Part 2. *Rehab Optom* 2(3)12-14, 1984.
5. Park WL, Unatin J, Hebert A: A driving program for the visually impaired. *J Am Optom Assoc* 64:54-59, 1993.
6. Lippman O, Corn AL, Lewis MC: Bioptic telescope spectacles and driving performance: A study in Texas. *J Vis Impair Blind* 82:182-187, 1988.
7. Taylor DG: Telescopic spectacles for driving: User data satisfaction, preferences and effects in vocational, educational and personal tasks. *J Vis Rehab* 4(2):29-61, 1990.

## ADDITIONAL READING

American Medical Association and American Association of Motor Vehicle Administrators: *Proceedings of the National Conference on Telescopic Devices and Driving.* Washington, D.C., June 11-12. Morton Grove, IL, Health and Safety Associates, 1976.
American Optometric Association, Low Vision Section: The use of bioptic telescopes for driving. *Rehab Optom* 1(2):8-10, 1983.

Bailey IL: Driving with bioptic telescopes—a position paper. *Rehab Optom* 1:9-11, 1984.

Bailey IL: Bioptic telescopes (letter). *Arch Ophthalmol* 103(1):13-14, 1985.

California Department of Motor Vehicles: *The Accident Record of Drivers with Bioptic Telescopic Lenses.* Sacramento, CA, author, 1983.

Danielson RW: The relationship of fields of vision to safety in driving. *Trans Am Ophthalmol Soc* 54:657-680, 1956.

Davidson T: Disaster or not? Telescopics for distance vision in mobility. *Low Vis Abstr* 1(2):3-8, 1972.

Faye EE: Driving with telescopes. *Nearpoint,* summer, 1975.

Feinbloom W: Recent developments in bioptic aids for driving, in *Proceedings of the National Conference on Telescopic Devices and Driving.* June 11-12, 1976. Arlington Heights, IL, American Association for Automotive Medicine, 1976.

Feinbloom W: Driving with bioptic telescopic spectacles. *Am J Optom Physiol Optics* 54(1):35-42, 1977.

Fonda G: Bioptic telescopic spectacles for driving a motor vehicle. *Arch Ophthalmol* 92(4):348-349, 1974.

Fonda G: A bioptic telescopic spectacle: Advantages and limitations. *Sight Saving Review* 48(3):125-128, 1978.

Fonda G: Bioptic telescopic spectacle is a hazard for operating a motor vehicle. *Arch Ophthalmol* 101:1907-1908, 1983.

Fonda G: Legal blindness can be compatible with safe driving. *Ophthalmol* 96(10): 1457-1459, 1989.

Goodrich GL: Driving and telescopic aids: A bibliography. *J Vis Rehab* 2(2):21-30, 1988.

Huss CP: Model approach—Low Vision Driver's Training and Assessment. *J Vis Rehab* 2(2):31-44, 1988.

Huss CP: A multidisciplinary approach to driving for the visually handicapped. *Rehab Optom* 2(2):10-11, 1984.

Johnson CA, Keltner JL: The incidence of visual field loss in 20,000 eyes and its relationship to driving. *Arch Ophthalmol* 101(3):371-375, 1983.

Jose R, Ousley BA: The visually handicapped, driving and bioptics—some new facts. *Rehab Optom* 2(2):2-5, 1984.

Hellinger GO: A cautionary view of driving with telescopes, in Faye EE, Hood CM (eds): *Low Vision.* Springfield, IL, Charles C. Thomas, 1975.

Janke M: Accident rates of drivers with bioptic telescopes. *J Safety Res* 14:159-165, 1983.

Janke M, Kazarian G: The accident record of drivers with bioptic telescopic lenses. Report #86. Sacramento, CA, State of California, 1983.

Jose RT, Butler JH: Driver's training for partially sighted persons: An interdisciplinary approach. *New Outlook for the Blind* Sept:305-307 and 311, 1975.

Jose RT, Carter K, Carter C: A training program for clients considering the use of bioptic telescope for driving. *J Vis Impair Blind* 77(9):425-428, 1983.

Keeney A: Field loss vs central magnification: Telescopes and the driving task. *Arch Ophthalmol* 92(4):273, 1974.

Keeney A: Practical concerns in driving with subnormal vision: Criteria for introducing new devices, in *Proceedings of the National Conference on Telescopic Devices and Driving,* June 11-12, 1976. Arlington Heights, IL, American Association for Automotive Medicine, 1976.

Keeney AH, Weiss S: Operational limitations of driving with telescopes, in Faye EE, Hood CM (eds): *Low Vision.* Springfield, IL, Charles C. Thomas, 1975, pp 204-207.

Keeney AH, Weiss S, Silva D: Functional problems of telescopic spectacles in the driving task. *Transac Am Ophthalmol Soc* 72:132-138, 1974.

Kelleher DK: Experience of a low vision patient driving with a bioptic telescope, in Faye EE, Hood CM (eds): *Low Vision.* Springfield, IL, Charles C. Thomas, 1975.

Kelleher DK: Adaptation and other considerations in driving with low vision, in *Proceedings of the National Conference on Telescopic Devices and Driving,* June 11-12, 1976. Arlington Heights, IL, American Association for Automotive Medicine, 1976.

Kelleher DK, Mehr EB: Motor vehicle operation by a patient with low vision: A case report. *Am J Optom & Arch Am Acad Optom* 48:773-777, 1971.

Kelleher DK: Driving with bioptics—a personal viewpoint. *Rehab Optom* 2(2):8-9, 1984.

Keltner JL, Johnson CA: Mass visual field screening in a driving population. *Ophthalmol* 87:785-790, 1980.

Keltner JL, Johnson CA: Visual function, driving safety, and the elderly. *Ophthalmol* 94(9):1180-1188, 1987.

Levin M, Kelleher DK: Driving with a bioptic telescope: An interdisciplinary approach. *Am J Optom Physiol Optics* 52(3):200-206, 1975.

Lippmann O: Driving with telescopic aids, in *Proceedings of the American Association of Automotive Medicine.* 1976, pp 204-216.

Lippmann O: Automobile driving with telescopic aids (letter). *Arch Ophthalmol* 98(5):930, 1980.

Newman JD: A rational approach to license drivers using bioptic telescopes. *J Am Optom Assoc* 47:510-513, 1976.

Padula W: The use of bioptic telescopes for driving. *J Rehab Optom* 1(2):8-10, 1983.

Padula W: The issue of driving with bioptic telescopes. *J Rehab Optom* 2(1):22, 1984.

Safety Management Institute: *Report on Conference on Telescopic Lens Systems and Driver Licensing.* Albany, Department of Motor Vehicles, Contract No. C54385, State of New York, 1975.

Smith DP, Layland B: A report on telescopic spectacles and automobile driving. *Austr J Optom* 58(9):337-339, 1975.

Spitzberg LA: A patient's experience on driving with a bioptic. *J Vis Rehab* 5(1):17-21, 1991.

Tallman CB: A positive approach to driving with telescopic glasses, in Faye EE, Hood CM (eds): *Low Vision.* Springfield, IL, Charles C. Thomas, 1975.

Tallman CB: Bioptic telescopic spectacle: A hazard for operating a motor vehicle (letter). *Arch Ophthalmol* 102(8):1119-1120, 1984.

Taylor DG: Telescopic spectacles for driving: User data satisfaction, preferences and effects in vocational, educational and personal tasks: A study in Illinois. *J Vis Rehab* 4(2):29-59, 1990.

Vics J: Low vision drivers wearing bioptic telescopic spectacles. *Optom Weekly* 66: 1145-1149, 1975.

Vogel GL: Training the bioptic telescope wearer for driving. *J Am Optom Assoc* 62: 288-293, 1991.

Wyatt WJ, Swick DR, Huss CP: The psychologist's role in low vision driver evaluation. *J Vis Rehab* 2(2):39-53, 1989.

# NONOPTICAL AIDS FOR ACTIVITIES OF DAILY LIVING

*A frequent chief complaint expressed by patients who are visually impaired is inability to perform routine activities of daily living (ADL) such as personal grooming, shopping, cooking, cleaning, and matching clothes. This complaint may not be completely resolved with the prescription of optical devices, but there are many nonoptical devices that may prove helpful. These nonoptical devices can be ordered from sources provided in Chapter 31. Since most clinicians do not want to have a large inventory of these devices, it is perfectly appropriate to provide catalogues to patients and their families so they may order their own. It is a good idea, however, to have some examples for demonstration as well as some of the particularly popular items. The latter include signature guides, reading guides (typoscopes), felt-tip pens, and large print playing cards.*

*Some patients who require more than assistive devices must be referred to a rehabilitation teacher. Such teachers have special training in adaptive techniques for those with visual impairments. An occupational therapist might also provide this service if he or she has had suitable training in the special techniques required for those who have visual impairments. The most likely source for locating a rehabilitation teacher is each state's department of vocational rehabilitation. The following sections review some adaptive tools and techniques for ADL.*

## COOKING

Stove markings can be made visible and/or palpable with special pens that deposit a thick colored "ink" (Hi-Marks™, available from the New York Lighthouse). A simple code can be devised such as an increasing number of dots for higher temperatures. Some microwaves are now available with large print markings. Favorite recipes can be copied onto notecards in large print. There are also large print cookbooks (see Resources, Chapter 31). Cans or jars can be labeled with miniature plastic models of the enclosed food, marked with raised letters, or placed in designated spots once an organizational scheme is formulated for the kitchen pantry. An inexpensive marking device is the rubber band. A specific number of rubber bands placed around jars or cans may be used to identify different foods.

Fluid levels in cups or bowls can be monitored with an electronic detector that gives an audible alarm when the level reaches its two probes, completing the electric circuit to the alarm (Figure 24-1). Other items that may prove helpful are large print timers, a cutting board with a chute to direct the food into the next receptacle, elbow length oven mits, slicing guides, and plates with a recessed center to keep food from being pushed off the plate.

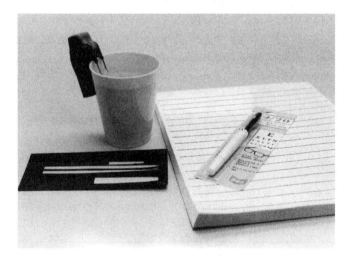

**Figure 24-1.** The "Say When" liquid level indicator emits an audible tone when the fluid level reaches the two probes and completes an electrical circuit. It is available from the New York Lighthouse (see Resources, Chapter 31). Also shown are bold line writing paper, a felt-tip pen, and a check writing guide.

## SHOPPING

A common problem in shopping is identification of paper money. One technique for "marking" one's own money is to fold each denomination in a characteristic manner. It is also possible to carry only one denomination (such as all one-dollar bills or to ask that change be given in all one-dollar bills). This avoids the frequent problem of being shortchanged by unscrupulous or incompetent clerks. It may not win any popularity contests, but the visually impaired shopper can always hold up the bill, turn to other shoppers, and announce loudly, "She said this was a ten dollar bill. Is it?" A portable electronic identifier was recently introduced that may become more popular as the price becomes more reasonable. Other items that might prove helpful are talking calculators and large print checks.

## PERSONAL SECURITY

Personal security is a mounting concern for everyone and is heightened by aging, living alone, and visual impairment, all of which often accompany each other. Things that might be suggested are portable personal alarms, large print telephone dials, programmable telephones, portable door guards, and home security alarms.

## RECREATION

A number of games are available in large print and Braille versions, including playing cards, bingo, dominoes, and Scrabble. Chess and checkers sets exist that use pegs on the pieces and holes in the board to keep the pieces from being bumped out of place. Chess sets can be purchased in a large variety of sizes. An increasing number of books are available in large print and recorded versions. Most people can learn to operate any cassette player tactually, but there are some players that are easier to operate than others. Television can still be enjoyed even if the picture is not very visible, and many people are pleased to rediscover radio. In some areas of the country, the Public Broadcasting System offers the Radio Reading Service. This service utilizes a sideband to the local FM station, and broadcasts can be picked up by a special receiver. The programming differs from standard radio in that a variety of newspaper and magazine articles are read over the air. This gives the listener access to versions that would ordinarily be available only in printed form. The local PBS station can be contacted to learn of the availability for a given area.

It is easy to adopt a sedentary and solitary lifestyle following the loss of vision if one feels confined to the home, but this is unnecessary. Recreation outside of the home will be enhanced by ensuring that the individual has good travel skills, which may require the services of an orientation and mobility instructor.

## ENVIRONMENTAL ADAPTATIONS

There are many environmental adaptations that can assist people who are visually impaired by enhancing their use of residual vision. The easiest areas to address are lighting, color, and contrast. These areas can be reviewed in the form of information sheets that can be given to patients and their families. The following sections include examples of such sheets. This information can also be provided in audible form in standard cassette tapes.

---

### SAMPLE INFORMATION SHEET

#### Lighting

You may find that it is harder to see at home or at work than it was when you were in the doctor's office. One possible reason is that the doctor used the best possible lighting along with high quality printed reading cards. Most common books, newspapers, and magazines do not have the same quality of print and paper and are therefore harder to read. Also, many people have low wattage light bulbs in their lamps at home or at work even though much stronger ones are available. Of course, sometimes too much light can also be a problem since it can cause glare or possibly eye discomfort. Each person must experiment with the lighting at home or at work in order to find the best possible arrangement.

If you think that more light helps you to see better, the following hints may help you have better lighting at home.

1. Change your light bulbs to a higher wattage. Light bulbs are readily available up to 300 watts.
2. Sit closer to the lamp when reading. The amount of light from a lamp decreases dramatically when you are farther away.
3. Adjustable bulbs such as "three-way" bulbs may be helpful if you prefer different levels of light for different tasks. An adjustable

---

rheostat for the lamp may also be helpful since it can be used to raise or lower the amount of light with great precision.

4. Change the shade on your lamp to one that is white or light tan. Any lamp may seem brighter if the lamp shade is changed to a lighter color. Dark color shades absorb light from the light bulb and do not reflect it into the room. This light is lost.

5. If you have difficulty getting close enough to the lamp, try an adjustable lamp. Adjustable lamps allow you to position the light in the best location. Some people may need to adjust the lamp so the bulb is just a few inches from what they are reading.

6. Try different types of lamps and light bulbs to determine what type works best for you. Some people prefer lamps with fluorescent bulbs since regular bulbs may be too hot when they are nearby. For some people, a combination of lamps works better than just one; for example, a lamp with a fluorescent bulb combined with one having a standard incandescent bulb may provide a better light source than either one alone. Some light bulbs use special filaments to create light that is similar to daylight. These bulbs may work better than the traditional types.

7. Natural daylight is an excellent light source, so you might try to establish a reading area near a window.

8. If changing lamps and light bulbs does not seem to help enough, you might consider other changes in the home; for example, heavy, dark curtains or drapes that don't open completely might block a significant amount of light from the window. Adjust curtains so they can be opened completely. If necessary, replace drapes with new ones that are lighter in color. Light colors reflect more light and make a room seem brighter. This is also true of the paint on the walls. If a room has darkly colored walls, they will absorb light instead of reflecting light back into the room. Repainting the walls in one or more rooms can significantly improve a person's ability to function visually. As a general rule, the lighter the shade, the more light will be reflected into the room off the walls.

When bright light seems to be a problem, the following hints may be helpful.

1. Glare may be experienced when a light source is directed into the eye at a specific angle. This can often be avoided by changing the angle of the lamp or by adjusting your position with respect to the lamp and/or window.

2. Glare or discomfort from bright lights may be reduced by blocking some of the light. This can be accomplished by wearing a visor or a hat with a large brim. This may be helpful indoors as well as outdoors.

3. Different types of lamps and light bulb types should be tried to find the best combination. Read the suggestions given above for increasing light, and modify the ideas to find the best light levels for your own situation.

4. Tinted lenses can be prescribed by your doctor to help block some light from reaching the eyes. Although many tinted lenses are available without prescription in various stores, the single best source for information about what is best for your eyes and situation is your doctor. Tinted lenses may be useful indoors as well as outdoors. Some people have several pair of tinted glasses, each of which is used in a different situation.

## SAMPLE INFORMATION SHEET

### Color and Contrast

When a person becomes visually impaired, it often affects his or her color perception as well as the visual acuity. Together, these losses make it difficult to perform ordinary daily activities. Visual function, however, may be enhanced with some simple adjustments around the home or work place. Color and contrast are two key areas that should be considered when making adaptations at home and at work. A simple definition of contrast is the difference in visibility between an object and its background; for example, dark gray print on a medium gray piece of paper has low contrast and is hard to see, while dark black print on white paper has high contrast and is more visible. The following hints will help you to think about adjusting color and contrast around the home or work place in order to use your vision more effectively.

1. Many people with a vision impairment express difficulty with eating because it is hard to identify the food on their plate or on the table. By paying attention to color and contrast, you can make some tasks easier; for example, imagine white milk in a clear glass sitting on a white tablecloth. That would have low contrast and be hard to see, as would carrots on an orange plate or black cof-

fee in a black mug on a navy blue tablecloth. It is much easier to see milk in a clear glass if the tablecloth or place mat is dark. The solution then is to serve foods in and on surfaces with contrasting colors. Most foods contrast well with a white plate, but you might try a variety of colored plates, place mats, and tablecloths and use them in the combinations that make each meal most visible.

2. The same ideas about color and contrast can be used around the house. Throw rugs that are hard to see may cause people to stumble but are easier to see if they contrast in color with the surface they are against. Furniture slip covers may be used to make a chair or sofa contrast with the carpet.

3. Good lighting enhances contrast. Lamps and ceiling fixtures should have bulbs with high enough wattage to make each room brightly yet comfortably illuminated.

4. In the bathroom, some attention to colors may also help. Try colored toilet paper to contrast with the wall on which it is hung. Make sure that your toothpaste and toothbrush are different colors. If the toothbrush is hung against the wall, it should have a bright color that contrasts with the color of the wall. Towels are available in many bright colors that contrast with the walls against which they are hung. A washcloth of a different color from the towels makes it easier to find. Try different colors of soaps to see which is most visible in your shower or bathtub. Use a colored glass (preferably plastic) to make it easier to see and to avoid breakage.

5. Contrasting sheets, blankets, bedspreads, and pillowcases are easier to identify and assist in making the bed neatly.

6. When preparing food, applying make-up, or performing other activities that involve using many small items, it may be easier to keep track of them if you spread a brightly colored towel or place mat out and then be sure to place the items on it each time they are used. If it becomes difficult to find a small item that you have been using, at least you know that it is somewhere on that colored surface.

7. Some other items to consider for color and contrast are: shelf paper, doorknobs, keyholes, table covers, telephones, lamp switches, wall switches, wall plugs, kitchen utensil holders, pens and pencils, key cases, pillboxes, napkins, and clothes. Look around the house and work place. Anything that you have trouble seeing may be easier to find and use if it, or its surroundings, are changed in order to increase contrast.

## SUMMARY

There are many activities of daily living that can be made easier to perform with the appropriate assistive devices. These devices can be identified in catalogues available for people with special needs. The single best source for assisting people who are visually impaired is a rehabilitation teacher, especially if the teacher is available for a home visit.

## ADDITIONAL READING

Branch L, Horowitz A, Carr C: The implications for everyday life of incident self-reported visual decline among people over age 65 living in the community. *Gerontologist* 29(3):359–365, 1989.

Breuer J: *Handbook of Assistive Devices for the Handicapped Elderly: A New Help for Independent Living*. New York, Haworth Press, 1982.

Dickman IR: *Making Life More Livable: Simple Adaptations for the Homes of Blind and Visually Impaired Older People*. New York, American Foundation for the Blind, 1983.

Hiatt LG, McQueen C: *Review of the Literature on Vision, Hearing, and Memory in Old Age With Implications For Self-Help and Environmental Design*. New York, American Foundation for the Blind, 1982.

Lee PN, Ingman SJ, Guarcello FP: Non-optical aids: An important part in low vision rehabilitation. *Rev Optom* 116(9):73–80, 1979.

Mehr EB: The typoscope of Charles Prentice. *Am J Optom Arch Am Acad Optom* 46(11):885–887, 1969.

Null RL: Kitchens designed for the low vision elderly. *J Vis Rehab* 2(4):45–53, 1988.

Ponchillia SV, LaGrow S: Independent glucose monitoring by functionally blind diabetics. *J Vis Impair Blind* 82(2):50–53, 1988.

# GENETIC COUNSELING

*A significant percentage of legal blindness results from hereditary disorders, and many hereditary disorders have ocular manifestations, even though they do not result in legal blindness. For these reasons it is important for a vision specialist, especially one who works with patients who are visually impaired, to have a good grasp of the principles of medical genetics. Legal precedents mandate both the recognition of genetic aspects of disease and the provision of genetic counseling when a hereditary disease is diagnosed.*

*Genetic counseling can take place only after an exact diagnosis and a complete family history are obtained. Part of the family history includes the construction of a pedigree showing both affected and unaffected family members. One might argue that genetic counseling is a logical part of the ocular health assessment. This has merit, yet experience shows that it is often ignored or performed in a perfunctory manner. The patient also may bear a psychological burden[1] associated with genetic disease that affects the rehabilitation process. It is therefore reasonable to consider genetic counseling in the context of vision rehabilitation.*

## GENETIC DISORDERS AND VISION

Approximately 15% of legal blindness stems from hereditary disorders. The most common cause of hereditary legal blindness is the group of disorders known as retinitis pigmentosa, which accounts for 5% of the prevalence and 3% of the incidence.[2] There are also many genetic disorders that cause ocular abnormalities and/or visual disabilities but do not necessarily cause total or legal blindness; for example, color vision disorders are quite common, affecting approximately 8% of males and 1% of females.[3] While these disorders are not typically considered severely debilitating, the clinician should keep in mind the fact that all disabilities are perceived differently by individuals and that it is the patient or other family members who decide how a disorder impacts on their family. Oculocutaneous albinism is one such disorder. There is at least one example of a couple electing to terminate a pregnancy after prenatal diagnosis confirmed that the fetus was affected.[4] The couple was of Middle Eastern origin and believed that in their society the offspring would suffer severe social and economic disadvantages due to the decreased skin pigmentation. Another example of the difference in individual perception of disability that the author has experienced in his practice occurs among families with retinitis pigmentosa. When there are many affected family members, the disorder is often considered an inconvenience rather than a handicap. On the other hand, if only a single family member is affected, it may be perceived by other family members as a severe handicap.

Many hereditary ocular abnormalities have been assigned to specific chromosomal locations; however, it is important to realize that new techniques of molecular analysis are resulting in a rapid increase in the identification of genetic loci and that any listing is virtually out of date as soon as it is published. Ocular abnormalities are also associated with chromosomal abnormalities and other patterns of malformation.

## LEGAL PRECEDENTS GERMANE TO GENETIC COUNSELING

Claims for damages may be made for both *economic harm* and *noneconomic harm*. Examples of noneconomic harm are emotional pain and suffering. Although courts were initially reluctant to allow damages for such claims because of difficulty in allotting a dollar value to an abstract condition, that is no longer the case. Economic harm is less difficult to value. Some examples of claims that have been made for recovery of economic loss include recovery of medical fees, cost of rearing a handicapped child, cost of institutionalization, and funeral expenses.[5]

Claims may be made by both the parents of a child born with a genetic disorder and by (or on behalf of) the child. The former is called *wrongful birth,* and the latter, *wrongful life.* The concept of wrongful life has been difficult for courts to accept, but this claim has been upheld by the supreme courts of both California and Washington. The potential for a major judgment is great since a suit may be brought by both the parent and the offspring and, in each case, for both economic and noneconomic harm. The medicolegal aspects of genetic counseling have been reviewed in detail by Milunsky and others.[6, 7, 8, 9] Several selected examples follow.

*Failure to Provide Genetic Counseling.* An obstetrician was successfully sued for failure to inform a patient, at increased risk for having a child with Down syndrome, of the availability of amniocentesis for detecting an affected fetus.[10] An affected child was born, and, following appeals, the supreme court of New York upheld the concept of wrongful birth on behalf of the parents but denied the claim of wrongful life brought by the infant.

*Misdiagnosis.* An audiologist was successfully sued for both wrongful birth and wrongful life when a couple gave birth to a second child who was totally deaf, after having been falsely assured that their first child had normal hearing.[11]

*Failure to Identify High Risk.* After they had a second affected child, the parents of a child who died of polycystic kidney disease brought suit against their physician for failure to identify the high risk associated with each pregnancy and for failure to provide them with appropriate genetic counseling.[12]

*Failure to Identify Ethnic Risk.* A couple gave birth to a child with Tay Sachs disease and alleged that their physician did not inform them of their special risk, as Ashkenazi Jews, to be carriers for this disorder. They sought damages for emotional injury and mental distress caused by having to endure the gradual and painful demise of their child.[13]

## PEDIGREE ELICITATION AND CONSTRUCTION

A pedigree is a pictorial representation of the patient's family and relatives. Traditional symbols are shown in Figure 25–1. Much of the counseling session centers on the information in the pedigree, which must be complete and accurate.

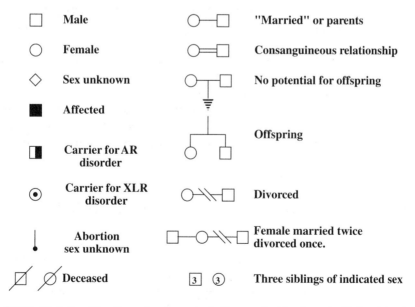

**Figure 25–1.** Traditional pedigree symbols. The symbol for "married" should not have a strict interpretation. It actually represents a couple that has produced, or may produce, offspring, and this does not necessarily imply marriage.

It can be difficult to obtain a complete pedigree since our mobile population spreads families over large geographical areas. It is not unusual for an individual to have little knowledge of previous generations or even contemporary relatives. Additionally, many people do not share personal medical information even with close relatives. Complete ascertainment may require phone calls, letters, solicitation of medical records, and examination of other family members.

Eliciting a pedigree is an art and must be learned through practice. A useful means of acquiring practice is to construct a pedigree for every new patient during the portion of the initial interview devoted to the family medical history. Medical conditions, age, and cause of demise, if appropriate, can be noted next to each symbol in the pedigree. In addition to providing practice, this might reveal hereditary or familial disorders that would otherwise be missed. This initial pedigree may be confined to first degree relatives (parents, siblings, and children); however, when a genetic disorder is suspected, the pedigree should include as many family members as possible, both affected and unaffected.

Delving into family relationships and medical histories may raise some sensitive issues. Therefore, it is best to explain, in advance, why such information is needed. Some potentially embarrassing situations can be avoided by thoughtful and tactful questioning; for example, a woman need not reveal infidelity or children born out of wedlock if the clinician asks about her "child's father" rather than her "husband" (they are not necessarily the same). Consanguinity can be broached casually by asking if there is any chance the couple might be *distantly* related, such as "10th cousins." It is normal to feel awkward and/or uncomfortable asking such personal questions, yet it is precisely this information that must be elicited from patients, on their behalf, to give them ethical and competent care.

A systematic approach to drawing the pedigree helps to avoid confusion. The clinician should ask the size of the family before writing, in order to know how much space is required. Space should be left so it will not be necessary to "squeeze in" additional symbols if some family members are inadvertently forgotten. As much information as is possible should be gathered about each person, as they are drawn, to avoid confusion from jumping back and forth from one person to another.

## CONFOUNDING FACTORS IN COMPLETE ASCERTAINMENT

Several pitfalls await the budding clinical geneticist. One of the easiest to overlook is *nonpaternity.* Accurate genetic counseling depends on establishing true blood relationships, and this is precluded by unrevealed nonpaternity. It is commonly estimated that 10% of all offspring are not the product of the presumed father, but others have questioned the validity of this percentage and have found estimates in the literature ranging from 1.4% to 30%.[14] A recent study[15] found a nonpaternity rate of 2.8% and noted that this compared favorably with previous reports of 5%[16] and 2.3%.[17] The message for the genetic counselor, regardless of the actual value for a given population, is that it is not zero. Nonpaternity therefore remains an issue to be considered. The investigation of nonpaternity has led to some interesting reports including dizygotic twins born to separate fathers,[18] one appearing in the literature as early as 1810.

Hereditary disorders are occasionally masked in affected individuals. Some autosomal dominant and autosomal recessive traits show such considerable variation in *expressivity* that an individual might be so slightly affected as to be clinically indistinguishable from normal without a rigorous and invasive evaluation. Autosomal dominant traits can be *nonpenetrant.* This means that the individual has the gene, but for some reason it does not manifest itself at all. A trait is said to show *reduced penetrance* if, in some families, individuals who have the gene do not manifest the trait. This is distinguished from *decreased expressivity,* in which the affected person does manifest the trait but to such a small degree that it escapes clinical attention.

It is extremely important to elicit consanguinity in a childless couple anticipating pregnancy. *Consanguineous relationships* have a substantially increased risk for offspring to have autosomal recessive disorders. If the couple has already produced an affected offspring, then they are each an obligate carrier. The elicitation of consanguinity is pointless with respect to that trait but is necessary for the consideration of other possible disorders in their offspring. If a couple denies consanguinity, the clinician should ask about birthplaces, nationalities or countries of origin, and shared family names. These areas might reveal a closer relationship than the couple originally believed or admitted.

When reviewing a couple's children, one must not assume that they are all the biological result of that couple. With the high divorce rate in the United States and modern sexual freedom, it is reasonable to assume that some or all of a couple's offspring may have come from a union other than theirs, or that they may be adopted.

The patient's description of affected family members may allow for the confusion of hereditary versus familial disorders and hence should not be taken as medical fact. An apparent history of hereditary macular degeneration might actually be a familial affectation by an environmental agent such as *Histoplasma capsulatum.* Neel and Schull[19] offered the following indicators of a hereditary disorder:

1. It occurs in definite proportions in people related by descent when environmental causes can be ruled out.
2. It does not occur in associated but unrelated lines, for example, in-laws.
3. There are characteristic and relatively consistent clinical findings.
4. There is greater concordance in monozygotic than dizygotic twins.

When one side of the family is identified as the source of the proband's disorder for a dominant trait, it is tempting to ignore the spouse's family history, but this invites the disaster of overlooking another hereditary disorder that might surface in their offspring at a later date. Additional areas that should be investigated are the family history of disorders other than the proband's as well as miscarriages, stillbirths, neonatal death, chromosomal abnormalities, mental retardation, or anything else "out of the ordinary." It is often surprising how much information is revealed by careful questioning after an apparent noncontributory history at the start of the examination.


## MODES OF INHERITANCE

Single gene disorders may be transmitted through several traditional modes of inheritance, the three most common being autosomal dominant (AD), autosomal recessive (AR), and X-linked recessive (XLR). Approximately 5,000 loci for single gene disorders are either confirmed or suspected.[20] These loci have been identified primarily by mendelizing phenotypes. The relative proportions are summarized by mode of inheritance in Table 25–1.

Many eye disorders may be inherited in more than one way, retinitis pigmentosa being a good example. The pedigree helps make the differential diagnosis between the modes of inheritance as well as between conditions with a similar clinical phenotype but different modes of inheritance. When the clinician is confronted with a patient who has a disorder that is known to be inherited in a particular manner but the pedigree is atypical, several possibilities should be considered: the disorder may be inherited in more than one manner; the pedigree may be incorrect or incomplete; the diagnosis is incorrect.

One of the less frequently encountered modes of inheritance is maternal inheritance, which has received ophthalmic interest following the report of Wallace et al.,[21] who described a replacement mutation in mitochondrial DNA (mDNA) that was linked with Leber hereditary optic neuropathy (LHON) in multiple families. For many years LHON had been thought to be XLR since affected families showed a preponderance of affected males and no male-to-male

**TABLE 25–1. Single gene disorders in man adapted from McKusick.[20] Suspected loci are those that seem certain but have not been fully identified or validated.***

|  | Autosomal Dominant | Autosomal Recessive | X-Linked Recessive | Total |
|---|---|---|---|---|
| Confirmed | 1,864 | 631 | 161 | 2,656 |
| Suspected | 1,183 | 923 | 175 | 2,281 |
|  |  |  | Grand Total | 4,937 |

*The numbers in this table should be considered an approximation only. Any such table is virtually out of date the moment it is composed because of the rapid development in identifying gene disorders.

transmission; however, confusion persisted because the pedigrees were atypi-cal in that females were often affected and males did not appear to produce car-rier daughters. The inheritance of mDNA is maternal, in the cytoplasm of the egg. This explains the lack of male-to-male transmission as well as the fact that females can also be affected since mDNA is passed by the mother to both male and female offspring.

There are several sources of error in pedigree construction to which the clinician should be alert. One source of error is the misunderstanding of family relationships, such as cousins, by the layperson. A pedigree with the correct cousin relationships is shown in Figure 25–2. Family members who are identi-fied as affected by the information giver, but who have not been examined per-sonally, should be considered "suspected" rather than confirmed. Failure to do so represents another potential source of error. When establishing the apparent mode of inheritance, the clinician should be sure to indicate on the pedigree who has been examined personally, or confirmed by medical reports, in order to give proper weight to both those who are affected and those who are un-affected.

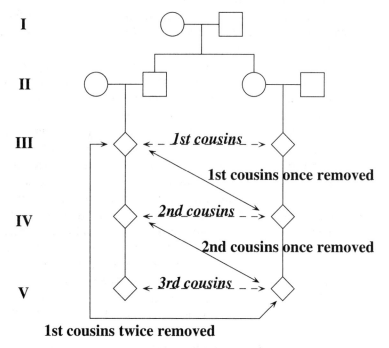

**Figure 25–2.** Cousin relationships are often misunderstood by lay persons. The correct relationships, as illustrated here, should be elicited rather than accept-ing the interviewee's interpretation.

Even the best obtainable pedigree may leave some doubt as to the exact mode of inheritance in that family because of incomplete penetrance, reduced expressivity, missed information, misinformation, and unavailable information. A thorough understanding of the modes of inheritance with their respective possibilities and impossibilities, allows the clinician to extract the maximum information from each pedigree. Genetic counseling should only be given after obtaining the best possible pedigree and establishing the exact diagnosis.

*Autosomal Dominant.* An autosomal dominant trait appears in successive generations (Figure 25–3A). Males and females are equally likely to be affected, and, on the average, one-half of the children of an affected person will also be affected. Noncharacteristic pedigrees do not exclude dominant inheritance. A dominant trait may not appear in the prior or succeeding generation. This apparent skipping of generations can occur because of decreased expressivity or decreased penetrance. The appearance of a known dominant trait with no previous family history may represent a new mutation.

*Autosomal Recessive.* The typical presentation of an autosomal recessive trait is a sudden occurrence of affected siblings in a family with no previous history of that disorder on either side (Figure 25–3B). When two people who are unsuspecting carriers mate, on the average, one-fourth of their offspring are affected, one-half are carriers, and one-fourth are neither. Males and females are equally likely to be affected. Successive generations will not have affected offspring unless those who are carriers or who are affected mate with others who are carriers or who are affected.

*X-Linked Recessive.* X-linked recessive inheritance is unique in that usually only males are affected, having received the gene from a female carrier (Figure 25–3C). It is possible for the female carrier to show minimal signs of the trait and in rare cases to have the full clinical manifestation. Both possibilities are the result of Lyonization,[22] and the latter may be referred to as unfortunate Lyonization. Lyonization in females who are carriers of an X-linked disorder is discussed further in the next section (see "Carriers" under Occurrence and Recurrence Risk Information). Another unique feature of XLR inheritance is that there is no father-to-son transmission. All of the female offspring of an affected male will be carriers. Male and female offspring of a woman who is a carrier are at 50% risk to receive the aberrant gene, with the males being affected and the females being carriers. Because there is only a 50% chance that any one male will be affected, apparent skipping of generations is a common finding.

*Maternal Inheritance.* A small amount of DNA is present in mitochondria, which is inherited maternally in the cytoplasm of the egg. As discussed above, defects in mitochondrial DNA have been established for some families with LHON.

*Other Modes of Inheritance.* Other forms of transmission exist that will not be discussed here. They include X-linked dominant, codominant, multifactorial, mosaicism, uniparental disomy, and genomic imprinting.

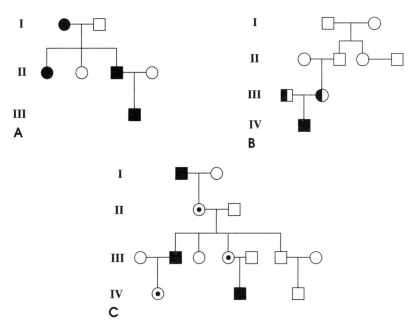

**Figure 25–3.** Three common forms of inheritance: (**A**) autosomal dominant, (**B**) autosomal recessive, and (**C**) X-linked recessive.

## THE COUNSELING PROCEDURE

Genetic counseling is more than the provision of occurrence or recurrence risk information. It must also include a review of the prognosis and alternative options as well as assistance in helping patients and families adjust to the difficulties they encounter. It is illogical to think that an individual professional could fulfill this complex role in each case. Common sense dictates that each clinician act within the realm of his or her own competence and access additional resources as needed.

The clinician must overcome the temptation to tack on the genetic counseling as an addendum to the examination, while exiting to see the next patient. The counseling session should be separate from the examination, and sufficient time should be allotted for questions by the patient. Since there are often gaps in the history recorded at the first examination, one approach to rescheduling the patient is to ask him or her to return after completing a thorough family history at home by calling or writing other relatives. It is also possible to indicate a desire to review the most recent literature about a condition before counseling the patient. This is always a good idea in any case.

No counseling can take place without an exact diagnosis. This may require additional testing such as physical examination, clinical laboratory studies, diagnostic imaging, electrodiagnostic procedures, and examination of other family members. Once the diagnosis is confirmed, the literature is consulted to determine the reported mode(s) of inheritance in order to determine risk information. If a complete pedigree has not been obtained, genetic counseling must await the gathering of the additional information, which may necessitate examining other family members and soliciting additional information, including medical records.

## Occurrence and Recurrence Risk Information

Risk information provides the numerical probability of having a first affected child (occurrence) or having additional affected children (recurrence). Numerical values should be given as accurately as possible. Statements such as "not much chance" or "chances are pretty good" are not easily interpreted and probably leave the counselor on weak legal ground if more exact statistics could have been cited. Risks are not always sought just for determining the probability of having an affected offspring. Many people want to know their risk for being a carrier of a disorder that appears in other family members or the risk that a spouse is also a carrier for the same disorder.

It is easy to lapse into the habit of quoting familiar odds such as a 25% risk for recurrence of an autosomal recessive disorder; however, there are more complex situations the clinician must be concerned with. Selected examples are given in the following sections.

***Other Genetic Disorders Within the Same Family.*** A family, or an individual, may have more than one genetic disorder. A careful case history and additional questioning during construction of the pedigree should reveal other disorders. A sample pedigree from the author's own experience that demonstrates this point appears in Figure 25-4. When other genetic disorders are discovered, they must each be addressed in the counseling session.

***Consanguinity and Incest.*** For patients seeking occurrence information, it is important to determine consanguinity since the risk for sharing the same genetic material is much higher in couples who are related. If a person is known to be a carrier for an autosomal recessive disorder, the risk of a first cousin to also be a carrier for that same disorder is 1/8. This is dramatically higher than the risk for an unrelated spouse from the general population; for example, the probability that anyone in the population at large is a carrier for autosomal recessive oculocutaneous albinism (OCA) is 1/50 (see Example 25-2), based on a prevalence of 1/10,000.

■ **Example 25-1.** Compare the risks (R) for having an affected offspring if a known carrier for OCA mates with a first cousin compared to an unrelated spouse from the general population.

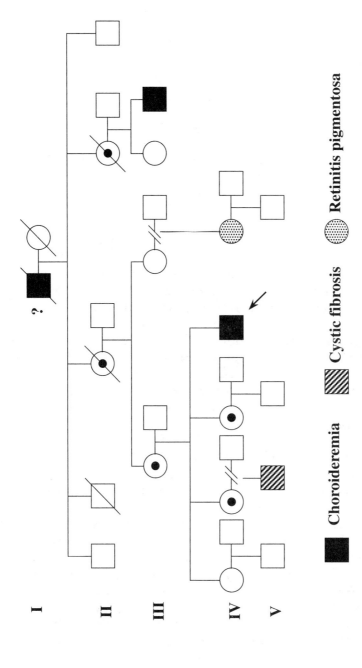

**Choroideremia**    **Cystic fibrosis**    **Retinitis pigmentosa**

**Figure 25–4.** A pedigree from the author's practice the illustrates the fact that more than one genetic disorder may occur in a given family. The proband (arrow) had choroideremia but had relatives with cystic fibrosis and retinitis pigmentosa. The diagnosis of (I,1) was unconfirmed, but he was reportedly blind at age 35. Two females, (IV,3) and (IV,5), are indicated as carriers, even though they are not obligate carriers, because they showed classic fundus signs of the carrier state.

If a known carrier for OCA mates with a person from the general population, the risk for an affected offspring is the probability that the first passes the gene (1/2), the spouse has the gene (1/50), and, if so, that the spouse passes the gene (1/2). The resultant probability is the product of the individual probabilities, and therefore:

$$R = 1/2 \times 1/50 \times 1/2$$
$$R = 1/200$$

If this same person who is a known carrier mates with a first cousin, the risk for an affected offspring is the probability that the first passes the gene (1/2), the first cousin has the gene (1/8), and the first cousin passes it (1/2). Again, the resultant probability is the product of the individual probabilities.

$$R = 1/2 \times 1/8 \times 1/2$$
$$R = 1/32$$

This particular consanguineous relationship increases the risk more than six-fold.

Incestuous relationships increase the risk for shared genes even more since the most common forms, father-daughter and brother-sister, involve a risk of 1/2 that one shares any deleterious gene present in the other.

**Pseudodominance.** A person with an autosomal recessive disorder who mates with a carrier for that same disorder has a 50% risk for each offspring to be affected, not the 25% quoted for a couple who are both carriers. On the average, because of the 50% risk, one-half of the offspring will be affected, and the inheritance appears to be AD. The term *pseudodominance* is therefore used to describe this unique situation.

**A Couple With the Same Genetic Disorder.** A couple, each of whom has the same AR disorder (that is, the same genetic defect at the identical locus) has a 100% chance that each offspring will be affected. The importance of an exact diagnosis is demonstrated by one couple, each of whom had AR oculocutaneous albinism (OCA). They received prenuptial genetic counseling from physicians and were informed that all of their children would be affected with OCA. The mother, upon becoming pregnant, was again told by her obstetrician that the child would have albinism. In fact, the mother gave birth to an unaffected offspring and was told that the child could not possibly be the offspring of her husband. Typing for numerous erythrocyte and serum proteins, antigens, and enzymes revealed no evidence of nonpaternity. It eventually became apparent that she and her spouse actually had a similar clinical phenotype but different disorders.[23] One had tyrosinase positive OCA, and the other had tyrosinase negative OCA. The clinical presentation is similar, but the genetic defects are different.

Every offspring of a couple, each of whom has the same AD disorder, is at 75% risk to be affected, not the 50% risk usually quoted for an AD disorder with only one affected parent. While this might seem a rare situation, it is not unknown. Institutional settings for people with vision disorders provide an increased opportunity for those who are affected to meet and marry someone with the same disorder. As shown with OCA, the couple must have the same disorder with the identical gene locus. If the loci are different and sufficiently distant so as not to be linked, the risk is 50% for each disorder.

*Nonpaternity.* If the clinician fails to identify nonpaternity, he or she may give incorrect counseling or even order unnecessary tests, such as prenatal diagnosis, for a couple in which the presumed father of an affected infant is not the biological father.

*Atypical Pedigrees for X-linked Recessive Disorders.* A hallmark sign of XLR inheritance is the lack of male-to-male transmission; however, it is possible for affected males to have affected sons if the spouse happens to be a carrier for that same disorder. Similarly, if a female is a carrier and a male is affected with the same disorder, they may have an affected female who is, in fact, homozygous.

*Carriers.* A person who is a known carrier for an autosomal recessive condition might present for counseling seeking to know what the risk is that the spouse, or prospective spouse, is also a carrier for that same condition. If the spouse is related or has a family history of the same disorder, it should be possible to determine the risk exactly. If the spouse has no family history and is not related, a calculation is still possible if the prevalence of the condition is known. In this case the risk, R, is calculated as follows if the prevalence is $1/p$:

$$r = 2/\sqrt{p}$$

■ **Example 25–2.** In the case of oculocutaneous albinism, the prevalence is approximately $1/10,000$; each of us therefore has a $1/50$ risk of being a carrier. This is determined as follows:

$$R = 2/\sqrt{p}$$
$$R = 2/\sqrt{10,000}$$
$$R = 1/50$$

In certain situations it is possible to know for certain that an individual is a carrier for the gene in question by examining the pedigree; for example, the following would all be carriers: daughters of a male with an X-linked recessive disorder, any offspring of a parent with an autosomal recessive disorder, and a female who has given birth to a male with an X-linked recessive disorder. These are all examples of *obligate carriers* since there is absolute certainty in each case.

Vision specialists are in a unique position to determine the carrier status for females with some X-linked disorders who may manifest signs that are distinguishable clinically. In each cell of a woman's body one of the X chromosomes inactivates.[22] This inactivation (Lyonization) occurs at random, and, if a sufficient number of those that remain active have the aberrant gene, it is conceivable that the woman can actually manifest the trait; however, the typical situation is that she shows some minimal signs, indicating her carrier status. Common examples of X-linked disorders and the ophthalmic manifestations in carriers are retinitis pigmentosa (mild pigmentary retinopathy), choroideremia (mild pigmentary retinopathy), Fabry disease (corneal whorls), and ocular albinism (patchy iris transillumination and/or patchy areas of light fundus pigmentation). When clinical examination is not revealing, another clue can be the number of unaffected male offspring for the woman at risk to be a carrier. Since each male offspring of a carrier would be at 50% risk to have the disorder, it seems intuitively obvious that if she had a large number of male offspring, none of whom were affected, her probability of being a carrier would be low. When there is only one, or a few, unaffected male offspring, the risk can still be calculated by Bayesian analysis,[24, 25] but this is typically beyond the training of the general practitioner. Carrier status may also be determined biochemically for selected inborn errors of metabolism and by molecular genetic analysis of tissue samples for a growing number of disorders.

In summary, the clinician must be careful to have a definite understanding of the genetic status of both partners in order to provide accurate counseling and risk figures. This information may come from pedigree analysis, clinical examination, and/or laboratory investigations.

## Prognosis

The patient must make decisions based on the risk estimates for occurrence or recurrence of the disorder; however, the key issue in interpreting the risk information is an understanding of the prognosis. The same numerical risk may seem smaller if the consequences are less significant and greater if the consequences are severe. Perhaps a good example is "Russian roulette." A 5/6 chance of success may seem pretty good, but the consequence of losing is dramatic. Not many of us are willing to take that chance. The prognosis, especially for a progressive disorder, helps to define the risk before it becomes apparent; for example, a severely affected baby may not seem that different from other newborns, but the disability will become more evident with age as significant milestones are missed. A clear understanding of the prognosis is important because the couple may make their decision about other offspring soon after having a first affected child and before the full impact on the family is apparent.

## Alternatives

There are many alternatives available to couples who are concerned that they might produce offspring with a genetic disorder. These must be reviewed as part of the counseling session. They are conveniently divided into preconception and postconception alternatives. Preconception alternatives include artificial insemination, surrogate motherhood, adoption, carrier testing, birth control, and "take a chance." Finally, with the rapid advances being made in medical genetics, it is possible that there will be new treatments, carrier tests, and diagnostic tests available within a few years for couples who may wish to wait. Postconception alternatives include prenatal testing, elective pregnancy termination, institutionalization of a severely affected offspring, and acceptance into the family. Prenatal tests may include ultrasonography, serum testing for alpha-fetoprotein (AFP) levels, amniocentesis, and chorionic villus sampling (CVS). Cells harvested from amniocentesis or CVS may be used to construct karyotypes, to perform biochemical testing for metabolic defects, or for molecular genetic studies. Amniotic fluid may be used for AFP levels or biochemical studies. The advantages of CVS are that it can be performed earlier than amniocentesis, typically around 12 weeks gestation as opposed to 14 to 16 weeks, and that results can be achieved faster through direct preparation without the necessity of cell culture.

## Language and Outcome

People with genetic disorders are just that—people. They should not be referred to as "albinos" or "Marfans" or by any other disease-related labels. Certain commonly used disease names with denigrating implications, such as "amaurotic idiocy" or "spastic ataxia," should be avoided when talking to family members.

With the exception of life-, family-, or health-threatening situations, the genetic counselor should not offer directive advice. The decision is the counselee's, not the counselor's. The patient might approach this issue obliquely by asking, *"What would you do in my situation?"* This and similar questions should be politely avoided, reminding the patient that each person approaches a situation differently based on personal and family experiences and goals, as well as ethical and religious beliefs.

The desired outcome is that the counselee will be able to make informed decisions and act in accordance with them. An additional aspect of the outcome is adjustment by the person or family to the disorder. This may require the combined effort of other professionals such as family, marriage, or personal counselors, although this should not be an assumed necessity.

## Follow-up

A follow-up letter, summarizing the topics discussed during the counseling session, provides permanent documentation supporting the information given to the patient. Patients should be encouraged to return if additional family information is uncovered as this may affect the counseling provided. For example, in a family that has only one male affected with retinitis pigmentosa, it is conceivable that he has the AR form or the XLR form or represents a new mutation of the AD form. The discovery of additional affected relatives may reveal the actual mode of inheritance and consequently alter the genetic counseling. Finally, the development of new diagnostic tests, based on techniques of molecular genetics, may allow diagnostic confirmation of phenotypically similar disorders such as the various types of RP, and these tests will enable the clinician to give more precise information. Several mutations in the gene for rhodopsin have been shown to be linked with retinitis pigmentosa in some families with the AD form.[26, 27] Presumably this mutation is the actual cause of the disorder, but that has not yet been established. Since different mutations may result in the same clinical phenotype, it is possible that they will have a somewhat different clinical course. This would affect the prognosis and would allow the clinician to give a prognosis based on a molecular genetic test.

## SELECTED ETHICAL ISSUES IN MEDICAL GENETICS AND GENETIC COUNSELING

### Other Affected Family Members Revealed in the Pedigree

One unresolved ethical issue is what to do about relatives who are identified as "at risk" to have affected offspring through the family pedigree. To contact these relatives would breach patient confidentiality, while to ignore the information might leave one liable for future suits, although there is no legal precedent for this. Until litigation proves otherwise, the most appropriate approach is for the clinician to inform the patient about other at-risk family members and ask that the patient contact them, suggesting that they seek appropriate follow-up. This should be recorded in the patient's file and further documented by inclusion in a follow-up letter.

### Effect of Counseling on the Patient and Other Family Members

When the clinician discusses alternatives with parents, affected children should not be present. If the parents wish to discuss the options of avoidance or elective termination of pregnancy, the affected child might wonder if they would have done the same with him or her if they had known about his or her condition in advance.

Parents who have children affected with genetic disorders may feel guilt for passing on the trait. Learning to deal with strong feelings of guilt may require management that is outside the domain of the primary eye care provider. Referral for personal, family, or psychological counseling should be considered.

It is possible that the clinical examination and/or counseling session will reveal that only one of the parents is responsible for passing a genetic trait to their offspring. If the couple had not considered this possibility previously, it might be an added burden on their relationship if one partner seeks to place blame for the event. This is most likely to be seen in examples of X-linked recessive disorders in which apparently normal carrier females pass the trait to their male offspring. If she were not an obligate carrier from having a previous offspring who was affected, the woman may have had no way of knowing that she was a carrier even though there were other affected family members.

## Predictive Testing and Adult-Onset Disease

The ability to diagnose genetic disease through molecular genetic techniques has introduced substantial ethical issues, one of which surrounds the ability to make a premorbid diagnosis of a severe genetic disease.[28] Huntington disease (HD), in an informative family (one for whom the test works), can now be diagnosed long before an affected person is symptomatic. HD is an autosomal dominant, progressive, neuropsychiatric disorder that is lethal and untreatable. Each offspring of an affected parent is at 50% risk to receive the HD gene. Since predictive testing is available in informative families, it is possible for an individual to know if he or she has the disorder before the onset of symptoms. Prior to deciding to be tested, each person must balance the possibility of great relief if the test is negative with that of potential devastation if the test is positive. Not everyone at risk will want to be tested.[29] Many individuals may not be emotionally or psychologically able to deal with the result. Since it is necessary to test multiple family members to determine an individual's risk, autonomy and confidentiality become important ethical issues. One concern with respect to autonomy is whether an individual will be coerced into taking the test by other family members who need to have that information in order to find out their own status. With respect to confidentiality, not everyone wants to know, or have others know, his or her test result. Ocular examples that are not necessarily life-threatening but for which family members may have similar concerns are late onset AD retinitis pigmentosa and LHON.

## SUMMARY

Knowledge in the area of medical genetics is increasing at a rapid pace, and up-to-date patient management requires an informed practitioner. It is the role of the clinician to be familiar with the scientific and clinical knowledge that has application to the management of genetic disorders of vision. The clinical application of new genetic information depends on the training and experience of the practitioner, and, as always, referral is the appropriate procedure when additional expertise is required. Primary providers of eye and vision care have a logical and important role in genetic counseling and in the clinical management of many genetic disorders.

Genetic counseling should be provided to the extent that the clinician feels comfortable with it. When this is not the case, there are many centers around the country that offer genetic studies and counseling. A list of referral centers can be obtained from the National Clearing House for Human Genetic Diseases (see Resources, Chapter 31); however, the experienced vision specialist has a better understanding of vision and vision disorders and can offer insights into the condition, and its prognosis, that other clinicians or counselors might not have.

In spite of the clinician's best efforts, patients may leave the counseling session without a clear grasp of the facts. Even if they do understand, the accuracy of their recall may fade quickly with time. A short summary letter allows them to review the information as necessary and also provides a permanent record of the provision of proper counseling.

The psychological ramifications of knowing that one has, or has passed on, a severe hereditary trait can be severe. The impact of the information on the patient should be assessed, keeping in mind the possible need for family, personal, psychological, or marriage counseling. Patients should be encouraged to return or call for further assistance whenever they have the need.

The practitioner should remain aware of the advances in genetics that may have an impact on the standard of care. For patients with an individual or family history of a hereditary disease that has been mapped, genetic studies may be available that can test for the carrier state or for an affected fetus. The patients must be made aware of this possibility and referred or given that option when appropriate. It is actually easy to meet one's responsibility in this area by taking advantage of a genetic referral center.

## REFERENCES

1. Hsia YE: The genetic counselor as information giver. *Birth Defects Original Article Series* 15(2):169–186, 1979.
2. *Vision Problems in the U. S.* New York, National Society to Prevent Blindness, 1980.
3. Nathans J: The genes for color vision. *Sci Amer* 260:42–49, 1989.
4. Eady RAJ, Gunner DB, Garner A, Rodeck CH: Prenatal diagnosis of oculocutaneous albinism by electronmicroscopy of fetal skin. *J Invest Dermatol* 80:210–212, 1983.
5. Shaw MW: Presidential Address: To be or not to be? That is the question. *Am J Hum Genet* 36:1–9, 1984.
6. Milunsky A, Annas GJ (eds): *Genetics and the Law I.* New York, Plenum Press, 1976.

7. Milunsky A, Annas GJ (eds): *Genetics and the Law II.* New York, Plenum Press, 1980.

8. Milunsky A, Annas GJ (eds): *Genetics and the Law III.* New York, Plenum Press, 1985.

9. Healey JM, Jr: The legal obligations of genetic counselors, in Milunsky A, Annas GJ (eds): *Genetics and the Law II.* New York, Plenum Press, 1980.

10. Becker v. Schwartz, 386 N.E.2d 807 (N.Y., 1978).

11. Turpin v. Sortini, 643 P.2d 954 (Cal., 1982).

12. Park v. Chessin, 386 N.E.2d 807 (N.Y., 1978).

13. Howard v. Lecher, 366 N.E.2d 64 (N.Y., 1977).

14. MacIntyre S, Sooman A: Non-paternity and prenatal genetic screening. *Lancet* 338(8771):869–871, 1991.

15. Le Roux MG, Pascal O, Andre MT, Herbert O, David A, Moisan JP: Non-paternity and genetic counselling. *Lancet* 340(8819):607, 1992. (See comments: Le Roux MG, Pascal O, David A, Moisan JP: Non-paternity rate and screening in genetic disease analysis. *Lancet* 341(8836):57, 1993.)

16. Edwards JH: A critical examination of the reported primary influence of ABO phenotype on fertility and sex ratio. *Br J Prev Soc Med* 11:79–89, 1957.

17. Ashton GC: Mismatches in genetic markers in a large family study. *Am J Hum Genet* 32:601–613, 1980.

18. Verma RS, Luke S, Dhawan P: Twins with different fathers. *Lancet* 339(8784): 63–64, 1992.

19. Neel JV, Schull WJ: *Human Heredity.* Chicago, University of Chicago Press, 1954.

20. McKusick VA (ed): *Mendelian Inheritance in Man,* 9 ed. Baltimore, The Johns Hopkins University Press, 1990.

21. Wallace DC, Gurparkash S, Lott MT, Hodge JA, Schurr TG, Lezza AMS, Elsas LJ II, Nikoskelainen EK: Mitochondrial DNA mutation associated with Leber's hereditary optic neuropathy. *Science* 242:1427–1430, 1988.

22. Lyon MF: Gene action in the X-chromosome of the mouse (*Mus musculus* L.). *Nature* 190:372–373, 1961.

23. Witkop CJ, Nance WE, Rawls RF, White JG: Autosomal recessive oculocutaneous albinism in man: Evidence for genetic heterogeneity. *Am J Hum Genet* 22:55–74, 1970.

24. Murphy RA, Mutalik GS: The application of Bayesian methods in genetic counseling. *Hum Hered* 19:126–151, 1969.

25. Nowakowski RW: Bayes' theorem and X-linked ophthalmic disorders. *Am J Optom Physiol Optics* 61:643–646, 1984.

26. Dryja TP, McGee TL, Reichel E, Hahn LB, Cowley GS, Yandell DW, Sandberg MA, Berson EL: A point mutation of the rhodopsin gene in one form of retinitis pigmentosa. *Nature* 343:364–366, 1990.

27. Sung CH, Davenport CM, Hennessey J, Maumenee IH, Jacobson SG, Heckenlively JR, Nowakowski RW, Fishman G, Gouras P, Finkelstein D, Nathans J: Rhodopsin mutations in autosomal dominant retinitis pigmentosa. *Proc Nat Acad Sci* 88: 6481–6485, 1991.

28. Huggins M, Bloch M, Kanani S, Quarrell OWJ, Theilmann J, Hedrick A, Dickens B, Lynch A, Hayden M: Ethical and legal dilemmas arising during predictive testing for

adult-onset disease: The experience of Huntington disease. *Am J Hum Genet* 47:4–12, 1990.

29. Quaid KA, Morris M: Reluctance to undergo predictive testing: The case of Huntington disease. *Am J Med Genet* 45(1):41–45, 1993.

## ADDITIONAL READING

Bhattacharya SS, Wright AF, Clayton JF, Price WH, Phillips CI, McKeown CME, Jay M, Bird AC, Pearson PL, Southern EM, Evans HJ: Close genetic linkage between X-linked retinitis pigmentosa and a restriction fragment length polymorphism identified by recombinant DNA probe L1.28. *Nature* 309:253–255, 1984.

Harper PS: *Practical Genetic Counseling,* 3 ed. London, Wright, 1988.

Hirschorn K: Medicolegal aspects of genetic counseling, in Milunsky A, Annas GJ (eds): *Genetics and the Law.* New York, Plenum Press, 1976.

McKusick VA: Mapping and sequencing the human genome. *NEJM* 320:910–915, 1989.

Mets MB, Maumenee IH: The eye and the chromosome. *Surv Ophthalmol* 28:20–32, 1983.

Milunsky A: Prenatal genetic diagnosis and the law, in Milunsky A, Annas GJ (eds): *Genetics and the Law II.* New York, Plenum Press, 1980.

Palca J: Human genome organization is launched with a flourish. *Nature* 325:286, 1988.

Parkman R: The application of bone marrow transplantation to the treatment of genetic diseases. *Science* 232:1373–1378, 1986.

Riccardi VM, Kurtz SM: *Communication and Counseling in Health Care.* Springfield, IL, Charles C. Thomas, 1983.

Rowley PT: Genetic screening: Marvel or menace? *Science* 225:138–144, 1984.

Sparkes RS: The genetics of retinoblastoma. *Biochemica et Biophysica Acta* 780: 95–118, 1985.

Thompson JS, Thompson MW: *Genetics in Medicine,* 5 ed. Philadelphia, W. B. Saunders Company, 1991.

# CHAPTER XXVI

# LOW VISION REHABILITATION FOR CHILDREN

*The principles covered in previous chapters apply to children as well as older patients, but there are also some unique differences. Because children have large amplitudes of accommodation, near devices may be used less frequently or may be prescribed to work in conjunction with the child's accommodation and hence have less dioptric strength. From a practical point of view, expensive and/or fragile optical devices are prescribed less frequently because of their short life expectancy in some young hands.*

*Children may resist using assistive devices because of peer pressure to conform and because other children may be less sensitive toward someone with a disability. With appropriate support, most children who are visually impaired can successfully compete in the public school setting; however, when academic performance suffers in the public school system because of the visual impairment, or when the social liabilities are significant, the residential school setting becomes a favorable option.*

*Children may be more difficult to examine for a variety of reasons, but most of the desired information can be obtained by modifying some test procedures. A successful examination begins with preparing the child before the visit, and that is where this chapter begins.*

*Finally, it is too easy to assume that the generalizations given above apply to every child; of course, that is not the case. Many children are easy to test, are mature beyond their years, and are good candidates for delicate optical devices.*

## PREPARING A CHILD FOR AN EYE EXAMINATION

A child is often apprehensive about an eye examination, but it is possible to reduce the associated stress through advance preparation. An eye examination involves bright lights and an unfamiliar adult performing close inspection or invasive testing well within the child's personal space. The examiner's appearance and surroundings may be reminiscent of other doctors who have caused the child discomfort in the past. The surroundings may be difficult to alter, but the white coat, a symbol associated with "ouch," can easily be abandoned. Parents and teachers may assist in preparing a child for the eye examination by creating games that involve playing with flashlights shined on and around the eyes. Games with lights can also be used to prepare for the examination of extraocular movements and visual fields; for example, the child may be encouraged to follow a blinking light to demonstrate eye movements and be taught to respond when the light comes into view from behind him or her. Advance preparation for visual acuity testing involves practice saying, signing, or matching symbols. The examiner may perform some tests with one eye covered; this too can be practiced with a "pirate's patch" or other type of occluder. During the examination eye drops may be administered as a mist from a spray bottle; this can also be practiced in advance with water by pretending that the mist is "fairy dust" or some other imaginative plaything.

A visit to the doctor's office prior to the actual day of examination will familiarize the child with a different environment and may serve to make the child less apprehensive on examination day. If other children are present in the office on the day of the visit as well as the day of the examination, it will seem more natural to the soon-to-be patient. The examiner can meet the child during a pre-examination visit and attempt to establish a friendly relationship. One approach to this familiarization step is to schedule the child for an introductory examination and perform only as much as is possible without causing the child to become upset. If that first visit turns out to be simply a familiarization visit, at least that purpose is fulfilled. If more can be accomplished, so much the better. The rule is to accustom the child to the surroundings and procedures in a gradual and systematic manner. The parents should understand this approach. A brochure explaining how to prepare a child for an eye examination is a good means of facilitation. The office staff should be skillful in techniques of making children comfortable. Of course, the ideal setting will have appropriate areas, toys, and reading materials for specific age groups. An excellent resource person for ideas on preparing children for medical procedures is a certified child life specialist at a local children's hospital. Certified child life specialists in a given area can also be located through the Child Life Council (see Resources, Chapter 31).

## ASSESSING VISUAL ACUITY

It is important to establish a child's visual acuity for all of the usual reasons (baseline data, prediction of magnification, and so forth) and also to determine school placement and the allocation of special resources. Acuity assessment in general, including techniques of preferential looking, was discussed in Chapter 4. The examiner should have a variety of acuity cards appropriate for testing children. If the child is not verbal, it may be possible for him or her to use manual signs to indicate the symbols or to match symbols. Matching can be accomplished by giving the child enlarged copies of the test symbols to hold in his or her lap and to point to when the corresponding symbol is displayed by the examiner. It may be necessary to train the child briefly, or over a period of time, in this technique. Children who sign may not use the exact sign, but this is not important; for example, if the sign for "rain" is used to indicate the symbol "umbrella," that works fine as long as it is used consistently since it is consistent visual recognition that is important, not the precise identification of the object.

It is not unusual for a child who is visually impaired to have had multiple eye examinations over a period of several years, all of which ended with the doctor saying something such as, *"It can't be determined exactly what Johnny sees. Come back in one year."* Yet if there is no plan for intervention, what will be different next year? Nothing. It is therefore important to establish a plan to facilitate getting more information at the next visit. The parents and/or teachers should be given a plan to teach the child activities that will help future evaluations; for example, they should be told about play activities that simulate portions of the examination in order to acclimatize the child to this experience. Another method is to provide a copy of acuity symbols such as those used on the Symbols for Children acuity card available from the New York Lighthouse (see Resources, Chapter 31). If the child can be taught to say, sign, or match these symbols (apple, house, and umbrella), it will be possible to obtain a visual acuity. The child should return whenever this is accomplished, whether it is one year or one month.

### Functional Vision Assessment

When exact visual acuities cannot be determined, a functional assessment can provide a reasonable estimate of a child's visual ability. While this can be accomplished in the office, the most useful information may come from long-term observation in the home and school settings. Teachers and parents may be given a list of behaviors to watch for and some ideas about how to record their observations. The following questions and observations can be used for assessing visual function.

1. Does the child perceive light? Different levels of light should be considered such as night versus day, indoors versus outdoors during the day,

room lights on versus room lights off, and smaller sources of light such as lamps or small flashlights.

2. Does the child attend visually to objects such as lights, faces, or toys? The observer must be careful to determine that the behavior is visual and is not elicited by another stimulus such as sound or smell. The presence of a person might be recognized by a particular smell such as perfume or cologne. Apparent visual attention to a toy might be a result of its making a particular sound. The size of the object and the distance at which it is seen can be used to estimate visual acuity. It may not represent an acuity as measured in the usual sense, but it does serve as a baseline visual behavior that can be monitored for change.

3. Does the child track a moving object? Objects such as lights or toys can be used to determine tracking ability.

4. Does the child appear to attend visually with both eyes or one eye only? If both eyes are used, do they appear to be used simultaneously or alternately? Does the child resist patching or blocking one eye more than the other? If so, this might indicate a preferred eye.

5. Does the child perceive colors? The assessment of color perception depends on an appropriately designed test. Teachers and parents may believe that a child can distinguish colors when he or she is actually responding to brightness and not hue. When color perception can be assessed accurately, it is important to do so since many school activities involve color-coded materials.

6. Does the child have a full visual field? Head turns may be indicative of a field loss when they are consistently used for viewing. If it has been established that a child has vision, two people can make a general estimate of a child's visual field if one stands in front to direct attention and the other moves a proven stimulus such as a toy or light from behind the child toward the front and records the locations in which it is first detected. When a light is used, it should have a discrete visible area; for example, a bare light bulb may cast a large amount of light in the general area, and the child may attend to that as opposed to the source itself.

7. Are there visual limitations to mobility? If the child is ambulatory, he or she should be observed for the use of visual clues in mobility. Observations such as whether or not the child can locate an open door or avoid obstacles in the path of travel are suggestive of a certain visual level.

8. Other visually related observations that can provide information about a child's eyes are the presence or absence of nystagmus, eye turns (strabismus), eye rubbing, eye poking, tearing, and eye movements.

Droste et al.[1] presented a functional assessment to be used when no response can be obtained from the low spatial frequency Teller card. Their proposed functional battery included observing for light perception, fixation, tracking, optokinetic nystagmus, ability to seize a red object, and an obstacle course. They concluded that the functional battery provided better discrimination of visual function than either the Teller cards or Snellen acuity for those with severe visual impairment and that Teller cards were most discriminatory in those with moderate vision impairment; however, their sample size for this study was limited. Until additional research establishes a particular battery of tests as best, any similar series of tests might be used to provide some baseline information for children or infants in whom a definitive acuity cannot be established. The results of a functional battery also serve as useful information even when acuities can be measured since performance often does not correlate with visual acuity.

Before a functional vision loss is considered proven, one must account for other physical and cognitive factors that might also interfere with performance. When a child has multiple disabilities, it is difficult to attribute particular behaviors to the presence or absence of a single sensory modality. It is important to have a thorough multidisciplinary evaluation of the complete child in order to make a confident visual assessment.

Some degree of clinical experience will allow a practitioner to make a reasonable assessment of visual ability based on the ocular pathology when acuities cannot be measured and a functional assessment is not adequate. An educated estimate may be necessary when placement or program acceptance requires a statement about visual acuity. When it will be helpful to the child and family, practitioners should not be reluctant to make such a statement but should be sure that the family understands both the purpose and the limitations of a clinical estimate.

The visual evoked potential (VEP) offers an objective means of determining additional information related to visual acuity (see Chapter 4). Some practitioners are willing to use the VEP to determine a recordable visual acuity, but this should be approached with some caution. There is at least one documented case of a person who had a normal VEP but no light perception.[2] A single such case should dissuade one from putting too much reliance on the VEP; however, it does offer useful information, and, in the author's experience, many parents are comforted by the fact that they know there is a recordable potential at the level of the visual cortex even though no judgment can be made about the child's actual visual level.

In some cases it is impossible to say with any degree of certainty what a child's visual capability is. When parents are eager for any bit of information, it is difficult to have nothing firm to tell them, but it is helpful to give them a very detailed explanation about what can and cannot be said with certainty. It is often the case that parents have taken their child for many evaluations and not only have received little information but also have had little opportunity to talk with the examiner(s). They have a difficult enough task caring for their child without being subjected to "too busy" or otherwise uncaring practitioners. If a child is evaluated on a day when it is not possible to spend sufficient time with the family to answer their questions, they should be reappointed specifically for a discussion of the findings and invited to prepare a written list of questions to be addressed at that visit.

## VISION STIMULATION

Infants and children who have significant vision impairment may benefit from a program of planned vision stimulation. Normal acuity develops in most people without any particular attention to stimulating the system, and visual exposure during everyday activities results in a normally functioning system. Vision stimulation would therefore be expected to assist a developing visual system that cannot obtain normal input in the traditional manner. It is well established that a lack of visual input can result in amblyopia in an otherwise normal eye, but it is not clear whether or not the same process takes place in an eye that is organically impaired. There is little doubt that vision stimulation can be helpful to some children in learning to utilize visual input more effectively. Therefore, it seems prudent to recommend active visual stimulation to assist a child in learning to use residual vision. Until there is adequate research, the clinician may also want to indicate that visual stimulation may help to prevent or reduce the risk of amblyopia overlay associated with various ocular diseases.

Considerable vision stimulation can be provided passively by ensuring that there are adequate sources of stimulation in the child's environment, such as pictures on the walls, brightly colored toys, a television, a mobile over the crib, and a window that permits an outside view. These considerations may be neglected if the parents assume that the child has no useful vision. When they can be applied, the techniques used in orthoptics are excellent and may be modified appropriately for the child with impaired vision. Teachers and parents who seek activities that can be performed at home and in the classroom can find several sources of such activities.[3, 4, 5, 6]

Improvement in visual acuity is not the only consideration in visual stimulation. There is also the matter of learning to interpret visual input in order to develop skills such as sitting up, walking, orientation, and feeding and to facilitate other types of learning. A discussion of this aspect of visual development is beyond the scope of the present work and has been covered elsewhere.[7, 8]

## LOW VISION DEVICES FOR CHILDREN

Children who are visually impaired will benefit from magnification. The principles are essentially the same as for adults, but the approach is modified based on the child's age, physical and cognitive abilities, and maturity. The ability to use a device effectively and to care for it is central to its success and longevity.

The social pressures of acceptance into one's peer group during childhood may eliminate the effective use of any device that makes the child seem different. This is less a factor in residential schools for children who are visually impaired, which makes such schools a preferred setting for some children. An optical device represents an additional piece of equipment to be carried, cared for, and kept track of. The effects of this additional burden should be considered before making a final recommendation.

A child who is phakic can typically accommodate adequately to achieve a high level of relative distance magnification. This means that a child can hold objects close enough to provide the required magnification and still focus adequately to achieve the clearest possible image. This reduces, to some extent, the necessity of providing microscopes or plus lenses for reading; however, there are circumstances under which these lenses should be considered. Prolonged accommodative effort can be fatiguing, so an add may be helpful. Performance may be better with a plus lens than with accommodation, and this should certainly be one of the deciding factors.

Physical ability may govern the choice between a hand and stand magnifier, just as it would with a person who is elderly. As a general rule, glasses are more common and hence more socially acceptable than hand-held devices. Optical assistive devices may become more useful in advanced grades since print becomes smaller and reading demands are increased. For school age children, it is helpful to have the parents bring samples of school materials to the examination in order to assess the need for magnification and the best manner in which to provide it.

A telescope is an excellent device for a child since it may become an object of envy as opposed to one of ridicule. Most children, visually impaired or not, seem to be fascinated with telescopes, and this makes their acceptance much easier. A telescope may not be required in the classroom if the child sits near the front of the room, but it can be very useful for field trips, mobility, and general spotting activities outside the classroom. If a child accepts a telescope and uses it effectively, even though it serves no immediate specific purpose, its use will initiate the adaptation to optical devices and magnification that will be necessary as the child grows older.

## Nonoptical Devices

The closed circuit television is an excellent device for children, but the lack of portability may make its use logistically difficult when the child must move to several classrooms during the day and study at home in the evening. Large print books seem as if they would be an excellent option, and to some extent they are; however, a single textbook in normal sized print may expand to several oversized volumes when set in large print. These volumes are heavy, are different from what everyone else has, and may not fit in the student's school locker. Other nonoptical devices that should be considered for children of all ages are reading guides, bold point pens, bold lined paper, writing guides, and high intensity lamps.

## THE RESIDENTIAL SCHOOL SETTING

Most children who are visually impaired should be able to succeed in the public school setting provided that the appropriate resources are available, which, unfortunately, is not always the case. The alternative setting is the residential school for those who are visually impaired, so named because most of the pupils reside there during the academic year. If a child is unable to succeed in the public school setting, either academically or socially, the residential school setting is an alternative to be considered.

There are both advantages and disadvantages to the residential setting. The major advantages are that the child is in a setting where the teachers are experienced in working with students who are visually impaired and that the social setting is more accepting since all of the students share, at least to some extent, the problems associated with visual impairment. The major disadvantage, apart from being away from home, is that the residential school represents a sheltered setting unlike what the child will experience as an adult, and parents may be concerned that the child will not be prepared to succeed in the sighted world. This is a legitimate concern but may not be a major concern if there is adequate opportunity during the school year to interact with children and adults who are not visually impaired. If the residential setting provides the environment that allows the child to succeed, it is the best choice for at least some period of time, although it may not be necessary for a child to attend the residential school for his or her entire academic program.

Parents often look to the clinician for advice on which school setting to pursue. This requires counseling that is most appropriately provided by an educator experienced in working with children who are visually impaired, but the clinician can provide additional support and insight that will help the parents make an informed decision. To this end, the clinician should be thoroughly familiar with the residential school(s) in his or her area with respect to the programs they offer and how their graduates compare academically with those who attend public schools.

## COMMUNICATING WITH SCHOOL PERSONNEL

A child in the regular school setting may benefit from a letter to each teacher explaining the nature of the visual problem, the performance limitations, performance nonlimitations, and suggestions to ensure success in the classroom. Forms provided by schools typically ask for the child's visual acuity, but it should not be assumed that this finding can be appropriately interpreted as a guide for special services. A written statement about the child's performance capabilities and limitations will be most meaningful.

Safety is a concern that should not be overlooked. Many forms have a question about "activities to be avoided," but this is not the only safety issue. A child with impaired night vision should have someone assigned to accompany him or her in the event of a blackout in the building or for activities such as assemblies or movies that may be conducted in a darkened environment. Sun exposure is a real threat to children with oculocutaneous albinism, and the school personnel may be unaware of the need to limit exposure time as well as to ensure that protective clothing and sunscreen are used. Children with restricted fields are at increased risk for injury by fast-moving objects from outside the field of view. This may preclude participation in certain sports. The clinician must balance the concern for safety with the importance of leading a normal childhood through participation in typical activities.

When one is asked if glasses are for full-time wear or not, some consideration should be made as to whether full-time wear is really necessary since the child may be subjected to unnecessary restrictions. The clinician should clearly specify activities during which the glasses may be safely put aside. This is particularly helpful for children who are not anxious to wear their glasses anyway and for those whose glasses are particularly heavy or cosmetically unpleasing. If a child uses one or more optical appliances, the teacher can reinforce their effective use if the clinician specifies the work distance and circumstances for use.

School personnel should be reminded to use materials and presentation techniques that provide the best contrast and are large enough to be seen comfortably. The low contrast purple print of the mimeograph machine is slowly vanishing thanks to the advent of modern copying machines, but it isn't gone yet, and mimeographed pages may be very difficult to see. Some copy machines can be used to enlarge print size and even to darken the output. A sample of letter sizes that the child can see may be helpful. This can be accomplished by photocopying the near acuity card and circling the appropriate row of letters; however, the letter size indicated should be that which can be read as continuous text.

Color-coded lessons are common and are a source of difficulty for those with impaired color perception. It is therefore extremely important to test color vision on all children and to report any abnormality with a statement about how it might affect performance in the classroom.

A child with a visual impairment may need additional time to complete examinations and assignments. A teacher might be falsely assured that the child has near normal visual function if acuity levels through optical devices are reported as normal or near normal. An example is reporting that a child can see 20/20 with a 3.0X telescope. This is not an accurate rendition of what is actually taking place. The child may read the equivalent of 20/20 but is doing so with the limitations imposed by the telescope. It should not be assumed that the teacher knows about the performance limitations caused by the small usable visual field or near work distance required with some optical devices. Again, a written statement is the best manner of communicating this information.

It is not unusual for a child to have had all of his or her psychoeducational testing performed prior to obtaining the best glasses or optical devices. It is also possible that test formats were used that were not appropriate for a child who is visually impaired. A discussion of this type of testing is beyond the scope of this work, but the practitioner should be aware that formats are available for testing children with a visual impairment; these have been reviewed elsewhere.[9] It may be necessary to request additional or repeat testing once the child's visual performance has been enhanced with assistive devices and appropriate training.

If the child has a progressive disorder or one with increased risk for complications, the clinician should specify behaviors that might indicate a worsening of the condition or the onset of a new problem that prompts an immediate referral. Teachers, in the author's experience, are often reluctant to make what they fear is an inappropriate referral. Therefore, it is important that a relationship be established in which they understand that all referrals are appropriate if they are concerned about a possible change in the child's vision.

## SUMMARY

Important aspects in the provision of services for children include the social concerns caused by peer pressure, the importance of early initiation of successful adaptation to a lifelong visual impairment, communication with school personnel, and, of course, vision preservation with safety glasses and periodic follow-up.

Communication with the school is best accomplished by providing detailed descriptive statements about the child's visual abilities as well as the vision problems and by communicating the circumstances that will allow the child to succeed visually in the didactic aspects as well as in the social milieu of the school.

## REFERENCES

1. Droste PJ, Archer SM, Helveston EM: Measurement of low vision in children and infants. *Ophthalmol* 98:1513–1518, 1991.
2. Bodis-Wollner I, Atkin A, Raab E, Wolkstein M: Visual association cortex and vision in man: Pattern-evoked occipital potentials in a blind boy. *Sci* 198(4317):629–631, 1977.

3. Barraga NC, Collins M, Hollis J: Development of efficiency in visual functioning: A literature analysis. *J Vis Impair Blind* 71(9):387–391, 1977.

4. Barraga NC, Dorward B, Ford P: *Aids for Teaching Sensory Development.* New York, American Foundation for the Blind, 1973.

5. Barraga NC, Morris J: *Program to Develop Efficiency in Visual Functioning.* Louisville, KY, American Printing House for the Blind, 1980.

6. Barraga N: Vision utilization, in Mulholland ME, Wurster MV (eds): *Help Me Become Everything I Can Be.* New York, American Foundation for the Blind, 1983.

7. Scott EP, Jan JE, Freeman RD: *Can't Your Child See?* 2 ed. Austin, TX, Pro-Ed, 1985.

8. Warren DH: *Blindness and Early Childhood Development,* 2 ed. New York, American Foundation for the Blind, 1984.

9. Bradley-Johnson S: *Psychosocial Assessment of Visually Impaired and Blind Students.* Austin, TX, Pro-Ed, 1986.

## ADDITIONAL READING

Brady HR, Hecke D, Culliton P: Spectacle-mounted telescopic lenses for children. *Annals Ophthalmol* 15(3):286–289, 1983.

Efron M, Lackey GH Jr.: The arithmetic test performance of low vision adolescents using two modes of magnification. *J Special Educators* 18(4):76–82, 1982.

France TD: Can my child see? The evaluation of visual function in children. *J Pediatr Ophthalmol Strabismus* 16(5):329–332, 1979.

Friedman G: Distance low-vision aids for primary level school children. *New Outlook for the Blind* 70(9):376–379, 1976.

Kelleher DK: A pilot study to determine the effect of the bioptic telescope on young low vision patients' attitude and achievement. *Am J Optom Physiol Optics* 51(3):198–205, 1974.

# REHABILITATIVE MANAGEMENT OF SELECTED DISORDERS OF VISION

*Each person is unique and requires an individualized prescription for vision rehabilitation; however, certain aspects may be generalized for selected vision disorders, and these are presented in the following sections. This chapter emphasizes treatment forms other than magnification and genetic counseling, which were covered in previous chapters. The disease management, apart from vision rehabilitation, is not part of the intended scope of this work and is therefore not addressed.*

## NYSTAGMUS

Nystagmus is more often an effect of the visual impairment rather than the cause of the visual impairment, but even in the former case it contributes to the overall level of impairment. When a null point exists, at which vision can be shown to be better, an attempt should be made to help the patient localize and maintain the null point for vision enhancement. Approaches to nystagmus dampening include alignment to the null point by prisms or surgery, feedback inhibition with contact lenses or biofeedback, and image stabilization.

## Optical Management

Dell'Osso[1, 2] has described the use of prisms to achieve a gaze and convergence angle that may result in an improvement of best corrected visual acuity for some patients with congenital nystagmus by achieving a desired version shift to a null point. For example, a gaze shift that requires $4^\Delta$ left and a convergence shift of $14^\Delta$ requires $4^\Delta$ base right O.U. and $7^\Delta$ base out O.U. The resultant prism would be $3^\Delta$ base out O.S. and $11^\Delta$ base out O.D. Dell'Osso argues that the prisms are preferred to simply turning the head and altering the gaze since there are social ramifications of not maintaining a straight-ahead head position. More importantly, the prism reduces the effort to see, which in turn reduces the nystagmus intensity.

## Biofeedback

Abplanalp and Bedell[3] reported an improvement in visual acuity from 6/35 to 6/25 using biofeedback with a patient who had oculocutaneous albinism. The patient learned to reduce the amplitude of the nystagmus by approximately 50% in response to auditory and visual feedback.

## Contact Lenses

Corneal contact lenses have been used to alter visual function[4, 5, 6] in persons with congenital nystagmus. Improved visual acuity through the use of contact lenses has been attributed to feedback inhibition caused by lid sensation from the contact lens edge. Evidence for this phenomenon includes a loss of beneficial effect with the instillation of topical anesthetic.[6] Other theories that seem less likely[6] have attributed the reduced amplitude to increased inertia or induced friction. Results with contact lenses are occasionally encouraging but often equivocal. As one might guess, if contact lenses worked well consistently, they would be an accepted and frequently used therapeutic modality, which they are not. Reports of success are often anecdotal and without actual measurements to verify any change in the amplitude of the nystagmus.

A trial with contact lenses for any patient with nystagmus is certainly worth consideration until research gives more definitive clinical guidelines. Another treatment consideration is combined therapy, such as contact lenses in conjunction with prism in spectacles or even a contact lens telescope, which might achieve some improvement from both the contact lens itself and the magnification of the telescope. For example, an improved optical interface resulting from a contact lens over an irregular corneal surface might explain cases of unexpected improvement, reported by some, that is beyond that predicted by the magnification of the telescopic system alone.

Controlled studies are required to validate the use of contact lenses for reduction of nystagmus amplitude. If the studies are successful, they will serve to distinguish nystagmus reduction caused by inhibitory feedback from nystagmus reduction caused by the patient assuming a head position that achieves the null point and hence reduces the lens-lid interaction (that is, the same end result for a different reason). Additional studies would also be useful to determine if magnification plays a role in nystagmus reduction and to determine the potential for improvement of visual function in isolated congenital nystagmus versus a secondary nystagmus associated with congenitally impaired vision as might occur with oculocutaneous albinism.

## Image Stabilization

An optical device that produces partial stabilization of retinal images can be created from a high plus spectacle lens in combination with a high minus contact lens, essentially a contact lens telescope.[7, 8] The theoretical concept is to utilize the spectacle lens to form a primary image near or at the center of rotation of the eye. The image would then remain relatively fixed in spite of eye movements. The contact lens puts the primary image in focus on the retina. Both polymethylmethacrylate and rigid, gas permeable (RGP) contact lenses have been used, but the high powers required make long-term use unlikely because of poor comfort.[9]

## Surgical Intervention

Surgery is an option for cases where intervention is considered mandatory and other approaches have been shown to be ineffective. Improvement in visual acuity, if any, is typically minimal. This may explain why a survey to determine the management of vertical or torsional head position in patients with congenital nystagmus and associated null point found that the overwhelming majority of respondents who saw patients with this problem reported "observation" as the treatment of choice.[10] Other potential surgical outcomes are reduction of the amplitude of the nystagmus (regardless of acuity) and alleviation of an unusual head posture that has been adopted to achieve a null point.

Retroequatorial recession of the horizontal rectus muscles has been reported to reduce the amplitude of manifest congenital nystagmus, improve the visual acuity modestly in some patients (about one line), and reduce anomalous head postures in some patients.[11, 12, 13] The head posture is altered by turning the eyes surgically in the same direction as the head turn. Although this surgery results in some limitation of ductions, this reportedly did not result in a functionally significant postoperative limitation of ocular motility in the references cited.

A new surgical method for nystagmus without a null point consists of placing a silicone encircling band around the globe over the four rectus muscles in the retroequatorial position.[14] This method reportedly did not have any ischemic complication of the anterior segment, nor did it cause any variation of intraocular pressure, probably because the silicone band was not tightened.

The potential advantages of this method are that it is reversible by cutting the silicone band and that it can be combined with recession-resection of the rectus muscles at the same time or at a later date.

Strabismus surgery and/or optical means may be used to convert manifest latent nystagmus to latent nystagmus in some patients.[15] Surgical or optical alignment of the eyes may reduce the nystagmus intensity and may also improve binocular visual acuity.

## RETINITIS PIGMENTOSA

### Light Deprivation and UV Protection

For some years it was hypothesized that light might hasten the progress of RP, based on the fact bright light had been shown to damage the retinas of rats with an inherited retinal dystrophy.[16] Occlusion of one eye of two patients with RP, each with a different hereditary mode of transmission, was performed by Berson[17] with an opaque scleral contact lens for six to eight hours per day for a five-year period. At the end of the study, the occluded eye had progressed at the same rate as the fellow eye in each case. Miyake et al.[18] reported a male patient with RP whose right eye had been occluded 42 years earlier by trauma, which had resulted in a corneal scar and a thick white membrane behind a pinhole pupil. They determined that his eye had been occluded with a 1.2 log unit density filter. The pupil was opened surgically, and it was shown that his RP was equally advanced in both eyes.

At this time there is no evidence in support of monocular occlusion for sight preservation in patients with RP. By the same token, the prescribing of UV filters may not be justified scientifically for protection against retinal damage caused by an assumed predisposition from RP; however, the mounting evidence that UV may cause some forms of cataracts and retinal damage makes it a reasonable clinical consideration. There may also be some subtypes among the many forms of RP that would benefit from light protection if they are pathophysiologically similar to the animal models, but this remains to be shown. Since posterior subcapsular cataracts are often found in association with retinitis pigmentosa, affected persons often prefer tinted lenses. The inclusion of a short wavelength filter should reduce some glare associated with scatter caused by the lens opacity.

### Psychosocial Aspects

Retinitis pigmentosa, regardless of the type, has unique characteristics that are particularly difficult for the individual to deal with: a known slow progression leading to severe impairment and possibly total blindness, a loss of mobility from decreased peripheral vision, and nightblindness exacerbated by seasonal changes in daylight hours and the artificial restrictions of Daylight Savings Time. When problems with personal adaptation interfere with achieving an acceptable lifestyle, a referral for counseling is appropriate.

## Orientation and Mobility Training and Field Enhancement

Training in techniques of orientation and mobility, primarily for night travel, should be initiated at an early age, even though it may not be needed for travel during daylight or in well-lighted areas until necessitated later by the constricted visual field. The introduction of technology that would intensify ambient light, such as used in the ITT Nightscope,[19] was heralded as an important advance for persons with nightblindness. The expectations were never fulfilled, perhaps because of the expense and the fact that it had to be used as a monocular in order to be as light and as cosmetically acceptable as possible. A bright flashlight for night travel is probably just as effective as an ambient light intensifier and costs considerably less. As a general rule, orientation and mobility training and field enhancement devices are most helpful when the visual field is less than 10° in widest diameter. The primary therapies to be considered for field enhancement are Fresnel prisms, concave lenses, and the reversed telescope. A hemianopic mirror is less likely to be useful since it may block a portion of the remaining field.

## Magnification

Due to the reduced visual field, it is difficult to prescribe magnification successfully for someone with RP since the enlarged image often exceeds the useful field of view. In general, devices designed for use at arm's length are more likely to be successful since the person's visual field is effectively larger at greater distances; for example, if one assumes that the housing of a stand magnifier leaves 2° of visual field on either side of the image, the linear distance encompassed by that 2° is greater at further distances from the eye. This may give the patient a functional improvement in its use (Figure 27–1). However, it should be noted that at greater distances from the eye, the magnification needed is also greater since there is a minification from the change in relative distance. Even though the magnification prescribed has to be greater due to an increase in relative distance, this may still offer a better functional approach than a microscope with its near work distance.

## OCULOCUTANEOUS ALBINISM

## Refractive Error

Significant amounts of hyperopic astigmatism are often associated with oculocutaneous albinism (OCA); however, the practitioner should not be surprised if

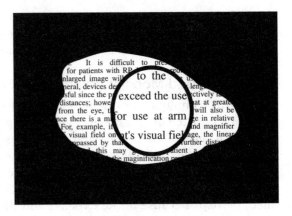

**Figure 27–1.** A person with a small central field of view will generally prefer a device that can be used at arm's length to take advantage of the maximum linear extent of the field. The device will be easier to use if there is some lateral field of view outside of the magnified area.

the patient rejects correction of the refractive error since it may make little difference subjectively. This is probably secondary to the macular dysgenesis, which renders better focus of little functional significance; however, since glasses will probably be prescribed for light protection, the refractive correction should be included if it affords even a small subjective or objective improvement. Bifocals may assist with maintaining a convergence point that minimizes the nystagmus. Prisms can be incorporated for the same reason.

## Light Protection

Ophthalmic filters that protect against UV and short wavelength visible light should be prescribed for outdoor wear even though persons with OCA are often not as photophobic as one would expect and may resist a tinted lens. The need for protection from ultraviolet light applies to the skin as well as to the eyes. A person with OCA is more susceptible to skin cancer and should therefore wear protective clothing and sunscreen and have periodic dermatological evaluations. The vision care provider should be alert to this potential problem and should include questions about skin lesions in the case history as part of the review of systems. Physical examination of exposed areas of skin should be included with the vision evaluation.

## Psychosocial Aspects

A person with OCA looks different. This is especially true for those who are of dark-skinned ethnic origin, and this may cause them problems with social acceptance and employability. When psychosocial problems interfere with the rehabilitation process or seem detrimental to the patient's well-being, referral for counseling is an appropriate management consideration.

## MACULAR DEGENERATION

### Eccentric Viewing

The primary hindrance to the successful use of residual vision by people with macular degeneration is the inability to view eccentrically with efficiency. It might seem intuitively obvious that a person would automatically learn to view eccentrically, but this is not always the case. The lifelong habit of central fixation is not easily abandoned by older patients. Eccentric fixation is a skill that can be taught, and improved, through systematic training (see Chapter 22).

### Magnification

Low vision devices are often successful in restoring useful visual function once eccentric viewing is reasonably efficient. Given that macular degeneration is primarily a problem associated with aging, microscopes are often preferred to hand-held devices for ease of manipulation.

### Activities of Daily Living

The association of macular degeneration with advanced age implies that adaptation will be more difficult because of other infirmities of aging and may make activities of daily living more difficult than might be expected based only on the loss of vision. Persons who are older will benefit from extended counseling about assistive devices and environmental adaptations. Nutrition is always an important consideration with aging. Because impaired vision may interfere with cooking, shopping, and food preparation, referral for assistance through senior centers and programs such as "Meals on Wheels" is potentially lifesaving.

## DIABETIC RETINOPATHY

Diabetic retinopathy is progressive and variable. It therefore has a poor long-term prognosis for visual rehabilitation because it is frustrating to the patient to try to adapt to worsening and variable levels of residual vision. A person with diabetes must play an active daily role in the management of the disease. This involves dietary control, exercise, self-monitoring of glucose levels, taking medications in the prescribed dosage at appropriate times, and, with peripheral neuropathy, monitoring the extremities for lesions. Each of these tasks becomes more difficult with reduced vision.

## Low Vision Devices

Dietary control involves shopping for appropriate foods, reading labels and recipes, measuring dry and liquid ingredients, cutting and slicing, and setting cooking times and temperatures. If the vision impairment is moderate, these tasks may be accomplished with routine optical devices. When the vision loss is severe, additional help may be obtained from nonoptical devices such as large print or Braille timers, cutting/slicing guides, scales with voice output, large print and Braille cookbooks, and stoves or microwaves with large print displays and raised or Braille markings (see Chapter 24 and Resources, Chapter 31).

Self-examination for lesions that might occur with peripheral neuropathy may be accomplished with a telemicroscope. A focusable unit is best since it allows easier examination without contortions. It may be necessary to utilize a mirror and adjustable lighting to view less accessible surfaces.

As a general rule it is wise to select devices that can be easily altered in accordance with the changes in residual vision; for example, an expensive, custom-designed device with fixed magnification is not a good choice unless the patient appears to have reached a relatively stable plateau.

Exercise and travel may be enhanced by training in techniques of orientation and mobility. Referral should be considered for those whose history or clinical evaluation suggests that the visual impairment restricts travel.

## Monitoring and Maintaining Glucose Levels

Optical and nonoptical devices to assist in maintaining glycemic control may play an important role in the patient's management. Oral medications can be sorted into compartmentalized boxes periodically by a care giver or by the individual with appropriate optical devices or even a CCTV. For those who must use insulin, there are a number of aids that assist a visually impaired person with diabetes in administering insulin properly, including prefilled unit dose syringes that do not have to be filled by the patient, syringes with an attached magnifier, and syringes that can be filled to a predetermined level by locking the depth of plunger withdrawal. The patient may have trouble ascertaining if he or she has infiltrated a vessel prior to injecting the insulin. The use of good lighting, a hand magnifier, and a light background may assist in making blood in the syringe more visible.

Monitoring blood glucose levels can be accomplished with a reflectometer that has a large digital meter or an auditory output. Spring-loaded devices for puncturing the skin may be used effectively since one can feel when they are in the correct location as opposed to having to manually pierce the fingertip with a hand-held lance. Patients should be warned not to share the spring-loaded device because of the possibility of transmitting other diseases such as hepatitis B, even though the lance is replaced with each use. Such transmission has been documented in a hospital ward in which the holder was not adequately cleaned between uses.[20] Even though the lance is replaced each time, blood may contaminate the end of the holder. The hepatitis B virus can remain viable in a dried blood sample for 10 to 14 days.

## Psychosocial Aspects

The reasonably well-informed patient with diabetes is usually knowledgeable of the potential for ocular and systemic complications soon after diagnosis. The onset of proliferative diabetic retinopathy has been shown to cause psychological distress by both loss of vision and other negatively experienced life events associated with the difficulties in adjustment to the retinopathy.[21] Wulsin et al.[22] found that diabetic patients often blamed themselves for vitreous hemorrhages that occurred within a short time frame of strenuous physical activity.

For some, the continual variability in residual vision is more frustrating than the adjustment to total blindness.[23, 24] Even effective treatment for retinopathy by photocoagulation may cause the additional visual problems of field loss, impaired dark adaptation, decreased visual acuity, and decreased color perception and may therefore contribute to the patient's psychosocial problems in adaptation to the visual impairment.

## SUMMARY

Each person who presents with a vision impairment has unique needs and unique potential that are based on individual differences as well as the etiology of the vision loss. For some etiologies, there are specific considerations such as night mobility for retinitis pigmentosa and seeing a glucometer for the person with diabetic retinopathy. These needs can be anticipated based on a knowledge of the pathophysiology of the disease, but the real needs, on an individual basis, are discovered from a thorough interview and from getting to know the person as an individual.

## REFERENCES

1. Dell'Osso LF: Improving visual acuity in congenital nystagmus, in Smith JL, Glaser JS (eds): *Neuro Ophthalmology*. St. Louis, C. V. Mosby Company, 1973, pp 98–106.
2. Dell'Osso L, Gauthier G, Liberman G, Stark L: Eye movement recordings as a diagnostic tool in a case of congenital nystagmus. *Am J Optom & Arch Amer Acad Optom* 49(1):3–13, 1972.
3. Abplanalp P, Bedell H: Visual improvement in an albinotic patient with an alteration of congenital nystagmus. *Am J Optom Physiol Optics* 64:944–951, 1987.
4. Abadi RV: Visual performance with contact lenses and congenital idiopathic nystagmus. *Br J Physiol Opt* 33:32–37, 1979.

5. Allen ED, Davies PD: Role of contact lenses in the management of congenital nystagmus. *Br J Ophthalmol* 67:834-836, 1983.
6. Dell'Osso LF, Traccis S, Abel LA, Erzurum SI: Contact lenses and congenital nystagmus. *Clin Vision Sci* 3(3):229-232, 1988.
7. Rushton D, Cox N: A new optical treatment for oscillopsia. *J Neurol Neurosurg Psychiatry* 50:411-415, 1987.
8. Leigh RJ, Rushton DN, Thurston SE, Hertle RW, Yaniglos SS: Effects of retinal image stabilization on acquired nystagmus due to neurologic disease. *Neurology* 38:122-127, 1988.
9. Yaniglos SS, Leigh RJ: Refinement of an optical device that stabilizes vision in patients with nystagmus. *Optom Vis Sci* 69(6):447-450, 1992.
10. Sigal MB, Diamond GR: Survey of management strategies for nystagmus patients with vertical or torsional head posture. *Annals Ophthalmol* 22(4):134-138, 1990.
11. von Noorden GK, Sprunger DT: Large rectus muscle recessions for the treatment of congenital nystagmus. *Arch Ophthalmol* 109(2):221-224, 1991.
12. Helveston EM, Ellis FD, Plager DA: Large recession of the horizontal recti for treatment of nystagmus. *Ophthalmology* 98(8):1302-1305, 1991.
13. Pratt-Johnson JA: Results of surgery to modify the null-zone position in congenital nystagmus. *Can J Ophthalmol* 26(4):219-223, 1991.
14. Fioretto M, Burtolo C, Fava GP: New surgical method for nystagmus without null point. *Ophthalmologica* 203(4):180-183, 1991.
15. Zubcov AA, Reinecke RD, Gottlob I, Manley DR, Calhoun JH: Treatment of manifest latent nystagmus. *Am J Ophthalmol* 110(2):160-167, 1990.
16. Dowling JE, Sidman RL: Inherited retinal dystrophy in the rat. *J Cell Biol* 14:73-109, 1962.
17. Berson EL: Light deprivation and retinitis pigmentosa. *Vision Res* 20:1179-1184, 1980.
18. Miyake Y, Sugita S, Horiguchi M, Yagasaki K: Light deprivation and retinitis pigmentosa. *Am J Ophthalmol* 110:305-306, 1990.
19. Berson EL, Rabin AR, Mehaffey L: Advances in night vision technology: A pocketscope for patients with retinitis pigmentosa. *Arch Ophthalmol* 90:427-431, 1973.
20. Polish LB, Shapiro CN, Bauer F, Klotz P, Ginier P, Roberto RR, Margolis HS, Alter MJ: Nosocomial transmission of hepatitis B virus associated with the use of a spring-loaded finger-stick device. *NEJM* 326(11):721-725, 1992. (*See comments:* Marcus DL, Lordi PF Jr.: Transmission of hepatitis B virus associated with a finger-stick device (letter). *NEJM* 328(13):969, 1993.)
21. Jacobsen AM, Rand LI, Hauser ST: Psychologic stress and glycemic control: A comparison of patients with and without proliferative diabetic retinopathy. *Psychosom Med* 47:372-381, 1985.
22. Wulsin LR, Jacobsen AM, Rand LI: Review: Psychosocial aspects of diabetic retinopathy. *Diab Care* 10(3):367-373, 1987.
23. Stern NG: Out of sight: Coping with diabetic retinopathy. *J Vis Impair Blind* 77(6):304-305, 1983.
24. Oehler JW, Fitzgerald RG: Group therapy with blind diabetics. *Arch Gen Psychiatr* 37:463-467, 1980.

## ADDITIONAL READING

Authors, *J Vis Impair Blindness* 72(9), 1978. This entire issue is devoted to articles concerning diabetes and aspects of vision rehabilitation related to diabetes.

Berson EL, Mehaffey L, Rabin A: A night vision pocketscope for patients with retinitis pigmentosa: Design considerations. *Arch Ophthalmol* 91:495–500, 1974.

Safran AB, Gambazzi Y: Congenital nystagmus: Rebound phenomenon following removal of contact lenses. *Br J Ophthalmol* 76:497–498, 1992.

# Selected Case Examples

The examples that follow are from actual patients. A complete discussion of the examination and management of each case is omitted in order to provide succinct examples that highlight the prescription of low vision devices in typical cases. The treatment plans presented certainly are not the only management options but rather are presented as illustrative examples of the principles in this text. The reader might try formulating his or her own treatment plan after reading the history, goal, and reference acuities and before reading the rest of the summary. This will assist in reinforcing the basic approach of determining the goal and then calculating the required magnification and the dioptric strength of the device that will provide it. The prescription of optical devices is not the only treatment option, so the need for nonoptical assistive devices should also be anticipated, as should management aspects unique to specific etiologies.

## OCULOCUTANEOUS ALBINISM

*Pertinent History:* Ms. "W" was 32 years old with relatively mild vision impairment from oculocutaneous albinism. Her chief complaint was decreased distance vision. She felt that her near vision was adequate for all her tasks.

*Goal:* She was a school teacher and desired improved distance vision for classroom activities. She expressed no concern with cosmesis related to the use of a low vision device.

*Visual Acuities:* Her best corrected distance visual acuity was 20/70 with each eye.

*Treatment:* A 2.75X hand-held telescope for occasional spotting of distant objects was prescribed. With this device she could read the equivalent of 20/25.

*Discussion:* A telescope was the only consideration since her near vision was acceptable to her. Although her distance acuity was rather good, it was not adequate for her needs. Two telescopes were demonstrated to her: a 2.75X hand-held model and a 3.0X designed to be spectacle-mounted. Although she preferred the spectacle-mounted model initially, she eventually decided that the hand-held telescope would be best for her.

Because her visual acuity was already quite good, it was reasonable to try a telescope that would let her read the equivalent of 20/20. The magnification of the telescope was determined as follows:

Magnification required = Reference size/Goal size
Magnification required = 70/20
Magnification required = 3.5X

The available telescopes in the diagnostic set were 2.75X, 3.0X, and 4.0X. She rejected the 4.0X model because of its size, and, of the other two, she decided on the 2.75X. Her predicted acuity with the 2.75X telescope was 20/25.5, which is almost exactly what she achieved. This was determined as follows:

Magnification = Reference size/Goal size
2.75X = 70/Goal size
Goal size = 70/2.75
Goal size = 25.45

Short wavelength filters were discussed, and genetic counseling was provided.


## AGE-RELATED MACULOPATHY

*Pertinent History:* Mr. "G" was an 82-year-old male with decreased central acuity secondary to macular degeneration. He had experienced decreasing vision for several years and had bilateral cataract extraction with IOL implantation, which, following a capsulotomy O.D., resulted in excellent vision. Subsequently, the vision with his right eye deteriorated, although he was unaware of it until it was demonstrated to him at a routine eye exam. Several years later, central vision was lost with the left eye also. He had undergone fluorescein angiography. Laser surgery was recommended, but he refused because he was unhappy with the retinologist, who, he said, had not explained what the fluorescein study meant or what the treatment was intended to do. He was a retired engineer who lived alone and reported no difficulty with daily activities. He was able to do his own cooking, and relatives provided him with transportation. He had been referred for vision rehabilitation by a local practitioner.

*Goal:* He wanted to see better at near in order to conduct his own affairs.

*Visual Acuities:* Best corrected distance acuities were 5/700 O.D. and 10/60 O.S. At near he could read 3M print at 40 centimeters with the left eye and a +2.50 add over best correction.

*Treatment:* A +8.00 D full-diameter microscope for the left eye was loaned to him to try at home for two weeks. With this device he could read 1M print. After the follow-up examination a +12.00 aspheric full-diameter microscope was prescribed for him.

*Discussion:* This patient had an excellent short-term prognosis for success. He was motivated, had a modest goal, and had relatively good vision with his left eye. He was not at all concerned with the near work distance required by a microscope. To see most printed materials he had to be able to read 1M print. The required magnification and the add that would provide it were determined as follows:

$$\text{Magnification required} = \text{Reference size/Goal size}$$
$$\text{Magnification required} = 3M/1M$$
$$\text{Magnification required} = 3X$$

$$M = rF$$
$$3 = (0.4)F$$
$$3/0.4 = F$$
$$+7.50\ D = F$$

A +8.00 full-diameter microscope was selected as the closest option in a prefabricated microscope that was available to loan to him. He was able to read 1M print with it as predicted. After two weeks he returned and expressed a desire to have something slightly stronger. Both +10.00 D and +12.00 D microscopes were demonstrated, and he preferred the +12.00 D. This was prescribed for him as a full-diameter aspheric lens for the left eye only since there was a significant difference in the acuity with the two eyes. He was not bothered by the unmagnified image with the right eye, so an occluder was not considered. He rejected the idea of a hand-held magnifier because he wanted his hands free. Telemicroscopes were not demonstrated since he immediately accepted the microscope and telemicroscopes would be more expensive, heavier, and bigger. As another consideration, his vision was not expected to be stable, and it would be less expensive to replace the microscope than a telemicroscope. He was counseled about the wisdom of obtaining another retinal consultation and was returned to the referring doctor for appropriate follow-up.

## HISTOPLASMOSIS

*Pertinent History:* Ms. "A" was a 34-year-old female who lost the central vision in her right eye secondary to histoplasmosis. She recalled being assured by her retinologist that her other eye would not be involved. Six months later the central vision in the fellow eye deteriorated. She was extremely despondent over her lost sight and when first examined was not willing to try assistive devices. She also had considerable difficulty with eccentric viewing that seemed related to her despondency since she lacked motivation to try to improve. She was a client of the State Vocational Rehabilitation Services (VRS).

*Goal:* Her VRS training goal was to operate a vending stand independently. That job required that she be able to see at arm's length to make minor repairs on vending machines and be able to see well enough at near to identify the various products, make change, and keep her own books.

*Visual Acuities:* Her best corrected distance acuity was 5/30 O.D. and 10/40 O.S. At near she was 0.25/2.5M O.D. and 0.15/1M O.S.

*Treatment:* The initial treatment plan was to teach her to view eccentrically with greater consistency. A program was initiated with large targets and progressed to smaller ones as her ability steadily improved. When she achieved a consistent level of eccentric viewing, the following permanent device was prescribed for her: a 2.2X spectacle-mounted full-diameter telescope for the left eye with a +3.00 cap. With the 2.2X telescope she achieved 20/40 O.S. With a +3.00 cap over the telescope she was able to read 0.5M print at 33 centimeters.

*Discussion:* Since she needed to work at an intermediate distance to repair vending machines and since this also required that her hands be free, a telemicroscope was the treatment of choice. Several telescopes were demonstrated, but she preferred the full-diameter option. It was mounted centered before the left eye with a black housing to reduce ambient light. With the cap she could see well enough at near to do her bookkeeping. The telemicroscope system was prescribed for her left eye since this was her better eye.

Because she could read 1M print at 15 centimeters but needed a greater working distance, a telemicroscope system that would still allow her to read 1M print was designed based on a 2.2X full-diameter model that had the largest field of view of those available in the inventory at that time. The power of the cap was derived as follows:

$$\text{Magnification required} = \text{Reference size/Goal size}$$
$$\text{Magnification required} = 1M/1M$$
$$\text{Magnification required} = 1X$$

$$M_{tms} = M_{cap} \times M_{ts}$$
$$1X = M_{cap} \times M_{ts}$$
$$1X = (0.15)F \times 2.2$$
$$1/(0.15 \times 2.2) = F$$
$$1/0.33 = F$$
$$+3.00 = F$$

With 1X magnification she should still be able to read 1M print, but at the new work distance of 33 centimeters by virtue of the telemicroscope system. In fact, she read somewhat better than predicted.

Although her vocational goal did not require a telescope, she was going to have one anyway in the telemicroscope system once the cap was removed. Her predicted distance acuity with the telescope alone was 20/36, and she achieved a result very close to that. This was calculated as follows:

$$10/40 = 20/80$$
$$\text{Magnification} = \text{Reference size/Goal size}$$
$$2.2X = 80/\text{Goal size}$$
$$\text{Goal size} = 80/2.2$$
$$\text{Goal size} = 36.36$$

It would have been possible to prescribe a telemicroscope system with a built-in cap and a fixed work distance and near magnification. The option of having a removable cap allowed greater flexibility since the system could be used as a telescope and several caps could be provided for different near tasks. A focusable spectacle-mounted telescope that could be used for distance and near was also considered. When she first used the telemicroscope at near, she felt uncomfortable seeing two different images. A clip-on occluder was tried over the fellow eye, and this offered relief. At her request, the right lens was then frosted. Several months later she asked to have the frosted lens replaced with a clear one, and that proved successful. She completed her training with VRS and acquired her own vending stand, which she was able to operate independently. She referred to her telemicroscope as "my miracle glasses."

This example demonstrates the fact that the predicted acuities are not necessarily what the patient actually achieves. They should, however, be close.

## OPTIC ATROPHY SECONDARY TO NEUROFIBROMATOSIS

*Pertinent History:* Mr. "L" had a history of optic glioma secondary to neurofibromatosis. Surgical intervention stabilized the optic atrophy, but he was left with decreased vision. He complained of difficulty seeing in school and eye fatigue with reading.

*Goal:* He desired improved vision for high school with the ultimate goal of attending college.

*Visual Acuities:* Best corrected acuities were 7/40 O.D. and LPO O.S. At near he could read 1M print at his preferred distance of 10 centimeters by accommodating.

*Treatment:* Two devices were prescribed: a 4.0X spectacle-mounted telescope for distance and glasses with protective lenses and a +4.00 add for the right eye to be worn full-time when the telescope was not being used. The telescope was mounted in spectacles with polycarbonate lenses, in the office, by drilling a hole in the right lens with a hole saw and a drill press.

*Discussion:* Since he was monocular, protection of the remaining eye became the first priority. His habitual reading distance of 10 centimeters led to a consideration of adds to relieve accommodative strain. He rejected adds higher than +4.00. Several telescopes were demonstrated to him, and he preferred 4.0X magnification. It was prescribed as a spectacle-mounted device so his hands would be free for writing and manipulating school materials.

His best corrected acuity at distance with the telescope was 20/25, which was very close to his predicted acuity of 20/28.57, determined as follows:

$$7/40 = 20/114.29$$

$$\text{Magnification} = \text{Reference size/Goal size}$$
$$4.0X = 114.29/\text{Goal size}$$
$$\text{Goal size} = 114.29/4.0$$
$$\text{Goal size} = 28.57$$

The +4.00 add would not be expected to provide any additional magnification since he was already reading with a +10.00 lens by accommodating to 10 centimeters. The add was prescribed simply to relieve his accommodative effort and was successful.

He completed high school and went on to college, although he was delayed by additional complications of neurofibromatosis that required surgery for increased intracranial pressure. Genetic counseling was provided based on his dominant family history.

## SUMMARY

These few examples illustrate some of the principles in the text and hopefully will serve to reassure the reader that it is easily within his or her ability to participate in this specialty area. A large inventory of devices is not necessary to provide appropriate care for many people who are visually impaired. The lessons learned from the previous chapters provide a systematic approach to the diagnostic trial and prescription of assistive devices. The vignettes in Chapter 30 include some additional case examples as well as insights into diagnosis and management.

# PRACTICE MANAGEMENT

*There is no mystery to providing low vision rehabilitation services. All it takes is a commitment to try. It is not necessary to have an expensive inventory of equipment to provide at least some services. In fact, it is possible to begin providing this specialized care with little additional equipment beyond that found in the typical practitioner's office. Additional equipment can be added as one's involvement grows. If specialized training is desired, it is available through continuing education courses, residencies, fellowships, and concentrated training sessions at selected facilities.*

## PROFESSIONAL TRAINING

Specialized training is most easily obtained through continuing education courses offered by national, state, and local associations. For those who have the time and want to obtain residency or fellowship training, there are a number of programs available. Several resources for information are given in Chapter 31.

## EQUIPMENT

It is possible for the practitioner to provide comprehensive low vision evaluations without purchasing additional equipment. There are several ways in which this may be accomplished. A novel approach used by the Vermont Commission for the Blind was to purchase a large inventory of diagnostic equipment, housed in a mobile van, that could be scheduled for use by selected practitioners throughout the state. A similar approach has been used in Alabama by the State Vocational Rehabilitation Service in which custom-designed kits of low vision devices were purchased by that agency for loan to practitioners. If such programs are not available in a practitioner's state, several practices might combine resources to purchase kits and share them on a prearranged weekly or monthly schedule. Practitioners may custom design their kits or, alternatively, buy standard kits. Finally, it may be possible to rent kits from a manufacturer of expensive devices that may be prescribed less frequently. Designs for Vision, Inc., has offered such a program in the past.

A considerable amount of low vision care can be provided with the equipment available in a typical practitioner's office. A standard trial lens set has high enough powers to demonstrate most microscope powers that will be prescribed. Additional equipment that is useful for examination of someone who is visually impaired includes one or more hand-held cross-cylinders of higher powers such as ±0.50 and ±1.00, a portable distance chart, a typoscope, and a variety of near cards, including some with continuous text. The near cards should be labeled in M notation. If this was not done by the manufacturer, the practitioner can label it as explained in Chapter 4.

A basic diagnostic set of low vision devices might include the following:

1. Several hand-held telescopes with powers of approximately 2.0X, 4.0X, and 6.0X. Examples that could also be mounted in spectacles would be more versatile.
2. One diagnostic telescope, in a trial ring, for a spectacle-mounted design. One of the most frequently prescribed telescopes in this category is the 2.2X FDTS from Designs for Vision, Inc. It is easy for patients to use since it is of low power and has a relatively large field of view. An alternate choice is the 3.5X expanded field telescope from Designs for Vision, Inc. This telescope is also relatively low in power but is perhaps more versatile since it is focusable.
3. Several hand-held magnifiers of various powers from +5.00 to +20.00 diopters.
4. Several stand magnifiers of various powers from +10.00 to +30.00 diopters. These should be labeled by the practitioner with the image location and enlargement factor.
5. Two types of microscopes: full-diameter lenses and prism-compensated half eyes. The half eyes can be purchased in sets of three or four powers. If individual prism-compensated half eyes are ordered, the available powers are +4.00, +6.00, +8.00, +10.00, and +12.00 D. There are also diagnostic sets of microscope lenses, mounted in trial rings, available from American Optical; however, if the prefabricated microscope spectacles are purchased, they can be dispensed and reordered. Recommended powers are from +8.00 to +24.00 D.

A basic diagnostic set, similar to the one described, can be purchased for under $1,500. Most of the items can be dispensed to patients, for cost recovery, if the practitioner decides not to continue providing vision rehabilitation care.

Several providers of low vision devices offer various diagnostic kits. The disadvantage of these kits is that they are not custom designed by the practitioner and therefore might include devices that will not be prescribed frequently, might not include an adequate range of powers, or might include more devices than desired. Prior to ordering any low vision devices, the practitioner should obtain catalogues from a number of sources in order to compare prices and ascertain the availability of diagnostic kits.

If the practitioner wants to maintain an inventory of devices for dispensing, there will be additional expense. While it is occasionally convenient to be able to dispense devices from an in-office inventory, it is not necessarily a good idea and certainly should not be considered a prerequisite to engaging in low vision care. There is a certain mystique about something that has been ordered specifically for the patient, and it is conceivable that the patient will respond better to a device that is not viewed as a stock item from the practitioner's "cupboard." One might argue that contact lenses are dispensed from an in-office supply, but contact lenses have always been perceived as a prescription device while hand-held low vision devices have not. It is fairly common for established practitioners to have an inventory of devices for loan to patients; however, to initiate and maintain this inventory requires additional expense.

## OFFICE DESIGN AND MANAGEMENT

### Office Design

People who are older or who are visually impaired are more likely to come, and return, to an office that facilitates their visit. This can be accomplished by making the office "friendly." Accessibility is important in that it creates a first impression. If steps are necessary to approach the entrance, they should be wide and clearly marked and have a good handrail. The waiting room should have good lighting, chairs with arms from which someone can rise easily, even if physically infirm, and large print books or magazines. One of the first things a patient is asked to do is to sign in. This can be made easier by providing a black felt-tip pen and a log sheet with broad, dark lines. Many of the suggestions made in the sample information sheets about environmental adaptations (Chapter 24) with respect to colors, contrast, lighting, and furniture are appropriate for the practitioner's office as well.

A display of assistive devices is a definite attention getter. Some magnifiers, large print playing cards, and similar items can be displayed in an obvious place with a sign that suggests that interested persons inquire about special services for those who are visually impaired. The author has a closed circuit television on the counter for assistance with signing in. This allows the person to accomplish an everyday task with an assistive device. It is also used to display the magnified image of the instructions on a medication bottle, which prompts people to think about other important applications. Many people enjoy experimenting with the unit even if they have no visual impairment. Brochures displayed in the waiting room are a good means of providing information and can be created to emphasize the practitioner's interest in working with those who are visually impaired.

## Patient Scheduling

Sufficient time should be scheduled for someone who is known to be visually impaired to allow for a slower pace, especially if the individual is older. A person presenting for a first visit will not necessarily be identified in advance as visually impaired. As soon as the clinician appreciates the fact that an extended evaluation will be required, it is best to advise the individual that a preliminary evaluation will be performed at that visit, related to the main goal, and that he or she will be rescheduled for additional special testing at another date. This allows the clinician to stay on schedule and prevents the patient from becoming disappointed at the end of the exam when his or her problems have not all been addressed.

Persons who are visually impaired may all be selectively scheduled on the same day of the week or month if the practitioner rents or shares a diagnostic kit of low vision devices and only has it available at selected times. This approach has been used in some states where a central agency invests in the diagnostic devices and makes them available to clinicians throughout the state. Selective scheduling on specific days may also assist in having a more smoothly running practice by establishing a routine for the day that is not interrupted with a variety of different patient types. A final advantage to this approach is the mutual support that may be established among patients and families in the waiting room when they meet others who share similar problems.

## Office Staff

The office staff must be sensitive to the problems of those with visual impairments. They can be trained to be helpful in anticipated areas of need and to display appropriate empathy, not sympathy. A majority of visually impaired patients are older and may have other traits—such as a hearing impairment, loss of short-term memory, physical instability, and other systemic disorders—that require patience from the receptionist or assistant. The office staff can be trained in the techniques of the sighted guide in order to assist visually impaired patients around the office. They should be taught to allow the patient to be as independent as possible and not to assume that everything must be done for someone who is visually impaired; for example, it is appropriate to ask if someone needs assistance in moving to the examination room or in filling out the appropriate forms rather than assuming that he or she needs it.

## Establishing Fees

There are two basic approaches to fee setting. The first is to charge on the basis of time spent or service provided per visit. This approach lends itself well to a relative service fee schedule.[1] For example, each encounter is charged at the practitioner's current rate for an abbreviated, intermediate, extended, or comprehensive visit. Some have argued that higher fees should be charged when the clinician practices at a higher skill level. To some extent this is accounted for in the present evaluation and management scheme that requires documentation of time spent with the patient and what portion of the time was devoted to specific activities such as counseling. A related example is the higher fee charged when the patient has been specifically referred for consultation by another health care provider with the appropriate documentation.

The second approach to establishing fees is to charge a global fee for a comprehensive plan. In this case the patient pays, usually in advance, for a "package" of services that are considered an integral part of the total rehabilitative effort. Such services may include a social interview, orientation and mobility evaluation, vision evaluation, prescription of low vision devices, and training in their use. This approach might work for a multidisciplinary practice but is less practical for the private practitioner; however, some private practitioners offer a scaled-down approach in which a global fee is charged for a smaller comprehensive plan. When third party reimbursement is sought, fees must be established and coded in a manner consistent with obtaining reimbursement. At this time, most third party plans do not pay specifically for vision rehabilitation visits or for optical appliances other than glasses for the correction of refractive error.

Fees will be the subject of considerable scrutiny and modification in the coming years as a national health plan is put in place and the ramifications of capitation and managed care are realized by the individual practitioner.

## ESTABLISHING A PATIENT POPULATION

The largest population of persons who are visually impaired is among the elderly, and many low vision practitioners provide screenings and vision care to residents of nursing homes. There are also many people who are visually impaired who are not elderly. One way to come in contact with these potential patients is to become a provider for the state vocational rehabilitation service. This requires meeting the local counselors whose caseloads include clients who are visually impaired and expressing an interest in working with their clients. Such state agencies can be located in the telephone book. Other agencies, commissions, or programs for those who are visually impaired may be located in the resource directory published by the American Foundation by the Blind (see Resources, Chapter 31).

Certain health care providers are more likely to have contact with visually impaired patients and may serve as a source of referral once a professional relationship has been established. Diabetologists and gerontologists are excellent sources, given that diabetes and aging are so closely associated with vision impairment. Physiatrists and others in rehabilitation medicine have contact with patients suffering vision loss from stroke and head trauma. Rehabilitation hospitals, nursing homes, and day care centers for the elderly are also excellent sources for the practitioner to approach. Virtually all of the equipment used for vision rehabilitation is portable, so the practitioner can assemble a kit in a carrying case when he or she provides care outside the office setting.

## HOW TO GET STARTED

It is easy to get started in low vision rehabilitation by approaching it incrementally. There are a number of other books and journal articles about vision rehabilitation, and it is a good idea to read some of these in order to get additional perspectives. Catalogues should be ordered from various suppliers, some of whom are listed in Chapter 31, in order to learn what is available and what it costs. The next step is to order a few devices that were suggested for a basic inventory, including a portable distance acuity chart and several near cards. It's worth repeating: label the near cards in M notation, have some cards with continuous text, and label any stand magnifiers with their image location and enlargement factor. The devices that should be obtained and tried first are those that are prescribed most often and those that are best received by patients. These are hand-held magnifiers, high bifocal adds, and microscopes (especially the prism-compensated half eyes in lower powers). The only thing missing at this point is the patient, but he or she will show up sooner or later. It will be sooner if attempts are made to facilitate referral or to make it known that the service is available (for example, with a display in the office).

## SUMMARY

Many vision rehabilitation services can be provided in the private practice setting. Simple office modifications can be made that will facilitate access for those who are older and/or visually impaired. There is a large and increasing population of people who can benefit from this specialty care. The typical office already has much of the required equipment. With the addition of a few additional examination items, a reasonable inventory of optical and nonoptical devices, and the knowledge gained from the previous chapters, the process can begin.

## REFERENCE

1. Jose RT, Ferraro JF: Developing a low vision fee schedule. *Rehab Optom* 1(2):1-7, 1983.

## ADDITIONAL READING

Appel S, Graboyes M, Brilliant R: A model patient care schedule for low vision services. *Rehab Optom* 1(3):11-12, 1983.

# REFLECTIONS ON LESSONS LEARNED

*After 19 years as the director of a large low vision clinic in an educational setting, I can recall many lessons that were reinforced in interesting ways, for both my students and myself. A few of them are presented in the following vignettes.*

## THE LESSONS

### Stereotypic Views

One day, early in my career, I looked in the waiting room and saw a couple filling in the patient data sheet. The male had extremely thick glasses and was holding the form very close to his eyes while writing. I thought to myself, "He must be really visually impaired." Yet when it was time for "his" appointment, it was his wife who sat in the examination chair. He had normal vision but was myopic; she had no refractive error but had less than 5° fields secondary to retinitis pigmentosa. None of us is immune to stereotyping or to being stereotyped, but we can learn to minimize its expression and its effect on our interaction with others.

### Visual Acuity and Legal Blindness

As a young practitioner, I was asked to provide a vision screening for the workers at a workshop for the blind. Being particularly eager to do a good job, I used the portable Feinbloom chart in order to measure everyone's acuity as precisely as possible. No "finger counting" or low contrast projected charts for me! Not too long after I completed the screening, the manager called and informed me that I had created a very big problem for the workshop. It seems that a number of the workers who had been previously categorized as legally blind by other practitioners were not legally blind by my report, and the workshop was therefore in jeopardy of losing its federal funding since 75% of the workers had to meet the definition of legally blind. What had happened was that everyone who had a visual acuity between 20/100 and 20/200 had previously been categorized as legally blind since the best they could read on the standard Snellen chart was 20/200. However, with a more accurate assessment their acuity was actually better than 20/200, and hence they were not legally blind by a strict interpretation of the definition. It was then that I learned to specify "20/200 by the standard Snellen chart" for those whose visual acuity fell in this intermediate range. I don't feel completely good about that compromise, but then I don't feel completely good about the definition of legal blindness either. In any case, the compromise certainly falls within the realm of customary practice since most practitioners use standard Snellen charts for measuring visual acuity.

## Prosthetic Eyes

Have I ever heard the "clank" of an intern's tonometer probe striking a prosthetic eye? You betcha! I'll even admit to trying retinoscopy on a prosthetic eye once (of course, I was a lot younger then).

Nobody likes to wait. One facility at which I had an affiliated clinic made a practice of having every new client—with no exceptions—receive a vision screening. One gentleman waited patiently until he couldn't stand it any longer and asked my technician why he had to be screened since he was completely blind and had two prosthetic eyes. She explained that we also evaluated people such as himself for comfort and cosmesis. He insisted that he was in a hurry and said, "I have another class to go to. Couldn't I just leave my eyes and pick them up later?"

## Visual Field Enhancement

I suppose everyone has used the old excuse, "My dog ate my homework," but how about the patient whose dog ate his glasses? There was a hole in the lens and multiple bite marks on the frame. The Fresnel membrane, placed for field enhancement, was long gone. I guess I'll never know, but sometimes, late at night, I still wonder.

My first patient with a field restriction had a partial right hemianopsia secondary to a brain tumor as a child. He had graduated from college and was a personable, handsome young male in his mid-20s. He had never driven a car and did not have an active social life since, as he explained it, he was confined to walking or riding his bicycle. He had come to our low vision clinic from another state, and I was sure I could help him. A Fresnel prism was demonstrated for field enhancement, but he really didn't appreciate the result. Nevertheless, he agreed to try it for a while and left the clinic to visit another friend in town. During that visit he was asked how the exam had gone. He said he was trying the prism but didn't feel it was particularly helpful. His friend, sitting to the side, asked, "Can you see me over here?" He replied that he could. His friend pointed out that he didn't think he could see that well to the side before and asked him to look without the prism. It suddenly became clear to him that the prism could enhance his visual field, and he got excited about trying it.

At follow-up he reported difficulty using the prism while riding his bicycle since some objects seemed to jump in and out of view. We developed a technique of scanning that would prevent him from missing objects that were hidden in the scotoma induced by the prism. That proved to be very effective. Soon thereafter he called and said he was learning to drive. He passed the vision examination and practical test in his state, purchased his own car, and drove to his next follow-up examination. By mutual request I rode with him and was convinced of his ability to drive safely. His entire life changed, not so much because of the field enhancement but because of the development of self-confidence that came with achieving a milestone he had previously thought was inaccessible. At his next visit I suggested that we go out for something to eat since it was the end of the day. He replied, "Sorry, not this time. I have a date." I asked, "How could you have a date? You don't live here and don't know any girls here." Well, it seems he was dating a young woman from his home state who was a stewardess and who had a stopover in our city. My, how things can change.

It would be wonderful if every clinical encounter resulted in a success story, but, of course, that is not the case. Every encounter does, however, offer the opportunity to assist someone in need, and even that attempt defines a certain measure of success.

## Predicting the Correct Magnification

One day I dispensed a hand-held telescope to a client in a residential vocational rehabilitation facility. I pointed out to him that even though there were two objective lenses, to make the system 6.0X or 8.0X, he only needed the lower power. "I know," he said, "but I still want the other one." "Why?" I asked. In a conspiratorial manner he whispered in my ear, "For the girls' dorm!"

## Avoiding False Expectations

A well-to-do older woman with macular degeneration went through an extensive evaluation and finally decided that the "HoneyBee" spectacle-mounted telescopes from Designs for Vision, Inc., were the best device for her needs. She was not the least bit deterred by their expense, and I thought we had reached an understanding about the appearance of the final prescription. At that time in my career, I would order a device with a 50% deposit, which she promptly paid. Several weeks later she presented for dispensing. She took one look at the prescribed lenses and said, "There's no way in the world I'm going to wear anything that looks like that!" She literally tossed them on a table and demanded her money back. I was a young practitioner staring a large financial loss in the face. Fortunately, Designs for Vision, Inc., worked out a mutually satisfactory exchange with us. I learned the value of repeating, numerous times, "Your glasses will look just like this!"

## Driving with Impaired Vision

One day a patient called the clinic and requested that we provide a letter certifying her legal blindness, which she would pick up later that day. She definitely had best corrected visual acuities less than 20/200 for each eye, and an intern prepared the letter. Just after she left the clinic, the intern realized that she had left something behind and hurried outside to see if he could stop her. When he returned, he ran up to me and exclaimed, "You know that lady who came by to pick up a letter certifying that she was legally blind? Well, I tried to return this package to her, but I was too late. She was already driving out of our parking lot!"

## The Central Scotoma

One woman informed us that she had spent a frustrating and unsuccessful period of time chasing a large insect around her kitchen with a fly swatter. Every time she looked at it, it moved and she could never hit it. It was later that she learned that the black "bug" was a central scotoma secondary to her macular degeneration.

Another lady told me of scrubbing a large spot in her sink until it disappeared. A moment later she was surprised to see that it had reappeared. Again she scrubbed it away and left to do some shopping. When she returned, much to her surprise, it had reappeared once more. This time in the course of her scrubbing she noticed that it occasionally vanished and came back. It was then that she first became consciously aware of the effect of her central scotomas.

## Training in the Care of Optical Devices

A young man with Usher syndrome (congenital hearing impairment with retinitis pigmentosa) received his new glasses and was very pleased with them. He worked as a kitchen helper at a rehabilitation facility. I was told a week later that he had had a frightening experience that caused him to think he had suddenly gone blind. It seems that he wanted to clean his new glasses and used an abrasive cleansing powder from the kitchen. When he put the glasses back on, his sight was gone! Apparently, it took quite a while to calm him down and explain, by sign language, what had happened.

A good friend who is a well-known cardiovascular surgeon called me one day to let me know how he was doing with his new glasses. He had wanted a particular frame, but it wasn't available in the dark color that he desired for his sun lenses. Another good friend, who is an optician, explained that it was no problem to dye the frame black, which he did, and everyone was happy at dispensing. One steamy summer day shortly thereafter the surgeon was on a shopping excursion in the sunny South and kept getting unusual stares from passersby. When he looked into a mirror, it was obvious why—the dye wasn't as permanent as we had thought, and he had a nice black ring around each eye! So what has this got to do with low vision? Well, he also owns several pairs of surgical loupes (telemicroscopes). Before surgery he has a nurse *warm* them in an autoclave so they won't fog over in the operating suite. Once the nurse forgot that he only wanted them warmed, and you can guess the rest. That was an expensive mistake—similar to that which one of my students made with a custom-designed spectacle-mounted telescope that he decided to adjust by first warming it in a salt bath. It came out looking rather like a Salvador Dali painting of a "melted" watch, but then so did the one a patient put in the oven to remove condensation that had collected inside the telescope!

## The Final Diagnosis

A middle-aged man was referred to me for low vision rehabilitation by a practitioner in another city. The patient was from out of state and had come to our state to visit his brother, who was a patient of the referring doctor and hence the eventual referral to me. He had very restricted fields, and ophthalmoscopically the retinal vessels were attenuated and the discs appeared pale. This was suggestive of retinitis pigmentosa, but the retina lacked pigmentary change. An ERG showed significantly reduced scotopic and photopic traces, but the patient did not consider himself to have ever had significant nightblindness. He expressed interest in the prognosis for his disorder and mentioned that his condition appeared stable subjectively and that he had been examined by several specialists, a few years earlier, in his home state without benefit of a diagnosis. I wrote to one and sent copies of his clinical summary, fundus photographs, and ERGs. I asked the specialist to compare them with his data and give me an impression about the relative change and his impression of the diagnosis and prognosis. The reply included that he had recommended a neurological evaluation, which I discovered our mutual patient had never obtained because of disdain for his original referring doctor.

Since the patient was returning to his home state and the diagnosis was uncertain, I urged him to obtain a neurological consultation and asked the specialist who had recommended it originally to follow up on the referral. Several weeks later I received a summary letter and read with pride that he had a pituitary tumor, which had been removed surgically in a successful operation. I read further, with increasing dismay, that during the hospitalization, his daughter had flown in to see him, and, while she and her mother drove to the hospital, they were involved in an accident in which the patient's wife was killed. When we act aggressively in what we believe is the patient's best interest, we must accept that there are certain consequences surrounding each action over which we have no control.

## The Correct Diagnosis or the Wrong Patient?

The chart said that the patient had oculocutaneous albinism, but the patient had dark hair and skin. The student was justifiably confused until, with closer examination, he discovered that the patient also had lot of make-up and dyed hair.

## Anatomical Confusion

It is often of interest to know what the patient thinks is the cause of his or her visual loss. One patient had a short right leg and optic atrophy of the left optic nerve. Her explanation of how this had happened was that, when she was very young, her father had dropped her, and the nerves from her left eye and right leg had become crossed, causing her contralateral disabilities. She may not have appreciated the clarification of this misunderstanding as much as her father did.

## Effective Communication

One of my first eye-opening experiences with doctor-patient communication took place with a patient who had a secret, although I didn't know it at the time. The secret was her diagnosis. After the initial examination I said, "Your reduced acuity is from loss of central vision that was probably caused by histoplasmosis," to which she replied, "I knew that. I just wanted to see if you could figure it out." Sometimes, or maybe always, what the clinician thinks of as "the patient examination" is actually a two-way street.

## Hidden Thoughts

This patient had optic atrophy with onset in the second decade. She had received numerous assessments by different specialists but still had no definitive diagnosis. She presented for vision rehabilitation, and, as part of the closing interview, I answered a number of questions. Finally, when asked if she had any other questions, she paused for a long while, and the conversation took the following turn:

> "Is it possible that this was caused by something that my mother took while she was pregnant?"

"Did you have something specific in mind?"

"Quinine."

"Do you know why she might have been taking quinine?"

"To prevent an unwanted pregnancy."

We had a long conversation.

## Whose Genes?

A five-year-old male with bilateral iris and retinal colobomas was brought to the clinic by his father. During the course of the examination, the father stated that he had told the boy's mother, "If we have another child like this one, I'm going to divorce you!" He was certainly surprised to learn that the trait is often dominant and that he might have the gene, but not the trait, due to decreased penetrance or expressivity. Since they desired additional children and wanted to know the risk for recurrence, it was decided that each of them would be examined to determine if one might show signs of a coloboma with decreased expressivity. Since both appeared entirely normal, it seemed that the son probably represented a new mutation, and they were informed that the recurrence risk was low. They now have a daughter with normal eyes and a son with not-so-normal eyes who is all boy, a good student, and, now, close to his father.

## Genetic Counseling?

A mother tearfully recalled her first experience with receiving "genetic counseling" several years earlier. Her son received an examination from a vision specialist. Her recollection was that he looked at her and said, "He is going to go blind, and you gave it to him." The diagnosis was juvenile retinoschisis. She was irreconcilably distraught and remains bitter over such a callous disregard for the emotional impact of this uncaring approach to communication of the diagnosis and its genetic implications.

## Eternal Optimism

A young man with retinitis pigmentosa has been a patient in my practice since the age of seven. He was all boy and enjoyed sports, including football and baseball, until such time that participation represented a physical threat to him. He, his parents, and I had many long discussions about his activities and tried to moderate our concern for his personal safety with his desire to be just like everyone else. He graduated from high school having competed successfully in a classroom with normally sighted peers, although he required a closed circuit television to do all of his reading. One summer during high school he got a job at a local hospital working in the laundry. He was already well beyond legal blindness on the basis of acuity and visual fields, yet he never told them and they never knew. Throughout his teenage years he hoped to be able to drive.

Each year he would come in for an eye exam just to see if he might meet the visual requirements. He knew he would not. I knew he would not. He knew that I knew he would not, and I knew that he knew that he would not. Nevertheless, it was as if it were a rite of spring, and we did our ritual dance.

When his inability to drive legally became an accepted fact, he refused to give up on the normal goals of young men. One day he called to discuss the possibility of joining the Marines. He had already been to see the recruiter. We had another of our long discussions and decided together that it was probably not a viable option. A couple of years later he called me to let me know what he had been up to, and was I surprised. He had gone to a school to learn to be a professional wrestler and was then traveling around the country to perform. That lasted several years. Presently he works for a manufacturer of athletic equipment. He called the other day to ask if he could use my name as a reference. I can hardly wait to see what's next!

## SUMMARY

Those were just a few of the many wonderful, sad, and humorous experiences I have had in this field. I look forward to many more and hope that you will also.

If you made it to this point, and it seems that you have, there is no reason not to begin providing low vision care in your own practice setting. Go ahead and take those first steps outlined in Chapter 29. When the next person with a visual impairment presents, you'll be ready. Include the appropriate questions in the interview. Correct the refractive error. Calculate the power needed to read some smaller print size and demonstrate the magnification, all in the systematic manner you have learned. As the number of patient encounters grows and your skills improve, your scope of services will expand. It will continue to get more interesting and more rewarding, both for you and for those to whom you provide care.

# RESOURCES FOR INFORMATION, TRAINING, AND MATERIALS RELATED TO VISION REHABILITATION

*The following sections are a compilation of selected resources for information and materials related to vision rehabilitation. It is not physically possible to list every available resource, and inclusion here does not indicate an endorsement by the author, nor does exclusion imply the opposite. Every attempt has been made to verify the accuracy of the addresses and phone numbers as of the time of publication. The author has no financial or other interest in any of the organizations, companies, or products listed.*

## RESOURCES FOR ASSISTIVE DEVICES

American Optical Corporation
14 Mechanic Street
Southbridge, MA 01550
(508) 765-9711
(800) 225-7498

This company is a source for high plus aspheric microscope lenses mounted in frames or in trial rings, prism-compensated half eyes, and other optical devices.

American Printing House for the Blind
(APH)
1839 Frankfort Avenue
P.O. Box 6085
Louisville, KY 40206-0085
(502) 895-2405

APH is a national organization that produces literature and educational materials, including textbooks, for persons who are visually impaired.

Audio Editions®
P.O. Box 6930
Auburn, CA 95604-6930
(800) 231-4261

Audio Editions carries a large selection of books on cassettes.

Blazie Engineering
105 East Jarrettsville Road
Unit D
Forest Hill, MD 21050
(410) 893-9333

Blazie Engineering's adaptive technology, primarily for computers, provides access for those who are visually impaired.

Bollé America, Inc.
3890 Elm Street
Denver, CO 80207
(303) 321-4300

Bollé is a source for a variety of ophthalmic filters, including mirror coatings and frames with side shields.

Carl Zeiss Optical, Inc.
P.O. Box 2010
Petersburg, VA 23804
(800) 446-1807
(804) 861-0033

Carl Zeiss's products include a variety of optical devices for those who are visually impaired.

Corning Medical Optics
MP 21 2 2
Corning, NY 14831
(607) 974-7823

This company manufactures the Corning Photochromic Filters (CPF).

Descriptive Video Service®
WGBH Educational Foundation
125 Western Avenue
Boston, MA 02134
(800) 333-1203

This service offers movies on video with a real-time verbal description of the action, locations, costumes, and sets that does not interfere with the movie's dialogue or sound effects. The concept is similar to close-captioned television for those with a hearing impairment. The videos play on a standard VCR with no adaptive device required.

Designs for Vision, Inc.
760 Koehler Avenue
Ronkonkoma, NY 11779
(516) 585-3300
(800) 345-4009

Designs for Vision, Inc., manufactures custom-fabricated spectacle-mounted optical devices, including telescopes, microscopes, and telemicroscopes. The company was founded by Dr. William Feinbloom, one of the pioneers in designing optical aids for persons with impaired vision.

Edmund Scientific Co.
101 East Gloucester Pike
Barrington, NJ 08007-1380
(608) 547-8880

This company carries a large variety of optical devices, including hand and stand magnifiers.

Edwards Optical Corporation
P.O. Box 3299
Virginia Beach, VA 23454
(804) 481-6285

Edwards is the manufacturer of the BITA™ spectacle-mounted telescopes.

Eschenbach Optik
904 Ethan Allen Highway
Ridgefield, CT 06877
(203) 438-7471

Eschenbach has a very large variety of virtually all types of optical devices, both hand-held and spectacle-mounted, as well as lamps and other assistive devices. The main office can provide the name of a regional distributor.

Fresnel Prism & Lens Company
7975 North Hayden Road
Suite A106
Scottsdale, AZ 85258-3242
(800) 544-4760
(602) 596-3998

This company manufactures press-on Fresnel optics.

The Hadley School for the Blind
700 Elm Street
Winnetka, IL 60093-0299
(800) 323-4238

The Hadley School provides home study courses designed for those who are visually impaired.

Hewitt Printing Corporation
7320 North Milwaukee Avenue
P.O. Box 48455
Niles, IL 60714-0455
(708) 647-8833

Hewitt produces signature guides, telephone guides for rotary phones, and guides for writing letters and checks as well as addressing envelopes.

The Houston Lighthouse
3530 West Dallas
Houston, TX 77019
(713) 527-9561

The Houston Lighthouse is a source for the mirror stand magnifier. This device uses a mirror instead of a convex lens, allowing the user to view the image from the front rather than having to look through the top of the device.

HumanWare, Inc.
6245 King Road
Loomis, CA 95650
(800) 722-3393
(916) 652-7253

HumanWare offers adaptive computer technology to give those who are visually impaired access to printed material.

Independent Living Aids
27 East Mall
Plainview, NY 11803-4404
(800) 537-2118
(516) 752-8080

This company carries a large variety of nonoptical assistive devices.

Jardon Eye Prosthetics, Inc.
17100 West 12 Mile Road
Southfield, MI 48076
(810) 424-8560

Jardon manufactures clip-on hemianopic mirrors.

Keeler Instruments, Inc.
456 Parkway
Broomall, PA 19008
(800) 523-5620
(215) 353-4350

Keeler provides primarily spectacle-mounted optical devices, including telescopes and telemicroscopes that can be mounted in the office by the practitioner. Other devices and kits are also available.

The Lighthouse
36-02 Northern Boulevard
Long Island City, NY 11101
(800) 453-4923
(718) 937-6959

The Lighthouse publishes a comprehensive and informative catalogue of optical and nonoptical devices as well as an excellent variety of acuity cards. Many of the listings for magnifiers are grouped by power and include parameters such as true power, lens diameter, and work distance. The Ocutech spectacle-mounted telescopes are available here. Also available is a consumer catalogue of assistive devices, excluding optical devices, for activities of daily living.

LS&S Group, Inc.
Wholesale Division
P.O. Box 673
Northbrook, IL 60065
(800) 468-4789
(708) 498-9777

The LS&S catalogue includes a large variety of optical and nonoptical devices.

Mattingly International
938 K Andreasen Drive
Escondido, CA 92029
(800) 826-4200
(619) 741-0767

The Mattingly catalogue offers a large variety of optical devices.

The New York Times
Large Type Weekly
P.O. Box 5792
New York, NY 10087-5792

This weekly periodical in large type covers world and national news, business, the arts, editorials, and book and film reviews.

Nikon, Inc.
19601 Hamilton Avenue
Torrance, CA 90502
(800) 645-6678
(310) 516-7124

Nikon makes spectacle-mounted telescopes and telemicroscopes that can be mounted by the practitioner.

NoIR Medical Technologies
P.O. Box 159
South Lyon, MI 48178
(800) 521-9746

NoIR produces a large variety of UV and IR filters (specifically the NoIR lenses and UVShields) as well as a limited number of hand-held magnifiers with tinted lenses called "Contrast Magnifiers."

Orascoptic Research, Inc.
7 North Pinckney Street
Suite 305
Madison, WI 53703
(608) 256-0344

Spectacle-mounted telemicroscopes called Wide-Field Orascoptic Telescopes are available from this company.

Resources for Rehabilitation
33 Bedford Street
Suite 19A
Lexington, MA 02173
(617) 862-6455

This organization is dedicated to providing training and information to professionals who provide services to individuals with disabilities. Also available are large print brochures concerning various disabilities such as diabetic retinopathy, vision loss, macular degeneration, and so on.

Tech-Optics International Corporation
59 Hanse Avenue
Freeport, NY 11520
(800) OPTICS-7
(516) 546-7480

Tech-Optics manufactures microscopes and the new HI-45 full-diameter aspheric high plus lenses.

Telesensory
455 North Bernardo Drive
Mountain View, CA 90404
(800) 345-2256
(415) 960-0920
(800) 537-3961 (for technical service)

Telesensory is a source for closed circuit televisions, computer adaptive technology, and similar aids.

Unilens Corp. USA
10431 72nd Street North
Largo, FL 34647-1511
(800) 446-2020
(813) 544-2531

Unilens manufactures the UniVision series of light aspheric lenses, which can be mounted by the practitioner on the front surface of a spectacle lens in any position desired through the use of an adhesive ring. The mount is not permanent, and the lens can be removed or exchanged for one of a different power.

## RESOURCE DIRECTORY

*Directory of Services for Blind and Visually Impaired Persons in the United States and Canada,* 24 ed

American Foundation for the Blind
c/o American Book Center
Brooklyn Navy Yard, Building #3
Brooklyn, NY 11205
(718) 852-9873

This is the single best resource book and should be considered a "must have" for any vision rehabilitation practitioner. It lists services available in every state and in Canada and is produced in both print and electronic formats. The book is particularly helpful for advising patients who are moving to a new location or who have acquaintances in other areas in need of rehabilitative services. Included are extensive lists of resources.

## SPECIAL INTEREST GROUPS, ORGANIZATIONS, AND INSTITUTES

American Bioptic Certified Drivers
(ABCD)
23872 Innisbrook
Laguna Niguel, CA 92677
(714) 495-3334

This organization is dedicated to promoting the interest of individuals who use bioptic lenses for the purpose of operating a motor vehicle.

American Council of the Blind (ACB)
1155 15th Street N.W.
Suite 720
Washington, D.C. 20005
(202) 467-5081

ACB is an advocacy group for those who are visually impaired that promotes independence and effective participation in society. It publishes *The Braille Forum,* which contains a variety of information, including pertinent legislative and governmental updates.

American Foundation for the Blind
15 West 16th Street
New York, NY 10011
(212) 620-2000

This is an excellent source of material about vision impairment and blindness in printed form as well as Braille, audiocassettes, and videos.

Association for Education and Rehabilitation of the Blind and Visually Impaired (AER)
206 North Washington Street
Suite 320
Alexandria, VA 22314
(703) 548-1884

A professional membership organization dedicated to the advancement of education and rehabilitation of blind and visually impaired children and adults, AER was formed in 1984 by a consolidation of the American Association of Workers for the Blind and the Association for Education of the Visually Handicapped. Members receive a bimonthly newsletter and reduced subscription rates to several related journals.

Association for Macular Diseases, Inc.
210 East 64th Street
New York, NY 10021
(212) 605-3719

This association provides information and support, primarily for those with loss of central vision.

Bible Alliance
P.O. Box 621
Bradenton, FL 34206
(813) 748-3031

This organization provides the Bible on audiocassette free of charge and produces recorded books in many languages.

Child Life Council
7910 Woodmont Avenue
Suite 310
Bethesda, MD 20814-3015
(301) 654-1343

This organization is composed of child life personnel, hospital school teachers, and others who use play, recreation, education, self-expression, and theories of child development to promote psychological well-being and optimum development in children, adolescents, and their families in health care settings.

Council of Citizens With Low Vision (CCLV)
5707 Brockton Drive
#302
Indianapolis, IN 46220
(800) 733-2258

CCLV, an advocacy group for those who are visually impaired, publishes a newsletter called *C.C.L.V. News.*

The Institute for Families of Blind Children
P.O. Box 54700 (Mail Stop #111)
Los Angeles, CA 90054-0700
(213) 669-4649

The Institute's excellent newsletter is primarily concerned with retinoblastoma but is also very germane to how families and individuals cope with loss of sight.

The National Association for Parents of the Visually Impaired, Inc. (NAPVI)
P.O. Box 317
Watertown, MA 02272-0317
(800) 562-6265
(617) 972-4441

NAPVI is a source of information and support for parents and families with children who are visually impaired, including those with multiple disabilities. Information is provided through workshops and publications. NAPVI publishes a quarterly newsletter called *Awareness.*

The National Association for the Visually
Handicapped (NAVH)
22 West 21st Street
6th Floor
New York, NY 10010
(212) 889-3141

This nonprofit national organization is devoted solely to the partially seeing. Services include discussion groups, newsletters, public education, and counseling.

National Federation of the Blind (NFB)
1800 Johnson Street
Baltimore, MD 21230
(410) 659-9314

NFB is an advocacy group whose stated purpose is the complete integration of the blind into society on the basis of equality, through removing legal, economic, and social discrimination.

RP Foundation Fighting Blindness
1401 Mt. Royal Avenue
4th Floor
Baltimore, MD 21217-4245
(410) 225-9400

The RP Foundation actively supports research in the area of retinitis pigmentosa and other retinal degenerative disorders. It publishes a periodic newsletter and literature about RP. People who are affected may register with the foundation, and information about them is maintained in a national database.

## OPHTHALMIC STANDARDS

American National Standards Institute,
Inc. (ANSI)
11 West 42nd Street
New York, NY 10036
(212) 642-4900

ANSI standards for LV devices are available as a written document entitled "American National Standard for Ophthalmics—LV Aids Requirements" (Z80.9-1993).

## PROSTHETIC EYES

American Optical Corporation
Monoplex Eye Service
14 Mechanic Street
Southbridge, MA 01550
(508) 765-9711
(800) 225-7498

American Optical offers plastic prostheses and supplies. Copies of some back issues of the *Monoplex Eye Bulletin* remain available.

Oculo Plastik, Inc.
1170 East Boulevard Henri-Bourassa
Montreal, QC, Canada
H2C 1G4
(514) 381-1849

This company is a source for plastic prostheses and supplies.

## GENETICS RESOURCES

American Society of Human Genetics
9650 Rockville Pike
Bethesda, MD 20814
(301) 571-1825

The American Society of Human Genetics provides general genetics information and has a large membership of researchers, clinicians, and genetic counselors who meet annually. The associated journal is *The American Journal of Human Genetics.*

National Society of Genetic Counselors
233 Canterbury Drive
Wallingford, PA 19086–6617
(215) 872–7608

This society is a source for information about professional resources, genetic disorders, and genetic counseling.

National Center for Education in Maternal and Child Health
2000 15th Street North
Suite 701
Arlington, VA 22201
(703) 524–7802

This organization publishes a guide to voluntary organizations related to various disabilities.

*Mendelian Inheritance in Man,* 10 ed, 1992
V.A. McKusick, editor
The Johns Hopkins University Press
2715 North Charles Street
Baltimore, MD 21218
(410) 516–6900

This large text, a comprehensive listing of known and suspected single gene disorders with a brief description and list of references for each, is the definitive resource. It is also available on-line by computer and recently has become available on optical disc. Because of the rapid developments in genetic research, this resource is updated frequently, and new editions of the book appear frequently.

## TEXTS AND JOURNALS CONCERNING VISION REHABILITATION

Bier N: *Correction of Subnormal Vision.* London, Butterworths, 1960.

Faye EE: Low vision, in Tasman W, Jaeger EA (eds): *Duane's Clinical Ophthalmology,* Volume 1. 1990, Chapter 46.

Faye EE: *Clinical Low Vision,* 2 ed. Boston, Little, Brown and Company, 1984.

Faye EE, Hood CM (eds): *Low Vision.* New York, Charles C. Thomas, 1975.

Faye EE: *The Low Vision Patient.* New York, Grune & Stratton, 1970.

Fonda GE: *Management of Low Vision.* New York, Thieme-Stratton, Inc., 1981.

Fonda G: *Management of the Patient with Low Vision.* Saint Louis, The C. V. Mosby Company, 1965.

Freeman PB, Jose RT: *The Art and Practice of Low Vision.* Boston, Butterworths, 1991.

Jose RT: *Understanding Low Vision.* New York, American Foundation for the Blind, 1983.

Mehr EB, Freid AN: *Low Vision Care.* Chicago, The Professional Press, Inc., 1975.

Rosenthal BP, Cole RD (eds): A structured approach to low vision care, in London R (ed): *Problems in Optometry,* 3(3), 1991.

Sloan LL: *Reading Aids for the Partially Sighted.* Baltimore, The Williams & Wilkins Company, 1977.

Woo GC (ed): *Low Vision Principles and Applications.* New York, Springer-Verlag, 1986.

*Journal of Vision Rehabilitation* (formerly *Rehabilitative Optometry*)
Media Productions & Marketing, Inc.
2440 'O' Street
Suite 202
Lincoln, NE 68510

*Journal of Visual Impairment and Blindness*
Publications and Information Services Department
American Foundation for the Blind
15 West 16th Street
New York, NY 10011

*Protocols for choosing low vision devices—Consensus statement.* National Institute on Disability and Rehabilitation Research, 1(4), 1993. A government publication available from:

Department of Education
National Institute on Disability and Rehabilitation Research
400 Maryland Avenue S.W.
Washington, D.C. 20202-2646
(202) 205-9151

## RESIDENCIES, FELLOWSHIPS, AND CONTINUING EDUCATION

American Academy of Optometry (AAO)
4330 East West Highway
Suite 1117
Bethesda, MD 20814-4408
(301) 718-6500

The AAO has an annual meeting with continuing education programs on a variety of topics, including low vision.

There is a separate Low Vision Section that confers Diplomate status to individuals who successfully complete the requirements. There is a Section meeting held as part of the annual meeting.

American Optometric Association (AOA)
243 North Lindbergh Boulevard
St. Louis, MO 63141
(314) 991-4100

The AOA has an annual meeting with continuing education programs on a variety of topics, including low vision. There is a separate Low Vision Section that meets in conjunction with the annual general meeting.

American Academy of Ophthalmology (AAO)
655 Beach Street
San Francisco, CA 94109
(415) 561-8500

The AAO has an annual meeting with continuing education programs in a variety of topics.

Association of Schools and Colleges of Optometry (ASCO)
6110 Executive Boulevard
Suite 690
Rockville, MD 20852
(301) 231-5944

ASCO publishes a directory of graduate and residency programs in optometry. There are a number of residencies throughout the United States that offer specialization in vision rehabilitation. Residency programs may be accredited by the Council on Optometric Education.

# INDEX